The psychology of health

Health psychology is one of the fastest growing areas of the behavioural sciences. As such it occupies an increasingly important place in undergraduate and postgraduate courses. Students in other disciplines, such as nursing, physiotherapy and occupational therapy, also need to learn about the role of psychology in understanding health and the treatment of illness.

This new textbook provides an up-to-date and comprehensive introduction to health psychology which will be invaluable to students of psychology and of the related behavioural and health sciences, as well as health visitors, physiotherapists, nurses and occupational therapists. It brings together a team of contributors with wide experience, both in research and practice and in teaching psychologists and health professionals alike.

In the first part of the book the contributors introduce the basic principles, theories and methodologies of health psychology, and look in particular at the psychophysiological basis of health, stress and coping.

The second part discusses psychological studies relevant to the experience of illness and hospitalization and the management of disease. It deals with the process of illness from the first perception of the symptoms, through medical treatment, to rehabilitation and recovery. Finally, the contributors focus on a range of health issues, including important topics neglected by other books, such as AIDS, contraception and abortion, and the role of the family in promoting health. This section clearly illustrates the diversity of research in health psychology and indicates the wider familial, social and political pressures on health behaviour.

Marian Pitts is Principal Lecturer in Psychology at Staffordshire University, and Honorary Research Fellow at the University of East London.

Keith Phillips is Head of Psychology at the University of East London.

The psychology of health
An introduction

Edited by
Marian Pitts
and
Keith Phillips

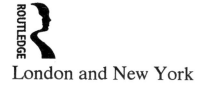
London and New York

First published in 1991
by Routledge
11 New Fetter Lane, London EC4P 4EE

Simultaneously published in the USA and Canada
by Routledge
29 West 35th Street, New York, NY 10001

Reprinted 1992, 1993, 1995

Typeset from the author's w-p disks by
NWL Editorial Services, Langport, Somerset

Printed and bound in Great Britain by
Mackays of Chatham PLC, Chatham, Kent

British Library Cataloguing in Publication Data
A catalogue record for this book is available from the British Library

Library of Congress Cataloguing in Publication Data
A catalogue record for this book is available from the Library of Congress

ISBN 0-415-04114-7
ISBN 0-415-04115-5 (pbk)

To
David, Tom and Megan
and
Julie, Clare, Rebecca and Amy

Contents

Figures and tables

Contributors

Mary Boyle Senior Lecturer in Psychology and Course Tutor for M.Sc. Clinical Psychology, Department of Psychology, University of East London.

Philip Evans Principal Lecturer, School of Biological and Health Sciences, University of Westminster.

Brenda May Associate Lecturer in Clinical Psychology, Department of Psychology, University of East London, and Honorary Clinical Psychologist, Great Ormond Street Hospital for Sick Children.

Jacky McGuire Psychologist at the Medical-Educational Evaluation Center, North Shore Children's Hospital, Salem, Massachusetts, USA.

Andrew Parrott Senior Lecturer in Psychology, Department of Psychology, University of East London.

Keith Phillips Head of Psychology, Department of Psychology, University of East London.

Marian Pitts Principal Lecturer in Psychology, Department of Sociology, Staffordshire University, and Honorary Research Fellow, Department of Psychology, University of East London. Formerly Lecturer in Psychology, University of Zimbabwe.

Preface

Health psychology is a rapidly growing field occupying an increasingly large place in undergraduate and postgraduate courses. Students of related professional disciplines such as nursing, physiotherapy and occupational therapy are also learning of the applications of psychology to the area of health. This book is introductory, designed to cover both the 'traditional' aspects of health psychology such as pain and coronary heart disease, and some newer areas of interest: abortion and contraception, AIDS and living with chronic disease. There has also been an attempt to broaden the areas of health concern for psychologists. To this end, chapters are included on the effects of psychoactive medicines, both wanted and unwanted; the psychopharmacology of addictive behaviours, such as smoking and drinking, and the role of the family in health education.

The contributors to the book are all teachers and active researchers in the area of health psychology. They share another common thread: at one time or another they were all colleagues at what was North East London Polytechnic, now known as the University of East London. Since the book's inception they have moved around and now span three continents. It is hoped that the book shows both the coherence of the original team approach they shared and the diversity of their current situations.

The book is in three parts. The first part aims to introduce the basic principles, theories and methodologies of health psychology. It considers especially the psychophysiological basis of health, stress and coping. The second part considers psychological studies relevant to the experiences of illness and hospitalization and the management of diseases. It covers the process of illness from the first perception of symptoms through medical treatment to rehabilitation and recovery. The third part focuses on a range of health issues. It builds on the basic principles covered in the first section and considers their applications. It attempts to illustrate the diversity of research in health psychology and to indicate the wider familial, social and political pressures on health behaviour.

The book is designed to provide the basis of a course of lectures on health psychology to undergraduates in psychology and related behavioural sciences.

It should, though, also be of use to students of other health disciplines and to postgraduates who need an introduction to specific areas of health research.

Acknowledgements

The editors would like to thank the contributors who, by and large, kept their earlier promises, and helped us in many ways throughout the preparation of this book. We would like to acknowledge the support given to us by many colleagues and friends in the Department of Psychology, University of East London and the Department of Psychology, University of Zimbabwe. In particular, thanks are due to John MacMaster of University of Zimbabwe who commented so usefully on several chapters, and to Martin Dunbar whose undergraduate dissertation was used as the basis for some sections of Chapter 5. All errors remain, unfortunately, our own.

The initial stimulus for this book came from the many students whose obvious enthusiasm for health psychology caused us to undertake its writing. Their contribution has been great and we hope that they will feel some satisfaction from realizing their part in its appearance.

We owe great thanks to our partners and families for their support too during the period of production of the book; their tolerance, good humour and general assistance throughout the project has done much to ensure its final delivery. Several friends acted as couriers between Harare and London, a much needed service, and our thanks go to Helen Jackson, Keith Cockcroft and Rodney Bickerstaffe.

We acknowledge permission to reproduce Figure 1.1 from Johns Hopkins University Press and Figure 1.2 from Elsevier Scientific Publishers Ireland Ltd. Finally we would like to thank David Stonestreet, of Routledge, for his initial encouragement and help throughout the production process.

Abbreviations

ACh	acetylcholine
ACTH	adrenocortico-trophic hormone
AIDS	Acquired Immune Deficiency Syndrome
ANS	autonomic nervous system
BAC	blood alcohol
BPL	blood-pressure level
BRS	Bortner Rating Scale
BSE	breast self-examination
C	cervical
CCU	coronary-care unit
CHD	coronary heart disease
CNS	central nervous system
CO	carbon monoxide
DA	dopamine
EEG	electroencephalogram
EMG	electromyogram
FTAS	Framingham Type A Scale
GP	general practitioner
HIV	Human Immunodeficiency Virus
5-HT	5-hydroxytryptamine
ICU	intensive-care unit
ivdu	intravenous drug user
JAS	Jenkins Activity Survey
MAO	monoamine oxidase inhibitor
MI	myocardial infarction
MMPI	Minnesota Multiphasic Personality Inventory
MS	multiple sclerosis
NA	noradrenaline
PNS	peripheral nervous system
PVC	premature ventricular contraction
RTW	return to work
SCI	spinal-cord injury

SI	structured interview
S-IgA	secretory immunoglobulin
T	thoracic
WCGS	Western Collaborative Group Study

Part I

Introduction

Part I is designed to introduce the reader to theories and methods of research which are found in this new and interdisciplinary area that links psychology and health. Chapter 1 considers the growth of health psychology and how health and illness behaviours have been investigated. Changes in the patterns of health and disease are considered and the contributions of protective behaviours for health are examined. Breast self-examination is used as a focus to illustrate the application of theories of health behaviour. Chapter 2 examines the psychophysiology of health. It considers the organization of the nervous, neuroendocrine and immune systems, methods and principles of recording responses within these systems and how these responses are relevant to the interpretation of health and well-being, and the aetiology and maintenance of disease states. Chapter 3 singles out the major issue of stress and coping and examines these constructs in detail. It considers the relationship between life events and stress and examines the methodological difficulties encountered in this area of research. This chapter also reviews the exciting area of psychoimmunological factors in the aetiology and development of disease. The chapters in Part I provide the background from which the student can consider the issues raised in respect of the particular instances of health and disease included in Parts II and III of this book.

Chapter 1

An introduction to health psychology

Marian Pitts

INTRODUCTION

Any activity of psychology which relates to aspects of health, illness, the health care system or health policy may be considered to be within the field of health psychology. Health psychology deals with such questions as: What are the physiological bases of emotion and how do they relate to health and illness? Can certain behaviours predispose to particular illnesses? What is stress? Can educational interventions prevent illness? and many others. One can formally date the beginnings of the interest of psychologists in these areas to the convening of a conference in 1978 and to the setting up of a section devoted to health psychology in the American Psychological Association in 1979. The British Psychological Society set up a Health Section only in 1986. Hence the recognition of health psychology as a clearly designated field is very recent; however, many of the ideas and basic concepts have been around psychology for a great deal longer than this. A widely accepted definition of health psychology is that put forward by Matarazzo in 1980:

> Health psychology is the aggregate of the specific educational, scientific and professional contributions of the discipline of psychology to the promotion and maintenance of health, the prevention and treatment of illness, the identification of etiologic and diagnostic correlates of health, illness and related dysfunction, and the analysis and improvement of the health care system and health policy formation.

This definition emphasizes the diversity of issues encompassed by the emerging discipline. There is also variety in the approaches brought to those issues. Some health psychologists would see themselves primarily as clinicians, others as psychophysiologists and others still as cognitive psychologists; what unifies them is their interest in the areas delineated by Matarazzo.

EARLY STUDIES

The relationship between mind and body and the effect of one upon the other has always been a controversial topic amongst philosophers, psychologists and physiologists. Within Psychology, the development of the study of psychosomatic disorders owes much to Freud. Psychologists such as Dunbar (1943), Ruesch (1948) and Alexander (1950) attempted to relate distinct personality types to particular diseases, with an implicit causation hypothesis. Work of this type has become more sophisticated in its approach and the chapters in the book on coronary heart disease and on chronic illnesses are illustrative, and critical, of this orientation. However, this psychosomatic approach has largely been abandoned by health psychologists in favour of a more behavioural or biological approach which seeks to employ interventions derived from behavioural medicine (see Chapter 8 on biofeedback, for example).

Another important aspect in the development of health psychology has been the changing patterns of illness and disease. Matarazzo (1983) points out that whereas contagious and infectious diseases contribute minimally to illness and death in the western world today, other illnesses have become more frequent and are of a different nature. Major breakthroughs in science have reduced the prevalence of diseases such as rubella, influenza, polio and tuberculosis in the western world; more deaths are now caused by heart disease, cancer and strokes. Recent studies and theories suggest that these diseases are, in part, a by-product of changes in life-styles in the twentieth century. Psychologists can be instrumental in investigating and influencing life-styles and behaviours which are conducive or detrimental to good health. The chapters in this book on AIDS and on essential hypertension (Chapters 10 and 12 respectively) illustrate areas where such interventions are being attempted. Increasingly, then, the major causes of death are those in which behavioural pathogens are the single most important factor.

'Behavioural pathogens' are the personal habits and life-style behaviours of the individual which can influence the onset and course of disease. It is not just the diseases of the 'developed' world which can be affected by behaviour and attitude: combating malaria, bilharzia and other diseases endemic in certain areas of the world can also be greatly helped by psychological input into publicity campaigns to change behaviour. As people the world over live longer, then the long-term effects of what Matarazzo calls (1983) 'a lifetime of behavioural mismanagement' can begin to express themselves in lung cancer, and heart and liver diseases.

HEALTH BEHAVIOURS

There has long been a common-sense notion that there exists a relationship between good health and personal habits. Plato said 'where temperance is, there health is speedily imparted'. Many groups have codified 'good' living habits into their religions and Matarazzo (1983) cites evidence of the outcome of healthy living and abstinence in such communities: Mormons in Utah have a 30 per cent lower incidence of most cancers than the general population of the USA, and Seventh Day Adventists have 25 per cent fewer hospital admissions for malignancies. Such statistics are powerful indicators that personal life-styles do much to ensure healthy bodies. This idea was first studied systematically by Belloc and Breslow (1972). They studied a sample of 6,928 people living in Alameda County, California. They examined several common health practices such as hours of sleep, regularity of meals, physical activity, drinking and smoking and they also investigated their respondents' health. They found that all adults who engaged in most of the healthy practices were in better health than those who engaged in few or none. The study was longitudinal in design, and Belloc further investigated the relationship between engaging in good health practices and health status over nearly six years. Belloc (1973) reports that the fewer good health practices a person reported engaging in during the first phase of the study, the progressively greater the risk that s/he would die during the next five and a half years.

Most research in this area incorporates the formulation of Kasl and Cobb (1966) of 'health behaviours'. These are defined as 'any activity undertaken by a person believing himself to be healthy for the purpose of preventing disease or detecting it in an asymptomatic stage'. These are distinguished from an 'illness behaviour' which is 'any activity undertaken by a person who feels ill, to define the state of his health or to discover a suitable remedy'.

Harris and Guten (1979) studied health-protective behaviours; those behaviours which people engage in to protect or maintain their health. They conducted an exploratory study of 1,250 residents in Greater Cleveland, USA. First, respondents were asked: 'What are the three most important things that you do to protect your health?' Subjects were then presented with statements on cards which described health behaviours and were asked to sort them into those that they did and those that they did not practise. Cluster analyses performed on these data produced categories to account for the various responses obtained by both methods. Categories of health protective behaviours thus found were:

- health practices – sleeping enough, eating sensibly and so forth;
- safety practices – repairing things, keeping first-aid kits and emergency telephone numbers handy;
- preventive health care – dental check-ups, smear tests;
- environmental hazard avoidance – avoiding areas of pollution or crime;
- harmful substance avoidance – not smoking or drinking.

Thus the kinds of behaviours which can be incorporated into a consideration of health psychology are varied and diverse.

Although most of us are familiar with the need to engage in preventive health behaviours, few of us actually do. Berg (1976) has stressed that most people are aware of what health behaviours should be engaged in, but they frequently do not engage in them and furthermore *do* engage in activities which they know to be harmful to their health. It is this cantankerousness which psychologists have spent a great deal of time examining.

A consistent focus has been on the role of knowledge in changing behaviours. Clearly, the argument goes, people need to be informed of the risks to themselves that certain behaviours (or non-behaviours) can engender. Having been appraised of the risks, they will then, in a rational manner, decide to modify their behaviours in the direction of greater health promotion and protection. Studies examining a range of issues relevant to health such as smoking, drug-taking, medical checks and adopting safer sex have fairly consistently shown that knowledge, by itself, does not lead to behaviour change. The example of seat-belt wearing provides a good illustration of this.

Kelley (1979) examined the role of the media in improving public health. He pointed out that the use of safety belts in cars greatly reduces the probability of death and injury following crashes. However, the availability of seat belts in cars does not guarantee their use. A study conducted in the USA in 1968 recorded only 6.3 per cent of car drivers wearing seat belts in a city area. Kelley attempted to design and execute a definitive test of mass media effectiveness in increasing seat-belt use. He was able to utilize cable television such that he could have a number of households which would receive advertisements concerning seat belt use, and another, equivalent number of households which would not. He used six different advertisements, produced professionally, and shown at specific times designed to target specific audiences. The advertisements were shown regularly over a period of nine months. He estimates that the average television viewer in the experimental group saw one or another of the messages two or three times a week over the test period. Observers positioned at designated sites within the area under study recorded seat-belt use and the car licence plate which enabled a trace to be made to indicate which of the two cable TV channels was available to that person's house. Kelley's conclusions were depressing: 'The results were clearcut. The campaign had no effect whatsoever on seat belt use.' There were no significant differences between drivers from households which had received the messages and drivers from the control households. Nor did the drivers from the test group change their seat-belt wearing at all across the test period. Kelley argues very forcefully from this study that mass-media campaigns are ineffective and an inefficient means of changing health behaviours. So what else is required, other than knowledge, to persuade people to look after their health? We will now examine suggestions for other factors which will influence health behaviour.

MODELS OF HEALTH BEHAVIOUR

Early studies of protective health focused upon demographic variables such as age, race and socio-economic class as determinants of the adoption and practice of health behaviours. This research resulted in descriptions of population groups which did or did not engage in preventive health behaviours. These findings were often contradictory and did not serve any great purpose – one cannot change one's age, sex or race. Consequently research has shifted to structural variables such as the cost or complexity of the behaviour, with a view to improving the adoption and practice of preventive health behaviours. There are several theories or models which have evolved in this context. Three of these have been particularly influential and are described below.

The health belief model

This model was proposed initially by Rosenstock (1966) and was modified by Becker and Maiman (1975). It attempts to explain health behaviour and compliance. It should be useful in predicting health behaviour before illness, such as screening for cancer, and compliance to medical regimens once ill. Therefore both sick role behaviour and preventive behaviours should be capable of being predicted. The model proposes that a person's likelihood of engaging in health-related behaviours is a function of several dimensions. An outline of the model is presented in Figure 1.1. It proposes that for a person to take a preventive action against a disease, the person must:

- feel personally susceptible to the disease (perceived susceptibility);
- feel that the disease would have at least moderately serious consequences (perceived severity);
- feel that preventive behaviour would be beneficial either by preventing the disease, or by lessening its severity (perceived benefits);
- that barriers, such as pain or embarrassment or expense, should not outweigh the perceived benefits of the proposed health action in order for the preventive health behaviour to occur.

The model has been used with some success to predict the adoption of several different health behaviours including vaccinations and screening for cancer (Janz and Becker 1984) though it seems that for some behaviours at least, perceived severity may be less important for preventive behaviours than either perceived vulnerability or cost–benefit considerations (Cleary 1987).

Self-regulating systems theories

Models of this type conceptualize the individual as an active problem solver whose behaviour reflects an attempt to close a perceived gap between current status and a goal, or ideal state. Behaviour depends on individuals' cognitive

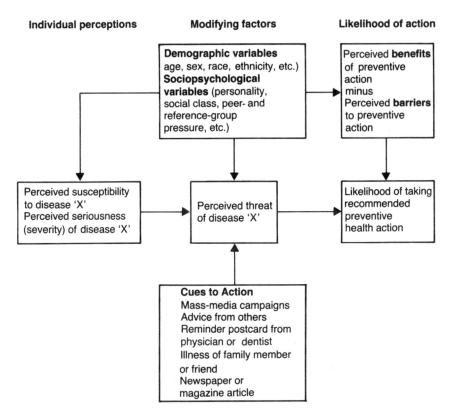

Figure 1.1 Health belief model
Source: Becker, M.H. and Maiman, L.A. (1975) 'Sociobehavioral determinants of compliance with health and medical care recommendations', *Medical Care* 13: 12. Copyright 1975 J.B. Lippincott Co.

representations of their current health status and the goal state, plans for changing the current state, and techniques or rules for assessing progress.

Leventhal's self-regulation model of illness (Leventhal and Cameron 1987) defines three stages which regulate behaviour. These stages are:

- the cognitive representation of the health threat, which includes any dimensions such as perceived symptoms, potential causes or possible consequences;
- the action plan or coping stage in which the individual formulates and begins a plan of action;
- the appraisal stage in which the individual utilizes specific criteria to gauge success of coping actions, with perceptions of insufficient progress leading to modifications.

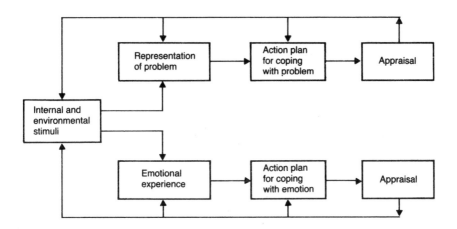

Figure 1.2 The self-regulatory model of illness behaviour.
Source: 'Behavioral theories and the problem of compliance' by H. Leventhal and L. Cameron, 1987, Patient Education and Counseling, 10, 127. Copyright 1987 by Elsevier Scientific Publishers Ireland Ltd. Reprinted by permission.

The model is presented in diagrammatic form in Figure 1.2. Emotional reactions can be evoked at any stage. Cultural or social differences, for instance in symptom perception or illness expectations, can lead to differing representations and different coping structures.

An attractive feature of this type of model is that it is active – it stresses the individual and how that single person can operate and reflect on his or her operations. This is also, though, its potential weakness; it has not been as generative of research and neat questionnaire construction as has the health belief model.

The theory of reasoned action

The theory of reasoned action derives from social psychology and seeks to explain the suggested relationships between attitudes and behaviours; it has become a major model for health promotion. The model identifies intention as the most immediate determinant of behaviour (Fishbein and Ajzen 1975). They argue that the immediate determinant of behaviour is a person's intention to perform that behaviour. Intentions are themselves a function of privately held attitudes towards the particular behaviour and socially determined subjective norms that represent a person's belief that others think she or he should behave in a certain way. The model attaches values to each of these factors. The particular values attached to each factor will depend upon the individual's beliefs and thus in many ways this model is similar to the health belief model.

One difficulty with this model is that it identifies a direct link between intentions and behaviours, but intentions are not always translated into actions. Even when an individual holds an intention towards some behaviour, action does not necessarily result. Also, other factors besides attitudes and social norms have been shown to influence behaviour. Bentler and Speckart (1979, 1981) for example, showed that habits can also have a direct influence on behaviour. To take account of these difficulties, Ajzen has extended the original theory to include an individual's perception of control or potential control which may modify behaviour directly or indirectly via the link through intentions. This modification is incorporated into the theory of planned behaviour (Ajzen 1985). There may be one or several reasons for not carrying out an intention to act in a particular way that is perceived as beneficial. The action may not be possible in a particular situation or at a particular time, it may be difficult or time consuming or it may simply be suppressed. From the point of view of the promotion of health behaviours, much greater consideration needs to be given to the impact of situational influences of this kind upon adherence to intentions to act in accordance with prevention.

There is a clear need for empirical studies that test these and other models for the adoption of preventive health behaviours since interventions based upon them have implicitly accepted their assumptions. If the determinants of precautionary behaviours could be identified this would be a significant step forward in campaigns against behavioural diseases such as AIDS, or smoking-related illnesses. There is little doubt that the principal variables identified by these models – perceived risk, perceived severity of the disease, perceived effectiveness of precautions and cost–benefit payoff – are important predictors of preventive health behaviours of many kinds (Janz and Becker 1984). However the value attached to each remains uncertain.

There have been several other models which are applicable to the area of health behaviour. The Subjective Expected Utility Model (Luker 1975) will be used as a framework for the discussion of contraception and abortion in Chapter 11: Bandura's theory of self-efficacy (1977, 1986) is likely to provide an interesting perspective upon health behaviours and especially on issues of coping with illness, and the adoption and maintenance of good exercise habits (see, for example, Biddle 1989). The topic of AIDS will be considered in Chapter 10 from the viewpoint of some of the models discussed so far together with some others. What is characteristic of these models of health behaviour is that research on their validities is correlational in design, and whilst significant correlations between pairs of variables are frequently reported, the amount of variance which any model accounts for in predicting the practice of health behaviours remains generally low. We will now look in rather more detail at one specific behaviour for preventive health and the factors which influence its practice.

BREAST SELF-EXAMINATION – A PREVENTIVE HEALTH BEHAVIOUR

A preventive health behaviour which has attracted much psychological interest and research is the practice of breast self-examination (BSE). This can be defined as the practice by a woman of examining her breasts in a systematic fashion for the purpose of detecting an abnormality. Breast cancer is one of the major health problems of women in the UK and elsewhere. Approximately 1 in 14 of all British women will develop breast cancer during their lifetimes. Each year in the UK 13,000 women die of breast cancer; it is the most common cancer in women and accounts for 20 per cent of all female deaths from cancer. An important factor in the prognosis for breast cancer is the stage of that cancer when discovered. The five-year survival rate is 85 per cent if the disease is discovered and treated at a localized stage; the survival rate drops to 53 per cent if the cancer has spread to the axillary nodes.

There are three main screening methods available in the UK for detecting breast cancer: these are mammography; physical examination by a health practitioner; and breast self-examination. Mammography is an excellent screening method as it detects non-palpable tumours. However, it is only available at present in the UK for older women in some health districts. For the vast majority of women, regular monthly BSE is recommended with physical examination by the health practitioner if any change or abnormality is noted.

BSE is a simple, safe and economical health-related behaviour which, it has been claimed, is effective in promoting the detection of breast tumours at an early clinical stage and of small size (Foster *et al.* 1978). Critics of breast self-examination have argued that it is likely to result in unnecessarily high levels of anxiety amongst women who find a growth and an increased likelihood of unnecessary surgery (Frank and Mai 1985). Nevertheless, it is widely promoted as a useful preventive health behaviour. Considering the potential advantages of regular BSE it is disappointing that relatively few women practise it. A National US Survey in 1973 indicated that although 77 per cent of American women knew of BSE, only 18 per cent had practised it monthly during the previous year. A follow-up survey carried out three years later found a figure of 24 per cent, while a government survey in 1980 found that 29 per cent of American women practised BSE monthly. Thus, in America there has been a gradual increase in the percentage of women practising BSE regularly. However, there remain about 70 per cent of women who do *not* practise BSE. Studies in Britain have found similar levels for BSE (Nichols 1983; Owens *et al.* 1987). Few studies have examined personality traits, intentions and other factors which may influence BSE. Obvious candidates for consideration have been those factors incorporated in the health belief model. It is interesting to note, though, that the relationship between BSE and breast cancer is complex. BSE does not result in a diminished chance of contracting breast cancer, and to practise BSE actually increases the likelihood of finding a lump and hence the possibility of surgery. Thus, the perceived benefits of BSE need to be qualified. Lowering a woman's susceptibility to breast cancer is not a feasible goal (benefit), but lessening the consequences of the disease may be.

Specific benefits which have been found to correlate positively with BSE are: a belief that if or when a lump is found something can be done, a belief in the advantages of BSE and a belief that a positive attitude towards BSE is possible. Barriers to BSE have been found to be the woman's confidence level (Edwards 1980), lack of knowledge concerning detection levels and the ability to detect a lump (McCusker and Morrow 1977), and lack of privacy to practise the behaviour (Zapka and Mamon 1982).

A scale of perceived benefits/barriers and susceptibility to breast cancer has been developed by Stillman (1977). Significant associations between BSE practice and the scale have been reported by Stillman (1977) and Hallal (1982). Stillman reported that 87 per cent of her sample of 122 women scored highly for perceived susceptibility – far higher than the 9–12 per cent who will actually contract breast cancer. Some 97 per cent thought BSE was beneficial, yet only 40 per cent practised BSE monthly. Rutledge (1987) studied 93 volunteer women. She again found perceived benefits/barriers to be directly related to BSE. She did not, however, find a relationship between perceived susceptibility and frequency of practice of BSE which is probably explained by the fact that BSE does not reduce *susceptibility* to breast cancer *per se*.

Calnan and his colleagues have also examined the health belief model and BSE (Calnan 1984). He found that the variables which contribute to the health belief model were amongst the best predictors of attendance at a class teaching BSE and at a clinic offering mammography, but that the amount of variance explained by these variables was small.

Hallal (1982) and Rutledge (1987) examined the relationship between self-concept and the practice of BSE. Hallal reported a positive association between self-concept and BSE, but Rutledge found it did not, of itself, contribute significantly to an explanation of variance regarding BSE. The factor of self-esteem is important in deciding which method of detecting breast lumps to advise women to undertake: a woman with low self-esteem who feels she will 'never be able to practise BSE' might be better advised to seek regular checks from a health adviser; similarly, advocates of BSE should stress that it *is* possible to learn the methods and that they should pay particular attention to those women who are expressing concern at mastering the technique.

Green (1970) suggested that variables such as the degree of social support available to a person may affect the practice of preventive health behaviours. Rutledge used the Norbeck Social Support Scale (Norbeck *et al.* 1981) to examine the role of social support in practising BSE. She reported no relationship and suggested that the scale did not measure the particular aspects of the social network which might affect BSE.

Finally, there has been regularly reported a negative association between age and the practice of preventive health behaviours – for example, Gould-Martin *et al.* (1982) and others. This finding has particular importance for BSE as the older a woman is, the more likely she is to develop a breast lump. Rutledge, however, failed to find any relationship between age and BSE practice.

The self-regulatory theory and the theory of reasoned action described above have not been applied directly to BSE. It is not easy to see how either theory would help us to predict more precisely who would engage in the practice, or, more important, how to increase the percentage of women carrying out the preventive behaviour. Both theories might, though, be of some help in planning education programmes on breast cancer and its detection.

Hobbs *et al.* (1984) review the evidence that teaching programmes on BSE can influence the opinions and knowledge of women about the advantages of early detection and treatment. They argue, however, that such changes in knowledge have little direct effect on the extent to which BSE is actually practised. It seems from the women's comments that the difficulties lie in knowing exactly what to do, and when and how often to do it. It is also the case that women are not particularly well informed about the risk factors associated with breast cancer; they are largely unable to make a realistic assessment of their own susceptibility to the disease and tend to overestimate the personal risks. Such overestimation may result in fear and denial as coping strategies. Further information which seeks both to reassure and educate women as to the actual incidence of breast cancer and the relative frequency of 'benign' lumps linked with detailed information on the practice of BSE could further reduce the number of women failing to carry out this procedure. However, as Kelley demonstrated with seat-belt use, more information or propaganda is unlikely, by itself, to change behaviour.

The lessons learned from the examination of the processes which influence the practice of BSE can be extended to other cancers. For example, testicular cancer can be cured if treated early and similar techniques of self-examination can be taught to men, or their partners, to enable abnormalities to be detected before they are at an advanced stage. Education about melanomas can also lead to the seeking of medical advice at an early stage of skin cancer.

CONCLUSIONS

Other chapters in this book will enlarge on much of what has been covered in this chapter. Specific problems and issues will be examined in detail in the light of the theories and models described above, and the area of breast cancer will be considered from the point of view of coping strategies which aid recovery in Chapter 9. However, having examined some of the areas of interest to health psychologists, we need to reconsider its future as a discipline. Marteau and Johnston (1987) have sounded a warning note about the development of the field. They caution that 'the relative neglect of psychological models and paradigms in work considered under the rubric of health psychology, results in approaches to problems in clinical and research contexts that owe more to a medical than a psychological perspective'. Johnston (1988) also suggests that at least five separate kinds of literature on health psychology appear to be developing, according to the problem studied and the journal in which the research is published. It is becoming increasingly difficult for any one person to keep abreast of the literature on the diverse areas of interest which are encompassed by health psychology. It must be hoped that, increasingly, research and theory building for one health issue will more clearly inform and guide research in other related topics and that psychological models of health behaviour will give rise to effective interventions for promoting health.

Chapter 2

The psychophysiology of health

Keith Phillips

INTRODUCTION

This chapter will describe briefly the structure and organization of the nervous, endocrine and immunological systems and their roles in the regulation of physiological responses and behaviour. The techniques involved in recording and measuring responses of these systems are considered, and finally their roles in the determination of health and illness are discussed. Those readers who are familiar with the basics of physiological psychology and psychophysiology may well wish to skip over the first two sections and move directly on to the psychophysiological aspects of health.

ORGANIZATION OF THE NERVOUS SYSTEM

The mammalian nervous system is made up of millions of individual nerve cells that are arranged in complex networks. Individual cells and groups of cells communicate with each other via special chemicals called neurotransmitters which trigger electrical events within these networks. These electrical events, called 'action potentials', are the code or language by which information is communicated within the system. In total the nervous system can be regarded as a highly sophisticated communication system that enables interaction between an organism and the physical world in which it lives. The individual elements of this system are arranged within a highly structured organization as one would expect of any communication network. A short but illuminating review of information flow within this system can be found in Boddy (1983).

When describing the organization of the mammalian nervous system it is usual to identify its central and peripheral components. The central nervous system (CNS) comprises the brain and spinal cord; the peripheral nervous system (PNS) is the collection of nerves from the CNS to the periphery and from the periphery to the CNS. These nerves may be further subdivided into somatic and autonomic components. Before we consider each of these components it is important to appreciate that these subdivisions are useful only for descriptive purposes: they are not separate systems in terms of their functional operations. The component structures are fully integrated with each other; changes that occur in the activity of the central nervous system will be accompanied by changes in the peripheral system and vice versa. The nervous system has evolved as a whole to allow behaving organisms to make successful adaptations to their environment. Ill health may be regarded as an indicator that successful adaption has not been achieved.

Central nervous system

The central nervous system is made up of the brain and the spinal cord. These are developed from the same embryonic nerve tissues, are entirely interactive and share an internal circulation of cerebrospinal fluid which protects against physical damage and provides a stable chemical environment to allow nerve cells to function. The CNS is enclosed by the bony coverings of the skull and vertebral column. In general terms the CNS can be thought of as having an executive role in the control and regulation of behaviour. It receives information from the outside world, integrates current information with past experiences and instructs the responses of agents or effectors that have effects upon behaviour. The obvious effector agents are the muscles of the skeletal system which cause our actions, but other effectors are the hormones secreted by the endocrine system and responses of the autonomic nervous system such as changes in cardiac activity or electrical signals from the skin. Though the CNS prepares the instructions for changes in the activities of these effectors it does not deliver them; that is the job of the peripheral nervous system. Similarly the PNS delivers to the CNS information from the outside world. Though the CNS may be considered to have an executive role, the regulation of behaviour is not entirely feudal since the operations of the CNS are influenced to a very large degree by feedback from the PNS.

Peripheral nervous system

The nerves of the PNS are divided into the somatic or autonomic nervous systems. The somatic system includes nerves from the sense organs (eyes, ears, skin, tongue and nose) which carry information from the outside world to the CNS. However the CNS is not simply a passive recipient of sensory information; it has nerves connected to the sense organs which actively and selectively filter out information. As well as sensory nerves, the somatic system also includes motor nerves that travel from the CNS to the muscles whose contractions result in actions (behaviour). Again this is not a unilateral operation as there are also sensory nerves from the muscles that relay the consequences of those actions back to the CNS. The interaction between the sensory and motor nerves of the somatic system and the CNS can be organized within the spinal cord alone, for example for simple reflexes such as the

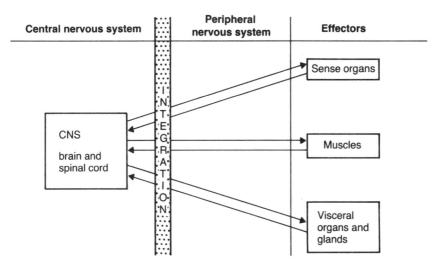

Figure 2.1 The organization of the nervous system.

knee-jerk reflex, but more usually it involves both the spinal cord and the various component structures of the brain.

The autonomic nervous system (ANS) is divided into two parts – the sympathetic and parasympathetic divisions whose actions are opposite though complementary. Usually, though erroneously, these two divisions are described solely in terms of their effector nerves which travel from the CNS to the organs and glands within the body. These innervations provide regulation of those visceral structures and hence regulation of the internal responses of the body. However, there exist in addition sensory autonomic nerves carrying feedback from the viscera to the CNS. This of course is how we become aware of sensations such as emotional states, hunger pangs or visceral pains. Thus, the somatic and autonomic systems are similarly organized (see Figure 2.1).

The sympathetic and parasympathetic systems have antagonistic actions yet play a combined role in regulating the internal environment of the body. Typically each organ receives inputs from both the sympathetic and parasympathetic divisions. However, the sympathetic system is diffuse and sympathetic nerves innervate several organs and glands. Thus, when activated, a generalized sympathetic reaction is observed in many of the body's internal organs. By contrast the parasympathetic innervation is more discrete and individual organs have their own particular innervation which allows more fractionated regulation of their responses. The sympathetic action causes mobilization of the body's energy resources preparing the body for action. It is accompanied by multiple response changes including increased cardiac output, sweating, inhibition of digestion, increased blood flow to the muscles and dilation of the pupils. These responses prepare the body for action. This pattern of sympathetic activation is often referred to as the 'fight-or-flight reaction' and is considered to represent a reaction to stress. (For further discussion see Evans, Chapter 3.) The parasympathetic division exerts an opposite effect. It acts to conserve the body's energy resources and its action is characterized by slowing of the heart, stimulation of saliva, digestive activities such as gastric secretions and intestinal peristalsis, and pupil constriction.

Response regulation via these two divisions is highly sensitive as they do not operate in an on–off fashion. Each division maintains some input to each of the various internal organs and the momentary response of any one organ is determined by the relative balance that exists between the two divisions at any moment. To take a specific example, the control of heart rate depends upon the relative inputs of sympathetic and parasympathetic innervations. When heart rate alters it is caused by a shift in the overall balance between the systems; a slowing of heart rate, for example, could be caused by increasing the parasympathetic stimulation or equally well by maintaining the para-sympathetic input at its current level but reducing the level of sympathetic input. The alterations of internal responding are sensed by internal sensory receptors which provide feedback to the CNS and may result in the initiation of behaviours by the CNS. For example, changes in gastric motility may be recognized as 'hunger', which may lead to initiation of actions to gather food whose consumption may eliminate the gastric contractions of the stomach: food-related behaviours will then cease. Within this closed loop there is no executive operator, simply mutual interdependence between the various components (see Brener 1981).

Despite its name it is also quite wrong to suppose that the ANS is an automatic system showing simply reflexive changes in activity. As the studies of operant conditioning of autonomic responses and biofeedback (see Chapter 8) have clearly demonstrated, the ANS is an adaptive system that is capable of learning to respond to the demands imposed by different environments (see Van Toller 1979 for further discussion of the roles of the ANS in behaviour).

NEUROENDOCRINE AND NEUROIMMUNOLOGICAL SYSTEMS

It is not the case that neural systems are the only mechanisms for regulating behaviour. The endocrine and immune systems are also involved and have prominent roles in health. These systems are well described by Rasmussen (1974) and Ader (1981) and are only briefly outlined here.

The endocrine system further extends the functions of the nervous system and their actions are fully integrated with reciprocal influences upon each other. The system controls several glands within the body that secrete into the blood stream chemical messengers called hormones which activate specific receptors in target organs which may show specific responses or may themselves be stimulated to produce other hormones which in turn act upon other organs, including the brain.

Secretion of many of these hormones is regulated by trophic hormones released from the pituitary gland which has a significant function in integrating the release of dozens of other hormones within the body. This highly complex chemical regulation system is itself regulated by the CNS and in particular the hypothalamus and limbic system, which are structures involved in the regulation of emotional and motivational states. The endocrine system is itself critically involved in basic biological functions including sexual differentiation and reproduction, metabolism and growth, emotional activation and reactions to stressors. It would be impossible to review all of the different endocrine actions that exist within the body but one example of its actions is the reaction of the endocrine system to stress (this is further discussed in Chapter 3).

In humans there exists next to each kidney the adrenal gland, which is made up of an outer cortex and an inner core, the adrenal medulla. Both of these are involved in the body's reaction to stressors. The adrenal medulla is innervated by the ANS and releases adrenalin and noradrenalin into the blood stream. These circulating hormones prepare the body for action by increasing cardiac output and stimulating respiration. It has been found both in laboratory studies and in real-life situations that psychosocial stressors, such as facing threatening stimuli, working under time pressure or admission to hospital, cause increased output of adrenalin and noradrenalin. It may be that the extent of this response varies between individuals according to how they react to environmental demands and it has been suggested that this differential response or reactivity may be associated with the development of certain diseases such as coronary heart disease (Cox 1983).

The adrenal cortex secretes the steroid hormones including cortisol, which has its effect on carbohydrate metabolism causing an increase in the blood glucose level. Regulation of the secretion of cortisol depends upon the complex regulatory mechanisms shown in Figure 2.2.

The trophic hormone adrenocortico-trophic hormone (ACTH), when released from the anterior pituitary gland, stimulates cells of the adrenal cortex to secrete corticosteroid hormones including cortisol which by its catabolic action releases energy from carbohydrate metabolism. ACTH is itself released in response to another hormone, the corticotrophin releasing hormone which is produced by the hypothalamus. Negative feedback loops exist at all levels of the system to self-regulate the production and release of these various hormones.

The endocrine system has long-acting influences upon the body. Once released hormones can circulate and activate receptors over substantial periods of time. Some act on receptors in the brain and influence behaviour directly; others have indirect influences via feedback from internal organs.

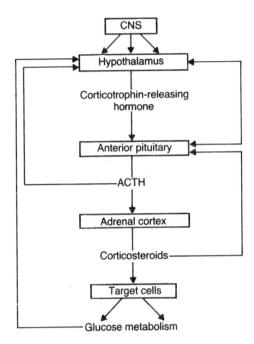

Figure 2.2 Pituitary–adrenal cortex response system.

The amounts of hormones circulating change in response to psychological influences and it has been established that the levels are associated with the development of disease and illness. For example, the opportunity to control an aversive stressor in rats influences the extent and duration of release of stress hormones by the pituitary-adrenal system (Dantzer 1989). Experimental studies with animals have shown that stress-induced increases of corticosteroid release are associated with the suppression of immune system activity (Cox and Mackay 1982). In humans these same psycho-endocrine mechanisms are implicated in the growth of some tumours such as breast cancer (Stoll 1988). It may be speculated therefore that between prolonged exposure to psychosocial stressors and the development of cancer there exists a link that may depend upon neuroendocrine mechanisms involving ACTH and their influence upon immunocompetence (Cella and Holland 1988).

The human immune system exists to protect the body against infection and diseases. Protection against harmful bacteria and viruses is provided by barriers including the skin and various mucous membranes of the mouth and nose, for example, as well as by active immunological processes including secretion of chemicals that can detect and inactivate pathogens, and activation of antibodies to give specific resistance to particular diseases. The immune system is continuously active but its effectiveness is sensitive to psychological influences including, for example, the effects of psychosocial stressors (Koolhaas and Bohus 1989). The relationship between psychological factors and the function of the immune system has been brought into prominence recently by the research upon Acquired Immune Deficiency Syndrome (AIDS) which shows that the immunosuppressive effect of the Human Immunodeficiency Virus (HIV) is influenced by co-factors including experienced or perceived stress (see Phillips, Chapter 10). Similarly there is good evidence that psychoimmunological influences are involved in the development and progression of cancers such as breast cancer (Cox 1988; Stoll 1988). There are indications too that recurrent infections with the genital-herpes virus are related to changes in immune-system function and those changes are themselves associated with experienced life stresses (Kemeny et al. 1989). Though much more research is needed on the precise mechanisms involved there can be little doubt that the competence of the immune system for resisting infection and disease is influenced by psychological processes and states such as stress, depression, major and minor life events. (In Chapter 3 Evans discusses further the significance of psychoneuroimmunology and health.)

RECORDING PSYCHOPHYSIOLOGICAL RESPONSES

Psychophysiology is concerned with the influence of psychological processes or changes in behaviour upon physiological responses. Unlike physiological psychology it is not concerned with identifying the substrates of behaviour, and its methods depend upon measuring responses in intact organisms (usually humans) during ongoing behaviours including the performance of challenging tasks such as solving problems, sleep, learning and so forth. The measurement techniques used to collect physiological data during these and other behaviours are often, though not always, non-invasive. Many researchers are content to use psychophysiological data as correlates of behaviours and to use them to index psychological processes such as attention, fear or stress. Others have argued that the data can be used more productively to identify and elucidate the processes linking physiology and behaviour (Obrist 1981; Phillips 1987). Only if the data are used in this way does psychophysiology as a discipline have significance for health psychology. The psychobiological approach demands that investigators move beyond simple assertions of the type, for example, that 'psychosocial stress causes hypertension' to true explanations that identify the processes involved in translating the impact of exposure to psychosocial stressors to disease states such as hypertension. This is more demanding since it involves much more than simply identifying psychophysiological correlates of hypertension but is all the more rewarding when successful, as the elegant studies of Obrist (1981) have clearly demonstrated.

Psychophysiological recording techniques have been developed that allow quantification of physiological responses of many different kinds including central nervous system activity (individual nerve responses, the electro-encephalogram or EEG), autonomic system activity (for example, heart rate), endocrine responses such as the blood levels of circulating stress hormones, and indices of immune-system function such as level of immunoglobulin in saliva. Each of these clearly requires specialized recording techiques whose description is beyond the scope of this discussion. Fortunately there are many good introductory texts that give an outline of the techniques involved in the measurement of these and other psychophysiological responses (Andreassi 1980; Hassett 1978) as well as comprehensive volumes that should be consulted by anyone wishing to make use of these techniques (Coles *et al.* 1986; Martin and Venables 1980). Some basic principles of recording are outlined below.

Recording bioelectric responses

Though the particular techniques used vary for different response systems, certain general features are common to all. These are illustrated in Figure 2.3.

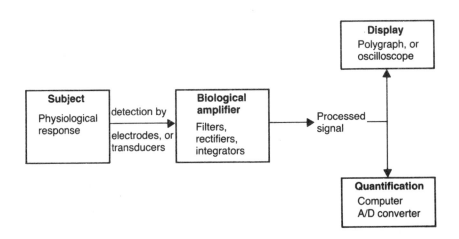

Figure 2.3 General features of a psychophysiological recording and measurement system.

The measurement of bioelectric signals can depend upon direct recording, indirect recording or the recording of transduced bioelectric signals. The differences concern the origins of the signals to be measured. Direct bioelectric signals originate in living tissues as a result of metabolic activity, and suitable electrodes placed on or near to those tissues detect those signals as electrical potentials. Good examples of this type of signal include the electroencephalogram which arises from cortical tissues, the electrocardiogram recorded from the heart and the electromyogram recorded from skeletal muscle fibres. Indirect signals are recorded indirectly from tissues by, for example, measuring the resistance offered by the skin to passage of a mild electric current presented via attached electrodes (skin resistance). Other signals are physical and non-electrical in origin, for example pressure or temperature, and special devices called transducers must be used to convert the physical signal into an electrical equivalent before they are recorded.

Once detected via electrodes or transducers the electrical signals generally must then be amplified since their magnitudes are small; many in the range of millivolts but some, such as EEG measures, in the microvolt range. In addition to simple amplification there may be further processing of the signals using electronic devices such as filters, integrators and rectifiers to isolate further the signal and to eliminate artefacts that can arise from the recording techniques. Once processed the signal is then available for display, which may be in real time using an instrument called the oscilloscope, or as a permanent written record on a paper chart by use of the device called the polygraph (literally 'multiple writer') which allows several response recordings to be displayed simultaneously on a single chart. For most applications it is usually necessary to quantify the changes occurring in the recorded signal. This may involve further processing such as the transformation of an analogue signal into a digital measure or sampling the response at fixed time intervals. Most quantification systems are now based upon microcomputers with purpose-written software packages. The basic assumption underlying the psychophysiological approach is that changes observed in the recorded signals correspond to psychological processes or behaviour that have significance for the subject or patient.

Ambulatory recording

The system for recording bioelectrical responses from living tissues described briefly above is employed in laboratory- and clinic-based investigations. Unfortunately it may be the case that subjects' or patients' responses in the laboratory or clinic do not compare to their reactions in other settings such as their work or home environments. This limitation has prompted the development of portable recording devices based upon instruments, using either radio-telemetry or portable data storage by cassette tapes or small microprocessors, that can be worn by individuals during their everyday lives.

Despite some reservations about their consistency and reliability, considerable progress has been made with these systems in recent years and there are now several ambulatory monitoring systems available. They have been used with some success to record responses over long periods of time during patients' everyday lives, including their home and work environments (Turpin 1985). The techniques have been used with some success, for example, to monitor changes in heart rates of patients who experience sudden onset of uncontrollable and unaccountable attacks of panic (panic disorder). In this context the technique has shown that the attacks are accompanied and perhaps preceded by sudden acceleration of heart rate above normal levels, suggesting that panic may arise from internal autonomic sensations which the person interprets in a catastrophic manner (Taylor *et al.* 1986).

Biochemical recordings

As pointed out in the first section of this chapter, psychophysiology is not only concerned with nervous-system responses. Equally important are the responses of the endocrine and immune systems and special biochemical techniques have been developed to measure the responses of these systems (Ader 1981; Christie and Woodman 1980). In some cases the biochemical measures provide data additional or complementary to those from electro-physiological recordings. In others such as diabetes the biochemical methods used to monitor the blood-glucose response (see Chapter 15) are essential for understanding the nature of the disorder and the opportunities for treatment.

Biochemical methods depend upon the analysis of one or more of the body fluids – saliva, blood, urine or sweat. These contain a variety of chemicals including salts such as sodium or potassium, metabolites including glucose, hormones such as adrenalin or noradrenalin, and indicators of the competence of the immune system such as immunoglobulin. The choice of fluid for analysis depends upon which chemical is to be screened. Analysis of chemicals from blood is a popular method since blood levels show the current status of metabolic function, unlike urine analysis which shows only the products of previous metabolic function. However, for psychophysiological studies blood analysis is not always appropriate since the techniques of collection – involving syringe and needle or pin prick – may themselves act as a stressor causing changes in biochemical reactions for some subjects at least. Collection of urine is a less stressful alternative but again there are problems. The constituents of urine vary considerably during the day and analyses may require collection of total urine output over twenty-four hours rather than analysis of a single sample. Clearly this can be problematic for subject and experimenter alike. Recently saliva has become a popular fluid for analysis. Salts, some hormones and immune-system indicators can all readily be measured from saliva though again there are procedural difficulties associated with its collection that can influence the analyses of content and confound interpretation of the data. The fluid secreted by sweat glands offers a further source of biochemical data though to date it has been less investigated than other body fluids.

PSYCHOPHYSIOLOGY AND HEALTH PSYCHOLOGY

The definition of health psychology given in the first chapter emphasizes the opportunities of psychology for promoting health, preventing and treating illness, identifying the aetiology of diseases, as well as informing health-care policies. Psychophysiology makes direct contributions to understanding the aetiologies of diseases and it suggests interventions that may be used to prevent and treat illnesses. The knowledge it brings about the links between psychosocial factors and disease indirectly assists strategies for health promotion and the planning of health-care policies. Its contributions, however, must be integrated with those from other types of psychological enquiry including social and cognitive approaches. The challenge facing health psychologists is to develop models that can take account of these different perspectives upon health and accommodate data derived from these different disciplines.

Epidemiological studies have established that illnesses are not randomly distributed. Psychosocial factors such as socio-economic status, social mobility and unemployment have been shown to be associated reliably with the incidence of several diseases such as coronary heart disease (for example, Brenner 1987; Marmot *et al.* 1978). Similarly, psychosocial factors encountered in individuals' work-places such as their authority over decisions and the opportunity to use and develop skills, which contribute to their decision latitude and sense of personal control, are associated with physio-logical responses such as changes in blood pressure and may contribute to ill-health. Broadly it has been found that the more decision latitude at work, the better the workers' health (Theorell 1989). Clinical studies have concentrated upon the relationships between adverse or significant life events and illness and find associations between life events and psychiatric disorders such as depression (Brown and Harris 1986). Other studies indicate that even the relatively minor life changes referred to to as 'uplifts' or 'hassles' predict changes in immune-system function and susceptibility to minor infections such as the common cold (Evans *et al.* 1988). At an individual level, research on the links between the Type A Behaviour Pattern and coronary heart disease (see Evans, Chapter 13) finds increased risk for those individuals displaying the behavioural characteristics that describe the Type A pattern. The demonstrations of these associations between psychosocial variables and illness or risk of disease pose fundamental questions for health psychology. How is it that psychosocial factors influence patterns of illness and disease within a population? Why is one individual but not another vulnerable to the effect of a particular psychosocial factor? Ultimately the links between psychosocial factors and disease must depend upon changes in neurological and biochemical responses. The challenge for psychophysiology is to identify the mechanisms involved and demonstrate the processes that give rise to illness and disease.

Clinical psychophysiology

Psychophysiology has come to occupy a central position in Health Psychology and has provided the techniques that are central to what might be called psychobiological models of health and illness (for example, Feuerstein *et al.* 1986; Weiner 1977). In recognition of this development, there has emerged a subdiscipline called 'clinical psychophysiology' which is defined by Turpin (1989: 7) as 'the application of psychophysiological techniques, concepts and theories to the explanation of psychological factors which influence health behaviours and risks'.

It would be quite wrong to suppose that the use of psychophysiological techniques is simple or that the interpretation of the data collected is straightforward. The potential problems are numerous and substantial. They have been well described by Turpin (1989), who identifies several critical issues – the appropriateness of different research designs, the selection of relevant or valid measures, situational factors that affect the measures recorded, the appropriate methods of data manipulation and analysis, and not least the interpretation and reliability of psychophysiological data. To take account of all of these issues psychophysiological studies must be planned with considerable care. Despite the difficulties and when care is taken, psychophysiological data provide a wealth of clues into the mechanisms maintaining health or underlying the aetiology of disease states.

Psychophysiological techniques have been used simply as correlates of either pathological states such as brain damage or psychological states such as anxiety. Although the former can be useful for identifying the physiological substrates of disorders and the latter for labelling the psychophysiological symptoms associated with states, neither of these applications is entirely useful for explaining the processes of health. For that, psychophysiological techniques must be used to unravel the mechanisms by which dysfunctional states originate and are maintained. This means that studies of health must consider and take account not only of physiological responses but also their relationships to social and psychological factors. The relationships between them are critical for health, and psychophysiology provides the means to identify the mechanisms by which they interact with each other.

Biopsychosocial models of disease

Within Health Psychology one model that has enjoyed considerable popularity is the 'stress-diathesis' model (Steptoe 1989), which may be called a 'biopsychosocial model' since it emphasizes the interactive effect of environmental and individual-vulnerability (genetic and psychological characteristics) factors upon health. Models of this type have been used to explain psychopathological states including schizophrenia (Turpin *et al.* 1988) as well as medical disorders such as coronary heart disease.

According to this model psychological and physical threats present demands upon an individual's resources and capacity for coping which give rise to physiological reactions involving the ANS, endocrine and immune systems of the body. The effects include both short-term and long-term components and these may have consequences for health depending upon the individual's predisposition or vulnerability to adverse effects. The physiological responses observed themselves may be entirely appropriate reactions to the demands faced and yet still pose threats to health. Sterling and Eyer (1988) have proposed the term 'allostasis' to describe the matching to demand of physiological resources that is provoked by the environment–individual interaction. Whether or not some or all of these responses have an effect upon health depends upon the individual's biological predisposition or diathesis. Vulnerable individuals develop chronic allostatic reactions such as reduced immunocompetence, or exaggerated sympathetic activation of the ANS, or increased secretion of adrenal hormones. Physiological reactions of these types have been implicated in the development of many disease states including cancers, cardiovascular diseases and susceptibility to infections. According to the stress-diathesis model there are several stages which lead finally to the development of a disease state. It is the interaction between the individual and the environment that is significant in giving rise to the necessary physiological reactions but it is the individual's biological vulnerability that finally allows those reactions to become translated into illness or disease.

Personal control and health

There are many factors that may be important in moderating the effects of the environment–individual interaction. Cognitive factors influence the way in which the environment is perceived and 'cognitive appraisals' frequently appear in models of stress and health. Amongst these various moderating variables, the concept of 'personal control' has become widely accepted as having significance for health (Steptoe and Appels 1989). The concept can be used at several levels of analysis from epidemiological studies, studies of occupational factors, and experimental studies of humans and animals engaged in laboratory tasks.

Despite problems in the definition of 'control' which has led to various classifications of types of control (Phillips 1989a) the concept has been instrumental in stimulating considerable research into the relationship between stress and health. From these studies it is clear that control or absence of control has predictable effects upon responses of the ANS, endocrine and immune systems. Moreover, individual differences exist in preference for control, the capacity and resources available for control, and strategies available for exercising control. These differences will, according to the stress-diathesis model, influence the pattern and extent of psycho-physiological responses required to meet particular environmental demands. Thus, 'control' can determine the allostasic responses that may themselves contribute to ill-health or its absence. The success or otherwise of these and similar models to explain illness and disease will depend upon the manner in which psychophysiological techniques are used to tease out the mechanisms involved. Simply labelling some response as a product of control or absence of control may superficially describe the relationship between psychological and physiological events but does not explain the processes involved. To identify those processes, much more elaborate and sophisticated investigations are necessary. These are not beyond the guile of psycho-physiologists as shown by the exemplary studies carried out by Obrist and his co-workers on the impact of behavioural demands for haemodynamic changes that give rise to hypertension (Obrist 1981).

Psychophysiological treatment of illness

In addition to providing the methods for unravelling the mechanisms involved in the aetiology of disease states, psychophysiology can also contribute to their treatment. The knowledge gained from psychophysiological studies of illnesses can be used to develop clinical interventions to prevent or treat those disorders. Steptoe (1989) has described how behavioural medicine has adopted interventions based upon the the stress-diathesis model of disease. The interventions may act at different stages of the disease process. Thus, cognitive interventions may be used to modify an individual's psychosocial resources. If it were confirmed that hypertension develops as a result of exaggerated cardiovascular reactivity (see Chapter 12), then interventions designed to reduce reactivity in vulnerable individuals, for example through relaxation training or biofeedback (see Chapter 8), might well be effective. Or interventions may be adopted that alter an individual's biological vulnerability, for example exercise training. At the moment the effectiveness of these interventions is still being evaluated. Initial indications provide cause for optimism and as Steptoe (1989: 233) has pointed out, 'The treatment of medical disorders is an important aspect of contemporary clinical psychophysiology and the methods that have been developed are likely to have a major impact on health care in the future.'

CONCLUSIONS

The operations of the nervous and peripheral nervous systems are fully integrated with those of the endocrine and immune systems. Elaborate mechanisms exist for self- and mutual regulation within and between these systems, and ill-health certainly reflects dysfunction within these systems. The fundamental task for Health Psychology is to develop models that explain how and under what circumstances these dysfunctions arise and how they become translated into illness and disease. The techniques of psychophysiology have proved useful for investigating the aetiology of diseases and have contributed to biopsychosocial models of ill-health. Psychophysiological methods may be used also as interventions for the treatment of disorders that have a psychophysiological component.

Chapter 3

Stress and coping

Philip Evans

A QUESTION OF DEFINITION

Readers often, I suspect, find introductory sections concerned with definitions a trifle tedious, wanting to get straight into the factual content of a chapter. I have some sympathy, but in the case of stress there really are important definitional issues to be addressed. That is not to say that we need to tie up the construct of stress in a strait-jacket of rigorous usage criteria. We shall find anyway that it defies such attempts and is better left as something of an umbrella term. What is necessary, however, is to be aware of the definitional issues involved.

When a person in an everyday sense uses the word 'stress' in a psychological context s/he will often have one of two things in mind: either things in life that are happening or have happened *to* a person, or processes, mental or physical, which are happening or have happened *within* a person. In other words, sometimes people talk of responding to stress, sometimes they talk of suffering it. Each is an acceptable usage of the word stress in the English language but each usage has important implications. In the discussions below, we shall colloquially refer to these usages as 'stress outside' and 'stress inside' respectively.

Stress outside

When people say they are under stress, they will point to various pressures at work, difficult deadlines for example, or troubles at home, in order to make their use of the term 'stress' more concrete. In that sense the troubles are taken to be exemplars of stress. In an analogous way we may talk of structures, such as bridges, being subject to the stress of gale-force winds, extremes of temperature or abnormal weight of traffic.

This seems at first glance to be a promising way of looking at psychological stress, and indeed it has given rise to much research in the area. In the language of research design it invites us to treat stress as an *independent variable* which we may observe or even manipulate with a view to specifying its effects on an organism. Thus a variety of factors from major disasters to minor hassles, from cognitive overload to sleep deprivation, from over-crowding to isolation, from electric shock to aversive noise, have been examined for their supposed stressful effects on behaviour.

Whether stress, as an independent variable, has been manipulated or merely measured is of course an important factor in interpreting such research, since an unambiguous cause–effect relationship between a supposed stressful experience and subsequent behaviour can only be properly shown in a genuine experiment which does manipulate stress. In the case of major or prolonged exposure to stress, such experiments have largely been confined to animals. However, by measuring several variables simultaneously and by carefully timing events, it has been possible to support causative hypotheses in relation to human beings whose natural exposure to stress has been system-atically observed. Sophisticated work in this vein has the benefit of avoiding distressing work with animals, which is increasingly seen as ethically dubious and which in any event often presents problems in generalizing to the human arena.

However, treating stress solely as an independent variable – something out there – has one rather serious drawback. It ignores the important point that different people may react differently to exactly the same so-called stressful event. Do we say that one person is stressed and the other not stressed? Or do we say that both are stressed but their reactions are different? If one person's behaviour were to indicate a very positive response to the so-called stressful experience, we may feel that it is stretching semantics to say that s/he has nevertheless been under stress. But if we say that such a person has not been under stress, we are implicitly recognizing that the meaning of the word stress resides, partly at least, inside the person. We shall now consider the notion that stress is to be defined as something inside the person.

Stress inside

Put in its strongest form, this view suggests that if we can measure a certain pattern of 'stressful' responses within a person, this is the sole criterion of whether or not that person has been 'stressed', regardless of the nature of the experience undergone. From this perspective, an apparently very positive life event may cause stress, or equally an apparently very negative life event may not do so. In a sense, this way of defining stress should take priority over external criteria, since investigations of stress as an independent external variable focus on just those sort of variables which we may normally expect but not necessarily know will produce certain types of 'stressful' effect. If no evidence of 'stress inside' were ever to be forthcoming following exposure to a purported external source of stress, we can be pretty sure that such an external state of affairs would very soon not be viewed as stressful. However, the difficulty for the 'stress inside' view becomes one of specifying exactly what constitutes a stressful reaction.

7859

With regard to the physiology of stress, we shall see that to an extent it is possible to specify processes which can be identified as evidence of the occurrence of stress. The first major theory of stress as a physiological process was put forward by Selye (1956). Selye defined stress in terms of a general pattern of 'arousal' responding, involving a number of neuroendocrine mechanisms, whose chronic activation ultimately led to the 'exhaustion' of the organism and an inability to cope with further challenge. The trouble with this kind of model, as we shall see, is that the assumed processes are not so general as might first be supposed. There are individual differences in the way people react physiologically to stress. Moreover, in the case of some physical sources of stress involving pain, for example, local physical responses can at the very least muddy the waters when it comes to identifying an assumed general pattern of physiological responding associated purely with something called stress.

It is of course theoretically possible to look for evidence of stress in what might conventionally be called a person's mental state: episodes of anxiety or depression, for example, which are more pronounced and long lasting than the blips which occur on any baseline of ordinary mood states. In this case, however, there is a potential conceptual difficulty which arises: mental symptoms shade inevitably into episodes of what is conventionally labelled as psychiatric illness, and such illness episodes have often been used by researchers as distinct dependent variables, in the aetiology of which stress itself is investigated as a factor.

All in all, then, there seem to be problems in defining stress solely in terms of a range of specifiable external situations or in terms of internal responses to unspecified external stimuli. The approach of most modern researchers has been to adopt what might be called an interactionist position. Stress is seen as a transaction between the environment and the person and a good deal of emphasis is placed on how the person perceives the challenges which the environment presents. The perception of challenge is also taken as crucial to the business of coping (or failing to cope) with potentially stressful circumstances. We shall return to models of stress and coping when we have outlined some of the basic physiology of stress, notwithstanding some of the difficulties which we have just outlined.

THE PHYSIOLOGY OF STRESS

What Selye did establish was the importance of two physiological systems in reactions to a wide variety of potential sources of stress. The first involves the autonomic nervous system (ANS), the adrenal medulla, and the release of the catecholamines, adrenalin and noradrenalin. This system had already been given prominence in Walter Cannon's theory of emergency motivation. Sympathetic arousal, through its effects on a variety of internal organs, mobilizes the organism for what has commonly been called 'fight or flight'.

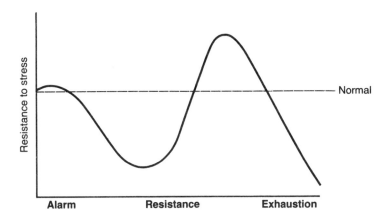

Figure 3.1 Selye's General Adaptation Syndrome.

The adrenal medulla, itself sympathetically innervated, secretes adrenalin and noradrenalin, which mimic the effects of direct sympathetic stimulation and provide a continuing back-up in the mobilization of the body's resources.

The second system is known as the pituitary–adrenocortical axis (see Chapter 2). The pituitary via the hypothalamus causes adrenocortico-trophic hormone (ACTH) to be circulated to the adrenal cortex. The adrenal cortex in turn produces corticosteroids of various kinds which help the adaptive process by, for example, providing muscles with long-term access to the body's energy stores.

The total adaptive response in Selye's original theory was seen as triphasic (see Figure 3.1). An original alarm stage gives way to a resistance stage during which the organism's resistance to stress is heightened, unless new sources of stress appear. If, however, the source of stress continues despite the organism's efforts to resist then the third 'exhaustion' stage ensues. Here harmful effects of high corticosteroid levels, such as ulceration and immuno-suppression, begin to become apparent, and overall resistance is decreased. If the process is allowed to continue, recovery is not possible and death is the final result.

Selye's original view was that the above represented a general response to stress of all kinds, as, indeed, is implied by the term General Adaptation Syndrome. As we suggested earlier this is in need of qualification, since not all people respond in the same way to identical stress sources and the same individual may respond differently on different occasions. This has led more recent commentators on stress (for example, Cox 1978; Fisher 1986) to emphasize the role that psychological processes play in mediating physio-logical effects. We also know that the physiological processes involved in adaptation are even more complex than envisaged in Selye's original model, involving, for example, the release of neuropeptides, with possible analgesic effects, and even neurally mediated effects on the organs of the immune system, although our knowledge in the area of psychoneuroimmunology, the hybrid science named by Ader (1981), is still in a state of infancy.

COPING AND CONTROLLING

Many recent models of stress implicitly or explicitly see it as the outcome of a cognitive process in which a challenge or threat is first of all perceived, the ability to control the challenge or threat is assessed, and finally a computation of discrepancy is made. Stress is thus seen as a consequence of perceiving a 'deficit' picture: uncontrollability, or helplessness. An example of a simple 'control' model of this type is illustrated in Figure 3.2. Although such models are attractive in that they seem to have a potential for great generality, they do tend to replace one tricky concept (stress) with another (controllability). Of course that is quite legitimate. What it means, however, is that we must now address the issue of controllability in more depth.

Seligman (1975) wrote a book on helplessness which did much to stimulate interest in the consequences of an organism learning that it lacks control over events. Various stressful and depression-like symptoms were shown to be associated with learned helplessness across a variety of species.

The original work of Seligman and his colleagues had come from the animal laboratory, where it is relatively easy to define control in an exact way. Usually some overt behavioural response is 'instrumental' in avoiding, escaping or otherwise mitigating the aversive event, usually electric shock. This kind of obvious control we shall term 'instrumental control'. In the case of human beings, however, instrumental control is only one of many kinds of more general control that people have, or, at least believe they have (see

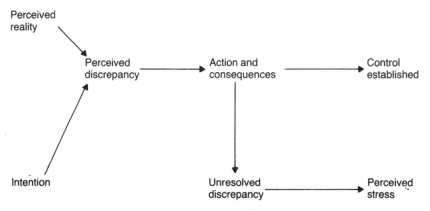

Figure 3.2 Cognitive control model of stress (after Fisher 1986).

Thompson 1981). Let us begin with that last qualification: 'or believe they have'. Note that the model in Figure 3.2 refers not simply to reality and discrepancy but to *perceived* reality and *perceived* discrepancy. In the context of our current discussion, this means that the control a person actually has is unimportant: it is how much control people believe they have which really matters. This allows for all sorts of stress-reducing stratagems on the part of individuals. For example, someone may respond well to a potentially stressful situation if s/he believes that his or her prayers have prevented a worse tragedy happening. Much superstitious behaviour can be rationalized by the agent as a form of 'magical' control, the main feature of which is the impossibility of falsification. However, we are still dealing here with a form of instrumental control, since the person involved is supposedly making some response in the belief that certain aversive consequences will be avoided or mitigated.

However, human beings are often differentiated from other organisms on the basis of their highly developed cognitive capabilities. In the area of stress, this means that human beings can show diversity in response to a potentially threatening situation according to how they cognitively *appraise* it. Much of the pioneering work in this area was carried out by Lazarus and his colleagues (see Lazarus 1974). In essence, they showed that physiological arousal prompted by exposure to a stressful film could be moderated by instructions given prior to the film. The instructions, in turn, were deliberately varied in order to encourage different appraisal processes, such as intellectualization or denial.

Thus, appraisal processes can be seen as ways of controlling and coping with potential sources of stress. This also raises the issue of individual differences. Presumably people learn characteristic ways of appraising threats, which may in turn be fairly general across many areas of their lives, or alternatively may be fairly specific to certain domains. Although instructions, as used by Lazarus and his colleagues, may modify people's appraisals, we may suppose that ordinarily, habitual appraisal strategies exist.

Individual differences also exist in the extent to which people appear to seek information about stressful circumstances. The link between information seeking and control seeking is not always simple. Information usually brings a measure of predictability. With regard to something like surgery, for example, the patient may learn when to expect certain types of pain, how long it will be likely to last and so on. A distinct preference for information about the course of aversive procedures is the general finding, certainly in the large number of studies which come from the animal laboratory (see Badia *et al.* 1979), which may lead us to suppose that predictability always entails a degree of controllability which in turn is stress reducing. However, in the case of human beings, matters are once again more complex. We shall see shortly that being informed about a forthcoming aversive event, for some people and in some circumstances, is far from being either a preferred or a stress-reducing state of affairs.

However, in general, and certainly in the case of the animal studies, predictability is sought, and there are persuasive theories which can explain why, for example, predictable aversive stimuli are generally preferred to unpredictable ones even though the predictable stimuli may be more intense or more frequent. The major theory in this area emphasizes the role that predictability plays in signalling periods of safety. In an important series of experiments Badia and his colleagues have shown that preference for information about impending electric shock is clearly demonstrated when warning signals are *necessary* but *not sufficient* conditions of shock (i.e. no shock is ever given without a prior warning signal but some 'false alarms' may be given): they are not however preferred when they are *sufficient* but *not necessary* (i.e. no 'false alarms' are given but some shocks may be delivered without warning). Put more simply the evidence indicates that the important factor is the safety which is guaranteed by the absence of a signal, rather than the certitude of shock in the event of a signal. It is arguable that being able to separate periods of danger and periods of safety enables an organism to optimize, in terms of time allocation, a variety of competing goal-seeking behaviours. Essentially, predictability confers controllability.

With regard to measures of stress, we have tended so far to assume that perceived controllability is linked to stress reduction. There is of course evidence for such a view. Animal experiments once again have provided the clearest picture, in so far as they have been able to manipulate the principal variables. Weiss's work on stress induced gastro-intestinal lesions (Weiss 1977) is among the most compelling. When rodents are paired off ('yoked') so that the aversive experience of one member of a pair is made identical to that of the other member, and when only one member of the pair can exercise control over the aversive stimulus (electric shock), it is the other animal, the passive partner with no control, which develops more severe lesioning. Note that the exposure to the physical 'stress' is identical for both animals: when the controlling animal fails to respond, both receive shock. Thus, the two animals vary solely on the psychological dimension of being in control or not.

Even in the world of animal experimentation, however, the above findings need some qualification. Controlling responses require effort and Weiss found that effortfulness itself produces stressful reactions if it is too great. This may well explain the results of an earlier study of similar design by Brady (1958) in which monkeys were used as subjects. Here it was the active controlling monkeys – the so called 'executives' – who suffered more ulceration. However, Brady's executive monkeys could only maintain control through highly effortful responding on a fatiguing time schedule, and this effortfulness was almost certainly a factor in producing Brady's results. Thus, controlling may often be a stress-reducing method of coping, but it is necessary to take the cost of the controlling itself into consideration.

A similarity exists here with respect to psychophysiological studies of coping by human subjects. Obrist and his colleagues have particularly looked at sympathetically mediated changes in tonic heart rate. Active coping, which often involves exercising control, is associated with increased cardiovascular arousal. The greatest increases in heart-rate activity, however, are elicited by tasks of moderate difficulty, neither very easy, nor next to impossible (Light and Obrist 1983). If one sees these experiments in terms of the probability of exercising effective control, it seems that maximal physiological arousal is obtained when maximal uncertainty exists about outcome (see Phillips 1989a). Contrarily, both very easy and very difficult task demands can lead to clear expectations of success and failure respectively.

Pursuing just this sort of theme, McGrath (1976) has argued that the potential for experiencing stress is greatest precisely when the perceived discrepancy between demand and coping resources is small. It is then that uncertainty of outcome is maximal. McGrath cites evidence from a study of baseball players (Lowe and McGrath 1971) where pulse rate was taken regularly throughout a whole batting season and examined in relation to players' perceived demand and outcome.

What certainly seems to be true is that the sort of active coping reliably associated with increased cardiovascular demand does have to be prompted, as it were, by a sufficient expectation of success. This does not mean to say, however, that expectation of failure in the face of threat or challenge is necessarily always less stressful. Indeed, such a theoretical position would seem somewhat to fly in the face of common sense. Cardiovascular arousal in any event does not on its own equal stress, and, as Cox (1978) points out, Lowe and McGrath badly confuse arousal and stress. Most people would find it appropriate to use the word 'stressful' to refer to certain states of low arousal (boredom or fatigue, for example) and most would also refer to some high arousal states as low in stress (for example, excitement). There is also empirical evidence for this assertion from factor-analytic studies of ratings which people give to various mood adjectives. Mackay et al. (1978) obtained two orthogonal factors akin to stress and arousal. Similar reasoning underpins the motivational theory of reversals (Apter 1982) in which hedonic tone (pleasantness–unpleasantness) is related to arousal by two curves rather than a single one. According to the 'meta-motivational' state of the person, high arousal may be felt as pleasant or unpleasant, and so may low arousal. If stress and arousal are independent we can envisage their combination to produce the four separate quadrants of Figure 3.3.

The active controlling coping which we have considered so far is typically associated with high arousal. What seems to be true, bringing all strands of our discussion together, is that total stress in such circumstances is best seen as a composite resulting from the magnitude of the external demand and partly from the uncertainty and effort involved in trying to meet the demand. In reality, however, we do have to admit that any precise weighting of these separate components is likely to prove an impractical proposition.

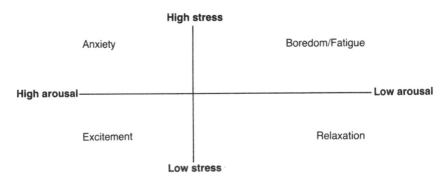

Figure 3.3 Mood states associated with the orthogonal dimensions of stress and arousal.

VIGILANT AND AVOIDANT COPING STYLES

As we have mentioned earlier, everybody does not always seek or desire information about an impending threat (see Chapter 5 for a discussion of this issue in relation to forthcoming surgery). Some would perhaps prefer to bury their heads in the sand and forget about the matter. Such coping strategies are often referred to as avoidant styles, in contrast to the vigilant style of behaviour which is usually required when obvious controlling responses are needed. In a variety of studies with human subjects, experimenters have tried to measure preference for information about aversive events by giving subjects a choice between monitoring for a warning signal and an alternative strategy: the opportunity to engage in a distracting (avoidant) activity of some kind. In all such studies it has been found that a percentage of persons favours a distraction strategy and a percentage favours vigilance.

The exact percentage of so-called 'monitors' and 'distractors' varies according to the particular contingencies of the experiment. For example, people are more likely to monitor, the more effective the control available (Averill *et al.* 1977; Evans *et al.* 1984). However, even when no control over the aversive event is possible, some subjects prefer to engage in monitoring. Equally, when total monitoring would permit complete avoidance of an aversive event by detection of a warning signal, some subjects will still choose the distracting activity. It is interesting to ask why.

With regard to active coping involving exercising controlling responses, we have stated earlier that total stress is likely to be a function not only of the magnitude of the threat but also the effortfulness and uncertainty of exercising effective control. In the kind of experiment just described, it is generally found that monitoring is associated with higher autonomic arousal than is distraction whether arousal is measured by skin conductance (Miller 1979a) or heart rate (Evans *et al.* 1984). If vigilant coping inevitably involves a certain amount of stressful arousal, it is likely that the degree of such arousal differs from subject to subject, perhaps depending on such factors as a native or learned tolerance of ambiguity or uncertainty. For some people, therefore, it may well be the case that total stress is reduced by relinquishing control. However, whether we describe such ostrich-like strategies as distraction, denial or as control-relinquishing becomes largely a matter of semantics. By relinquishing uncertain control over a source of stress and avoiding needless worry by distraction, a person may in fact be exercising a kind of superordinate control and be minimizing the stress involved in the whole 'package deal' of threat and anticipation of threat.

Indeed, Miller (1979b) put forward a theory of control which does allow for such complexities. She calls it the minimax theory, which refers to its main prediction: individuals will act to minimize the maximal danger. In cases of simple instrumental control it makes the same predictions as, for example, the safety-signal hypothesis, which we mentioned earlier. However, by allowing concentration on the longer term, it is flexible enough to predict the relinquishing of control, if that guarantees less overall danger. One problem with minimax theory is that it is perhaps too flexible, but any more detailed discussion is beyond the scope of this chapter. The interested reader can find such discussion elsewhere (for example, Fisher 1986; Miller 1979b; Thompson 1981). Suffice it to say that there are plenty of everyday examples where we routinely surrender control to experts, who look after our lives in hospitals, on aeroplanes and in many other places. How much we simply surrender and relax, or still wish to be kept informed, has also been the subject of investigation in coping research.

Just as the laboratory experiments which we have considered distinguish vigilant and avoidant coping styles, so these are also found in real-life settings, such as the facing of surgery. We shall not go into the vast area of whether greater information in general helps or hinders patients as this is considered in detail in Chapter 5. We can, however, mention one study which suggests that the habitual coping style of patients themselves may be a crucial determinant of whether more detailed information about procedures will or will not be beneficial. Miller and Mangan (1983) gave a group of gynaecological patients a questionnaire prior to a surgical investigation. On the basis of the questionnaire results, they divided patients into 'monitors' and 'blunters', the latter being the researchers' way of referring to a person biased towards an avoidant style of coping. Although Miller and Mangan found that detailed information was not on the whole helpful, and in many cases led to more stressful experiences, the pattern of results did depend to an extent on the preferred coping style of the patient. Monitors fared better with information, blunters worse.

Surgery is just one of the many life events which we have on occasion to experience. Let us now turn finally to a consideration of life events in general, their role in creating or relieving stress, and the part that stress itself may play in the causation of physical illness.

LIFE EVENTS RESEARCH

Since Dohrenwend and Dohrenwend (1974) published a major book on life events and stress, there has been a continuing research impetus in this area. The focus has been on potentially stressful situations to which nearly everyone is exposed to some degree during the course of their lives: major upheavals such as marriage, birth of a child, divorce or bereavement, as well as minor everyday upheavals of all kinds, which are often referred to as 'hassles'. Physical illnesses, major and minor alike, have been linked to such life events – for example, heart disease (Theorell 1982), cancers such as leukaemia (Wold 1968), colds and influenza (Evans *et al.* 1988; Stone *et al.* 1988; Totman and Kiff 1980). Psychological illnesses such as depression (Brown and Harris 1978; Paykel 1974) have also been associated with life events. To the fore when we wish to review studies of life events and illness are considerations of methodology. There is now a vast amount of data, but their interpretation is by no means a simple matter.

A question of measurement

Measuring life events presents considerable problems. One of the first approaches to the question of measurement was to draw up lists of events, based on the judgements of researchers themselves. Criticisms of these early attempts could be made on several grounds. They sometimes lacked comprehensiveness, it being by no means certain that the events chosen were fully appropriate to the sampled populations. Non-events were typically ignored even though they may sometimes be very important to individuals, for example not being promoted at work. Some of the events were confounded with consequences which were also the subject of investigation. For example, an individual who loses his or her job may subsequently suffer from depression: however, it is possible that a detailed investigation of the circumstances of the job loss may reveal it to be tied up with early symptoms of depression. In other words the job loss may not be so much a cause of depression as an effect. Alternatively some third variable related to both job loss and depression may cause a spurious 'association'. However, the major criticism of early life-event 'scales' was that they were unidimensional. They only considered the quantity of life events and not the quality. This point needs expansion.

One of the most widely used early scales was the Readjustment Rating Scale of Holmes and Rahe (1967). A number of subjects were asked to rate items such as 'marriage' in terms of how much adjustment they entailed with reference to other items. Average ratings were then used to come up with general calibrations for future studies. The drawback of such averaging procedures is that there seems to be plenty of evidence of variability in the way that different target groups, not to mention individuals, perceive such events. In view of the models of stress which we detailed earlier in this chapter, it would seem a requirement of more precise research that a subject's own ratings of events are taken into account.

A similar consideration of more recent life-events research has been to explore other dimensions of events, such as perceived control and perceived desirability. We may note that undesirability does not necessarily equal stressfulness, since desirable events may involve adjustments from routine which may be partly stressful. Other aspects which may be important concern the domain in which the events occur (work, family and so on). Such refinements may accomplish various goals. They may increase the significance (by which is meant 'importance' rather than just statistical significance) of associations between events and illness measures. It has often been pointed out that most studies of life events and illness, despite their statistical significance, do not explain much of the variance in illness incidence. Second, refinement of life-events measurement may discriminate which factors are important in relation to illness, and which are not.

Methodological issues

There is general agreement among researchers that even unrefined life-event scales weakly predict a variety of illness episodes, and that illness episodes follow on from 'stressful' periods within a time span not exceeding two years (Chalmers 1982). Even such a limited conclusion, however, relies on taking a broad view of a number of studies and arguing from consistency of effects, since the problems of clearly interpreting individual studies are manifold, owing to a variety of methodological issues. We shall mention just a few.

Many early studies were retrospective. Thus, researchers would probe people about their life-events record after they became ill. This raises problems of recall accuracy, including the general difficulty with retrospective designs that people may well be motivated to 'find' causes for their present illness in preceding events. Even prospective designs have had to face the problem of recall accuracy, since they often involve the same process of trawling a past period (typically the previous six months prior to a follow-up period). Most researchers would nowadays recommend that designs should be prospective and that measures of life-events incidence should obtain ratings from structured interview procedures which allow detailed consideration of the accurate timing of recollections, clearly a vital matter.

Moderating variables

It has been emphasized throughout this chapter that individual persons and their perceptions of reality intervene between objective events and the experience of stress. It should therefore come as no surprise that some people who have high life-event scores sometimes show little or no illness reactions. Moderating variables, lying within the person or in his or her social context, have therefore been found to influence the impact of life events. In general researchers refer to the phenomenon as 'buffering'.

One variable that has received much attention is that of social support. In their study of depression Brown and Harris (1978), for example, found that the deleterious effects of life events could be attenuated if the person were, so to speak, socially embedded, and had a good network of social support within a community. Stone *et al.* (1988) and Evans and Edgerton (1989) have found that desirable life events ('uplifts') predict the onset of colds *by their absence* as much as *hassles* by their presence. Kobasa *et al.* (1982) have described a trait of 'hardiness' centred on the individual's belief in the controllability and normality of challenge, which seems to predict resistance to illness in the face of life-event stress.

General versus specific theories

The discussion of life events so far has echoes of Selye's general-adaptation theory of stress. Although some researchers have chosen to look at specific illnesses, while others have looked at general illness susceptibility following stress, the implication of both sorts of evidence has been that stress as measured by life events predisposes to illness in general. No doubt such a position would also attach to itself a vague working hypothesis which might be called 'somatic weakness', whereby, in certain individuals, certain somatic systems might be weaker than others and like a car that is driven too hard, the bits that fail will be those which were weakest to start with.

Suggestions have been made, however, which countenance different routes to different types of disorder depending on a more refined analysis of how a person may characteristically respond to the potential stress of life events. In particular Fisher (1986) pulls various strands of evidence together in a tentative attempt to identify two possible routes to illness, depending on the coping resources of the individual. It is argued that situations which lead to effort and challenge but which are not obviously distressing lead to physiological arousal but operate primarily via the traditional catecholamine route, which was mentioned earlier. Activation in this case may put a person at risk of what Fisher calls 'somatization', whereby persistent abuse of the biological systems leads to anatomical changes, which in turn increase the risk of disorders such as coronary heart disease. The second route becomes relevant when coping is less effective, and when effort is accompanied by distress. The mechanism here is thought to depend upon greater involvement of the adrenocortical system and involves lowered immune-system efficiency and thus heightened susceptibility to infectious and perhaps cancerous illnesses. Discussion of sympathetic arousal in relation to coronary heart disease can be found elsewhere in this book (see Chapter 13). In the final section of this chapter, therefore, we shall examine the evidence that life events and stress can be linked to impaired immunocompetence and increased vulnerability to infectious disease and cancer.

PSYCHOLOGICAL INFLUENCES ON IMMUNITY AND DISEASE

One technique of investigation has been to measure the efficiency of the response of lymphocytes (immune-system cells) in subjects who have been exposed to some major stressful event. The event of bereavement was used in two key studies (Bartrop *et al.* 1977; Schleifer *et al.* 1983). Compared with matched controls in the first study, and compared with pre-bereavement scores in the second prospective study, it was found that bereavement produced significantly lower levels of immune response. As Baker (1987) points out in a review article, this lends some substance to an observation recorded in the *British Medical Journal* of 1884 to the effect that bereaved persons are abnormally prone to infection.

In a another review of psychoimmunological research, Kiecolt-Glaser and Glaser (1986) report on their own research on marital disruption. Poorer immune function on a set of measures, including lymphocyte responsiveness, was shown by separated and divorced women compared with matched controls. Amongst the sample of married women, poorer immune functioning was associated with poorer state of marriage and greater depression.

Jemmott and his colleagues have investigated the effects of stress on measures of secretory immunoglobulin (s-IgA), which is contained in the secretions that coat the mucosal surfaces and constitutes the immune system's first line of defence against infections, notably those of the upper respiratory tract, gastro-intestinal and genito-urinary systems. Jemmott and Magloire (1988) demonstrated lower concentrations of s-IgA in students during an exam period compared to control periods before and after exams. Moreover, s-IgA concentrations paralleled reported stress levels.

The links between stress, immunocompetence and infectious illness are likely to be of importance over a short period of time. It is interesting to note in this context the recent work on susceptibility to upper respiratory infections such as colds, which has already been mentioned (Evans and Edgerton 1989; Evans *et al.* 1988; Stone *et al.* 1988). These three studies all used a prospective within-subjects design, in which subjects filled in life-event scales daily for several weeks. Among those subjects who succumbed to colds during the investigative period, the researchers found a quite pronounced change in desirable or undesirable event reporting around four days prior to onset of illness episodes. Given the consistency of the time lag across all three studies, it is significant that such a time scale maps exceedingly well on to a model which sees stress lowering s-IgA protection at just the time that viral exposure is likely to be taking place, given what is known of the incubation period for the common cold.

When we turn to cancer, the time scale for the development of disease is altogether much less certain. Researchers have found that natural-killer (NK) cell activity is impaired by examinations stress (Kiecolt-Glaser *et al.* 1984). NK cell activity is thought to be important as a defence against cancer.

However, definite links between stress and cancer in humans have not yet been fully established, although there is a considerable body of reports from experiments on animals (for a review see Justice 1985).

Although the role of life events is uncertain, what seems to be a feature of human-based research is the association between depression and cancer, and depression can arguably be linked via helplessness and control theory to the adrenocortical-immune system route in Fisher's binary model. Higher cancer mortality rates for bereaved spouses have been reported (Fox 1981), although a later longitudinal study (Jones *et al.* 1984) only found suggestive statistics for breast cancer. Perhaps the most suggestive results on the link between depression and cancer come from a seventeen-year follow-up study of over two thousand factory workers in Cleveland, Ohio (Shekelle *et al.* 1981). All subjects were between 40 and 50 years of age and all completed the Minnesota Multiphasic Personality Inventory (MMPI). Among those scoring highly on Depression, the death rate from cancer during the follow-up period was twice the expected norm. The result was not explicable in terms of confounding variables such as age, smoking and so on.

The work of Greer and his colleagues with breast-cancer patients has also been illuminating with regard to affective processes. Initially, Greer and Morris (1975) showed that women who proved positive for cancer at biopsy were more likely prior to biopsy to report very little tendency to express anger. In a later study, Greer *et al.* (1979) reported on the progress of patients with breast cancer. The greatest mortality was shown by the group who exhibited a hopeless attitude to their illness, and the least mortality was associated with groups who showed either fighting spirit or denial styles of coping. Finally, Pettingale *et al.* (1981) reported on immunological measures during the course of treatment. The results were complex but suggested to the authors the importance of recognizing and treating symptoms of depression in such patients. With respect to cancer, then, an interim and tentative conclusion would probably emphasize the importance of styles of coping with events rather than the events *per se*. What seems to increase vulnerability may be a mixture of passive acceptance, hopelessness and depression; what may be protective is some form of active resistant type of coping style. Such an interim conclusion is however very tentative and based on an as yet slim collection of data.

SUMMARY AND CONCLUSIONS

We have seen that stress is a very broad term involving a transaction between an individual and his or her environment. Certain patterns of physiological activity are associated with 'being stressed' but important variation exists in such patterns. However, the physiology of stress is vital to our increasing understanding of how psychological pressures come to have pathological consequences for our physical selves. Cognitive theories of stress emphasize the way in which individuals both appraise potentially stressful situations and also evaluate their coping resources. Coping in turn is seen in terms of controlling. Human beings, however, can exercise control in subtle ways, including defensive forms of appraisal and psychological distraction, and the theoretical issues are, as we have seen, far from being simply stated.

Associations between stress and illness have been suggested by writers of every century. However, recent research on life events has given an empirical justification to such claims. Although life-events research in relation to illness has to face considerable methodological problems, there is now a considerable body of findings which supports the idea of 'psychosomatic' links. Finally, the new hybrid science of psychoneuroimmunology is beginning to show us more about the mechanisms by which psychological stress may come, partly at least, to cause physical illness of various kinds.

Part II

Patient behaviour and the management of illness

Part II examines the behaviour of people in medical settings and the management of illness. It begins with a chapter on the psychology of medical consultations which considers the issues of when people decide to take medical advice, how that advice is given and understood, and why the advice is sometimes not followed. A major topic for research, that of compliance, is examined; how compliance is defined and measured, what factors affect it, and how compliance rates might be improved. Chapter 5 moves into the area of the experience of treatment by considering the reactions of patients to hospitalization and to impending surgery. The role of preoperative interventions, and their effects on anxiety and stress for influencing recovery from surgery, are also discussed. Special emphasis is given to the methodological difficulties that research in these areas has encountered. Chapter 6 reviews the psychological and pharmacological effects of psychoactive medicines. It points out that psychoactive drugs are amongst the medicines most commonly prescribed by general practitioners and examines their target effects and unwanted side-effects. Factors such as personality traits and dosing regimens which affect their behavioural actions are also considered.

Chapter 7 provides a discussion of pain. It outlines theories of pain, discusses its measurement and has a particular emphasis upon the management of pain. The following chapter critically reviews applications of biofeedback which is one of the most commonly used and controversial management techniques in the field of health psychology. Chapter 8 describes its range of applications and assesses the success or failure of biofeedback as a clinical technique. Part II is completed with a chapter on research into recovery and rehabilitation. It examines key themes including the stage model of recovery. It also compares research into two chronic diseases – multiple sclerosis and Parkinson's disease – and evaluates the role of personality factors in the experience of living with chronic disorders.

Chapter 4

The medical consultation

Marian Pitts

Nearly everyone in western societies visits the doctor from time to time. How often a person visits and what s/he expects and gains from the consultation is the subject of this chapter.

SYMPTOMS AND THEIR MEANING

The consultation rate of patients to General Practitioners (GPs) in UK is about five times a year (Williams 1970) although there is considerable variation around this figure. The evidence suggests that the decision to consult or not involves complex psychological processes including patients' perceptions of their symptoms. Research has shown that the majority of symptoms of illnesses are not reported to a medical practitioner and Last (1963) coined the term 'illness iceberg' to describe this phenomenon. Morrell and Wade (1976) and Scambler and Scambler (1984) investigated the perception of symptoms in samples of healthy women. They both report a figure of about one medical consultation for about eighteen 'symptom episodes'. Hannay (1980) asked a random sample of people registered with a health practice to indicate on a symptom check-list whether or not they were currently experiencing a symptom and to rate its severity and the degree to which it was disabling. He reports that 26 per cent of people who rated themselves as suffering from at least one severe symptom did not refer themselves for medical treatment. Cunningham-Burley and Irvine (1987) interviewed fifty-two women with young children about their responses and treatment of their children's illnesses. They also collected diary data from the mothers. They found that on 49 per cent of the days for which data were collected, mothers reported a symptom in their children. For a large proportion of these symptoms no action was taken by the mothers. The most common symptoms for which no action was taken were respiratory symptoms (for example, a runny nose) and changes in behaviour, followed by sickness or diarrhoea. For the rest of the symptoms (cuts, grazes, coughs), some kind of action was taken, of which by far the most common was to provide an over-the-counter remedy for the child. Analgesics, such as aspirin, and cough mixtures were the most frequently used (56 and 52 per cent respectively of all medications administered). Mothers reported contacting a health-care professional on only 7 per cent of the days when a symptom had been noticed. Thus, the overwhelming response to noticing a symptom was not to seek 'outside' help immediately, but to self-treat or do nothing. Clearly, then, there is no one-to-one simple relationship between perceiving a symptom and seeking medical help. Pennebaker (1982) has carried out extensive research on the perception of symptoms and their interpretation. He has found that awareness varies greatly between people; and that people are more aware of bodily symptoms when they are bored and less aware when fully absorbed in a task. He has even used this finding to relate the incidence of coughing during a university lecture with its interest value.

Mechanic (1978) presents a simple model of health decisions which suggests that people attend to the number and persistence of symptoms that they experience; they decide if the symptoms are recognizable or familiar; they consider the possible disabling aspects of the symptoms and they may apply their own cultural and social definitions of illness. Other factors also play a part: there is considerable evidence that people experiencing psychological distress may use the health services more frequently and for different purposes than others (Tessler *et al.* 1976).

Thus, the decision to visit the doctor is usually taken after some analysis and possible discussion of the problem. The opinion of others is nearly always sought first. Scambler and Scambler (1984) report a ratio of eleven 'lay' consultations usually involving a spouse or close friend to every medical consultation. The opinion is then taken as some sort of trigger for the legitimate seeking of medical help. As Stimson and Webb (1975) report, there is a concern expressed almost universally 'not to waste the doctor's valuable time' and the opinion of others is regarded as an endorsement that the problem is not trivial. Another incentive or trigger to consultation may be when a minor problem persists longer than was anticipated. This 'wait and see' strategy has been commented upon by Locker (1981): 'any symptoms which last for a few days or more are seen to be of a more serious nature.' Locker also describes the 'critical incident' which can trigger a consultation: a sudden change in the nature of the symptom, an increase in pain level or the discovery that a previous interpretation was no longer appropriate are all possible critical incidents. Finally, the decision to consult is premissed by the expectation that the doctor can take some useful action; the recurrence of a symptom which the person has experienced previously and for which s/he has received no useful treatment may well not result in a further consultation – 'I think it's a waste of time because I've been through the pipeline before . . . so I don't really feel there's a lot of point going through that lot again' (quoted in Locker 1981).

There have been several investigations of the influence of social or demographic factors on self-referrals to primary care. Ingham and Miller

(1986) conclude that such variables play a very minor role in comparison with that of symptoms. In particular they report that the people who are most likely to consult are those who cannot say what is causing their troubles, followed by those who believe that there is an internal physical cause, rather than an external physical or a psychological cause of their trouble. Robinson and Granfield (1986) examined the characteristics of the 'frequent consulter'. They describe a picture of the frequent consulter as having a large number of symptoms which recur. These symptoms are of the kind which do not usually indicate major illness and are, in fact, often ignored by other people. They found that these frequent consulters also take many more self-prescribed medications; these include health foods and vitamin supplements, pain killers, inhalers and a wide range of other preparations. It would seem, however, that these preventive steps do not alleviate their ailments and they consult again.

Thus, there is a complex relationship between the perception of symptoms of ill-health, the responses to such symptoms and the decision to seek the opinion of a health professional. The next section examines the experience of a medical consultation.

CONSULTATION AND DIAGNOSIS

A medical consultation is not like an ordinary social encounter or conversation; Stimson and Webb (1975) describe it as a focused interaction which is geographically and temporally defined and which has a high degree of specificity – peripheral topics are only rarely mentioned – and in which there is a competence gap between doctor and patient. Both patient and doctor bring to the meeting a number of expectations of how the encounter will go and what the outcome might be. It is of interest to see how different the set of expectations of doctors and patients are. The patient has first to describe a symptom or set of symptoms to the doctor who, in turn, is expected to provide an explanation (diagnosis) and possibly advice or medication. The patient necessarily must be selective about what s/he reports and the decisions on how to present the problem can influence the doctor's response. As Blaxter (1983) describes it: 'a consultation presents incompatible obligations: to be brief and helpful, not waste time which is manifestly in short supply, and yet somehow to tell the story of a life in all its long detail'. Stimson and Webb report a great deal of anticipatory work before the encounter takes place; patients rehearse what they will say either simply to themselves or to others. In examining a series of 150 essays written by teenagers about 'going to the doctors' they found that 55 per cent of the content was given over to this anticipatory aspect of the encounter and only 36 per cent to the actual consultation itself. The rehearsal aspect may enable patients to present their concerns in the most appropriate light – but it may also be that such rehearsal changes the emphasis of what is being conveyed in ways which are not readily apparent to the doctor.

Patients choose the order in which to present their concerns: it may be that 'physical' problems are mentioned first, or it may be related to the perceived severity of the various problems to be reported. In this latter case it is not always (if ever) the most serious problem which is raised first. Patients frequently seem to need some time to work their way into the consultation and tend to 'save' their underlying concerns until they are confident of a sympathetic hearing. The absence of such reassurance may well result in a major concern not being mentioned at all. Korsch et al. (1968) reported in their study of consultations at a paediatrics out-patients department that 24 per cent of mothers failed to raise their major concerns. Ways of assessing areas of concern by the patients may themselves interact with such concerns. Stimson and Webb (1975) comment that questioning prior to the consultation may raise a problem to a level of awareness which affects the later interaction. They report a woman as saying while responding to a check-list of problems presented by the researchers: 'Now you've mentioned it I might ask him about that' – and she did! Patients do more than describe symptoms in neutral fashion; they often hint or suggest possible causative factors. Should the doctor fail to respond to these hints then the symptoms may be represented in a somewhat different manner. Due deference is made to the doctor's expertise; the doctor is questioned only as a representative of the profession with its fund of knowledge whilst his or her own knowledge is rarely directly questioned or examined.

One of the most important aspects of the consultation from the patient's point of view is the awareness that the doctor's time is 'precious' and limited. Stimson and Webb report that in at least one-third of their sample of interviews, some reference was made to the shortage of doctor's time and the necessity not to waste it. This perception also governs the number of concerns a patient feels able to raise. They report an average consultation time of around four minutes – given the brevity of the interaction there is a lot of pressure on both sides to complete the 'business' efficiently.

From the point of view of the doctor, s/he is required to solve a problem – by making a diagnosis or providing an explanation for the problems presented by the patient. One of the problems identified by researchers is that errors may result from a diagnosis made too early in the consultation. Given the likelihood that patients may not present their most serious concerns first then doctors can be led astray by early less central complaints. Wallston (1978) has reported that doctors systematically distorted information presented late in an interview in order that it be made to fit with an already established opinion or diagnosis.

Much work has considered the tendency on the part of problem solvers, doctors included, to seek confirmatory instances for their hypotheses. Wason and Johnson-Laird (1972), and many others since, have charted the penchant for looking for positive instances rather than the more efficient strategy of seeking negative instances to disconfirm tentative hypotheses. The work of Tversky has also shown that thinking probabilistically does not come any more easily to doctors than to the rest of us. McNeil *et al.* (1982) studied three groups of people, including a group of doctors who were presented with imaginary problems concerning choice of treatments for cancer. They were given information on immediate and longer-term risks and survival rates following the two treatments: radiation and surgery. They found that all groups of subjects were swayed in their choice of treatment by the labelling of the treatments and all groups also paid more attention to short-term risks of treatments than to longer-term survival rates. Diagnosis often involves the assessment of statistical risks; the study by Tversky and Kahnemann (1974) showed that people have difficulty in assessing the statistical relationship between symptoms that arise with differing incidence rates. There have been some attempts to improve the process of diagnosis, sometimes with technological aids such as computers. One such computer program is MYCIN developed by Davis *et al.* (1977) which has been designed to diagnose the cause of infections. It has a relatively high agreement rate with expert medical opinion, but it is unlikely ever to replace or even complement the GP in the typical local health centre. Furthermore, it still remains for the doctor to collect the information to be fed into the program and the interviewing skills required for such information gathering are considered next.

Weinman (1981) suggests that the generation and choice of hypotheses during diagnosis are governed by:

- the clinician's own concepts about the nature of clinical problems; i.e. the extent to which s/he espouses biological or psychosocial explanations of disorder will obviously guide the questions asked;
- the clinician's estimate of the probability of a given disease; and as we have already seen, probability estimates are subject to many influences;
- the seriousness and treatability of the disease. Here Weinman offers the example of acute abdominal pain in children: acute appendicitis would be considered early as a hypothesis because of the costs and benefits associated with correct diagnosis of that disorder – it is relatively easy to treat and not to treat would have serious consequences;
- personal knowledge of the patient; a person's past medical history but also past encounters with the GP will guide his or her decisions. The 'frequent complainer' is likely to generate different hypotheses from a 'rare attender'.

Eddy and Clanton (1982) analysed the psychological process by which doctors solve complicated diagnostic problems. They suggest the following six steps be taken to arrive at a diagnosis:

- the aggregation of groups of findings into patterns;
- the selection of a 'pivot' or key finding;
- the generation of a cause list;
- a pruning of the cause list;

- the selection of a diagnosis;
- the validation of a diagnosis.

At the first stage: a number of elementary findings are combined to form a higher-order aggregate. Then, one or two key findings are focused upon – this is the selection of the 'pivot'. After selecting a pivot, all other details of the case are temporarily ignored and a list of diseases is constructed which could have caused the pivot. The next step is to inspect the diseases on the cause list one at a time and measure them against the case noting the presence or absence of critical findings. This list is pruned by searching for the most probable diagnosis: this is not done statistically; rather, the doctor determines whether the pattern of findings in the case could have been caused by the disease under consideration – i.e. it is a comparison rather than a calculation. Then, possible diseases are compared two at a time throughout the pruned cause list. Eddy and Clanton (1982) remark: 'The beauty and power of this approach is that it allows selection of the most probable disease without requiring estimation of a single probability.' Finally, the clinical diagnosis is considered against all the findings of the case. This allows for a review of the diagnosis and the evidence in support or against it.

This account was derived from a consideration of clinicopathological exercises and it is not yet clear to what extent these stages are used by doctors in practice. Nevertheless, it should be recognized that diagnoses are not absolute entities; rather, they are predictions made with varying degrees of certainty about prognosis. These predictions can be changed as a result of new information or further developments of symptoms. This aspect of diagnosis is often felt to be unsatisfactory from the patient's point of view. The suggestion to 'come back and see me if it doesn't clear up in a day or two' is one that is perhaps seen as a 'fob-off' when a clearer statement of cause or prognosis is expected. This attitude is represented at its extreme by one of the doctors in Stimson and Webb's (1975) study who ignored a problem raised by a patient towards the end of the consultation. He remarked: 'Well, it obviously wasn't anything very important. And if it is, then he'll be back again before very long.'

A recent study by Tapper-Jones et al. (1988) examined GPs' use of written materials during consultations. They found that the majority had used some educational material, the vast majority using free-hand diagrams generated during the consultation; none had prepared any educational materials themselves in advance. Where prepared materials were used, the most common source was pharmaceutical companies. Very few doctors were aware that they could obtain educational materials for patients from local health education units. Most of the leaflets used explained diseases rather than advising on health behaviours; Tapper-Jones et al. conclude, 'many general practitioners think that they primarily provide curative rather than preventative care for their patients.'

The ending of consultations is another aspect of the interaction which is a matter for negotiation between doctor and patient. A doctor may signal that the consultation is drawing to a close by offering a summary, repeating a reassurance or set of instructions, or by physically distancing him/herself from the patient – pushing a chair back, closing a pad, putting down a pencil or even standing up. Quite often the issuing of a prescription is the main signal. The patient may seek to prolong the consultation by asking another question or by introducing a new topic, or by taking a longer time than necessary to gather clothes or belongings together – but these delaying tactics are unlikely to be particularly successful if the doctor has decided to terminate since s/he represents the 'powerful' half of the encounter.

PRESCRIBING

Doctors think that patients want pills and of course patients sometimes do. A survey in 1974 by the Consumer Council found that doctors estimated that four out of five of their patients expected a prescription, but Cartwright (1967) and others have found that this is likely to be an overestimate. Cunningham-Burley and Irvine (1987) found from interviews with fifty-four mothers that 'contrary to popular belief, these mothers did not expect prescriptions from their doctors.... They were wanting the doctor to check that everything was all right; thus an examination and diagnosis or an "all clear" became more important than a prescription'. Stimson and Webb reported that in nearly 70 per cent of the consultations they monitored some drug, medicine or dressing was prescribed and when these patients were interviewed prior to the consultation about two-thirds indicated that they expected a prescription. 'Expecting' does not necessarily mean that a prescription was wanted or indeed that the medication would be used.

The medical consultation is capable, then, of resulting in satisfied patients (consulters), and satisfied practitioners. What follows from a consultation is likely to be closely related to these satisfactions. The next section will consider people's behaviour after seeking medical advice.

THE PROBLEM OF NON-COMPLIANCE

Compliance is the behaviour of a person following medical advice or directions. Compliance tends to carry the connotation of a passive adherence on the part of the patient to the doctor's wishes and other rather more positive terms such as co-operation and collaboration are perhaps to be preferred since they imply a more active relationship on both sides. Nevertheless, it is compliance which is the term which has gained most widespread use in the literature. There is now a vast literature on the subject; Ley (1988) charts an increase from twenty-five publications on the topic in the 1950s, through 168 in the 1960s, to 744 in the first four years of the 1980s. Concern about the 'problem' of compliance is understandable. Non-compliance can at the very least be expensive in the wastage of expensive drugs and the use of hospital facilities, but it can also be potentially dangerous and lethal in its repercussions for the health of individuals.

Non-compliance can occur at any stage of the medical process. A person can fail to attend a clinic or hospital appointment; s/he can attend but fail to cash the prescription or fail to complete the medication prescribed; s/he can also fail to attend follow-up sessions or to follow specific regimens.

The measurement of non-compliance

Measuring what is, in essence, the absence of behaviour is particularly problematic. Some aspects of non-compliance are however more easily measured than others. Sackett is reported as saying, 'accurate measurement of compliance is not easy; easy measurements of compliance are not accurate' (cited in Haynes 1987). We will deal first with a relatively straightforward area – the non-attendance at medical appointments. Sackett and Snow (1979) reviewed several studies of attendance rates in the USA and derived figures of 50 per cent show-up if the appointments were initiated by health professionals, rising to 75 per cent show-up if the appointments were made by the clients themselves. There were seasonal variations and marked differences between clinics – antenatal clinics had the best attendance rates, and geriatric clinics the worst. The reasons for these differences are likely to be many and various: the degree to which attenders are self-reliant for transport to and from the clinic, are relatively well and fit, are aware of possible subsequent repercussions of non-attending, are attending for themselves or for others such as babies or children – all these are likely to be strong influences on the attendance rate. Many measures have been tried to improve these rates: Hochstadt and Trybula (1980) showed that a reminder in the form of a letter or telephone call improved appointment keeping substantially at a community centre. Many dentists now issue reminder postcards about a week prior to a six month dental check-up, again in the hope that this will improve attendance.

Compliance with medication regimens

Ley (1988) defines non-compliance for medication uptake as:

- not taking enough medicine;
- taking too much medicine;
- not observing the correct interval between doses;
- not maintaining the correct duration of treatment; and
- taking additional unprescribed medicines.

Again the implications of these failures to comply with medical advice are potentially extremely serious. The most popular method for assessing the extent of non-compliance with medication regimens is by patient interview. This method has many problems associated with it: there is some social pressure not to admit to forgetting or to failing intentionally to follow medical advice; in addition patients may simply forget whether or not they have taken the medication. It is therefore extremely important that information gathered by interview be collected in a manner most likely to elicit accurate responses. R.B. Haynes *et al.* (1980) began their interviews by saying, 'People often have difficulty in taking pills for one reason or another and we are interested in finding out any problems that occur so that we can understand them better'; the implication that this is a problem which occurs for most people is more likely to elicit answers than one which stresses how unfortunate it is that pills are not taken and then invites patients to 'confess their failures'. A recent study by Morisky *et al.* (1986) reports the development of a short series of questions which cover general aspects of compliance and they have claimed validity over five years in predicting blood-pressure control. This form of structured patient interview shows much promise.

A study reported by Roth (1987) examined patients with peptic ulcers for their intake of antacid medication. They compared patients' stated intake with the number of empty bottles of antacid they returned. For those patients who claimed to have followed directions 100 per cent of the time, the correspondence with returned bottles was extremely poor, varying from 2 per cent upwards, with a mean of 59 per cent. For those who indicated that they had missed the very occasional dose i.e. 80–90 per cent compliance claimed, the correspondence with bottles returned remained extremely poor. Only for those who reported taking no medication was the correspondence good. Roth concludes:

> when a patient states that the medication is taken regularly, it often is not. When a patient states that occasional doses are being missed, that is usually an understatement of the extent of deviation from the regimen. However, when a patient states that the drug is not being taken, this is usually corroborated.

It has been shown to be particularly pointless to use doctors' estimates of compliance. Both Davis (1966) and Caron and Roth (1968) found doctors to be very poor judges of the extent of non-compliance. Roth (1987) reports doctors overestimating patients' intake of medication by 50 per cent. They are also poor at identifying which patients in particular do not comply – indeed, the majority of GPs do not enquire about this aspect of the process at all, perhaps assuming that their responsibility ends with the writing of the prescription and the end of the consultation.

Other measures of medication uptake include pill counts, and blood and urine tests. Whilst these have the aura of greater objectivity, results from such studies also need to be treated with caution. Pill counts do not indicate when exactly the pills are taken; the fact that a pill has left a bottle does not necessarily imply that it has been consumed by the appropriate person, and even blood and urine tests do not guarantee that the same dosages were being consumed in the periods between testing as were being consumed immediately prior to testing. Only direct observation can really be regarded as approaching a reliable method and that in most cases is not a practical option.

When studies compare these various measures of non-compliance it is nearly always the case that both pill counts and urine and blood tests reveal higher incidences of non-compliance than patients report. Ley (1988) cites nine studies where both methods have been used and, overall, he finds that patients report an average of about 22 per cent non-compliance, while the 'more objective methods' from the same studies yield an estimate of 54 per cent.

Compliance rates of a number of specific groups of patients have been studied. Of particular interest are the studies which deal with elderly patients. There are many aspects of the aged which could lead to particularly poor compliance with medical regimens – they may have failing memory or sight and may have fewer people about to remind them. Kendrick and Bayne (1982) demonstrated that 13 per cent of a sample of older people could not open the flip-top pill containers, 53 per cent could not deal with the palm-turned caps and 65 per cent could not accurately line up the two arrows on cap and bottle. These problems are not confined to the elderly and many of us find 'child-proof' pill bottles to be 'person-proof' too.

In general, however, the search for demographic and personality characteristics unique to non-compliers has been singularly unproductive and it is worthwhile remembering that compliance among health professionals and doctors themselves is no better than that of people in general (Leventhal and Cameron 1987).

Most of this research regards non-compliance as 'a problem', and indeed it often is. But it can be argued that there is sometimes a rational basis for a patient's non-compliance; the patient may feel that the medicine is inappropriate, that it has been ineffective in the past or that the side-effects are more troublesome than the disorder under treatment. The important aspect is that GPs should be aware of these doubts at the time of prescribing and either alter the prescription or spend some time discussing the reasons governing the necessity for complying. Non-compliance is not simply a medical problem; all of us regularly receive advice about what might be in our best interest to do, from having the roof fixed to making a will; the extent to which we choose to follow such advice is part of our right as free individuals to take decisions for ourselves about our own affairs, even our own health and lives.

FACTORS INFLUENCING COMPLIANCE

Thompson (1984) reviews a number of factors which influence compliance with medical advice. He quotes Davis (1966) who found that 60 per cent of doctors and medical students ascribe non-compliance to the patients' 'unco-operative behaviour'. Whether this is the case or not, there is little that can be done to alter patients' personalities and it is more productive to examine other factors which can be manipulated to improve matters.

Satisfaction with service

A study by the Consumers' Association of the services offered by GPs found that access to the doctor was seen as a major problem; 26 per cent complained of long waits at surgery and 20 per cent of difficulty in getting an appointment. Geersten et al. (1973) looked at the relationship between time spent waiting to see the doctor and compliance. Sixty seven per cent of patients who had waited less than half an hour were compliant, 48 per cent who had waited from between 30 minutes and one hour and only 31 per cent who had waited longer than an hour were compliant with subsequent medical advice. This matches well with the study by Stimson and Webb (1975) who comment on means of controlling access to the doctor. Ancillary staff such as receptionists are placed between patient and doctor to control flow; they are, though, often seen more powerfully as decision makers on whether access to the doctor should be granted at all. They quote a mother:

> the receptionist always asks me what is wrong with the child. But I've got so used to her now that I've got a bit catty and I say, 'well if I knew that, I wouldn't be calling the doctor out would I?'.

Stimson and Webb also report numerous complaints from patients that their illnesses are supposed to match surgery hours – 'by the time you see him you are well.'

Arber and Sawyer (1985) surveyed over 1,000 adults about their experiences of receptionists. They concluded 'the hostility expressed by the public towards receptionists is grounded in the reality of receptionists' actions'. They found that large practices tended to operate by more rigid rules, and that parents with dependent children were those who expressed most antagonism about the receptionist's role as 'gatekeeper' – or, as Arber and Sawyer rather more vividly label it, 'a dragon behind the desk'.

A major study by Korsch et al. (1968) reported a strong link between patients' satisfaction with the consultation and compliance with advice stemming from that consultation. 'Satisfaction' was associated with:

– the doctor being friendly rather than business-like;
– the doctor seen to understand the patients' concerns;
– patients' expectations of treatment being met;

- the doctor being seen as a good communicator;
- the provision of information.

They conducted a series of studies at a Los Angeles out-patients' paediatric clinic and their findings have formed the basis of much subsequent work on satisfaction. Overall they found that satisfied mothers were three times more likely to comply with medical advice than dissatisfied mothers. They also found no relationship between length of consultation and satisfaction level – a finding which has since been disputed.

Buller and Buller (1987) found that patients' evaluations of the doctor's communication were associated strongly with patients' evaluation of the medical care that they received. A style of interaction which they describe as 'affiliative' received more favourable evaluation than a 'controlling' style. They also report a relationship between the amount of time spent waiting to see the doctor and the satisfaction with medical care.

The measurement of satisfaction is in itself very complicated: the phrasing and emphasis of the questions can influence greatly the levels of satisfaction found. Wolf et al. (1978) devised a medical interview satisfaction scale, which seeks to provide a valid measurement instrument for this rather broad concept. Ley (1972) reports a curvilinear relationship between time after discharge from treatment and level of satisfaction. In other words those studies which examine satisfaction immediately on discharge from hospital and those which measure satisfaction eight weeks after discharge are likely to find higher satisfaction than those sampling satisfaction three to four weeks after discharge. This needs to be remembered when comparing studies as only rarely has satisfaction been measured across several time periods. Finally, Mirowsky and Ross (1983) regard patient satisfaction and visiting the doctor as a 'self-regulating system'. They seek to account for the discrepancies between previous studies by this means. They find that satisfaction with the doctor increases the frequency of visiting the doctor, which, in turn, decreases satisfaction. This is presumably because there is an increased chance of an 'unsatisfactory' encounter as the number of visits increases. Nevertheless, patients' satisfaction is still held to be one of the most important influences on compliance.

Patients' understanding of medical instructions

Another major influence upon compliance is the knowledge which patients bring to a consultation and their understanding of what is said to them during the consultation. Boyle (1970) and Hawkes (1974) reported clear differences between doctors and patients in their understanding and use of anatomical terms. A phrase like 'sciatic nerve' will be interpreted differently when anatomical knowledge is sketchy or absent. Samora et al. (1961) took fifty common items of medical vocabulary such as malignancy, cardiac, tendon and so forth. and embedded them into sentences. When the sentences were given to patients to explain what was meant, fewer than thirty were correctly explained by the majority of patients. There are some indications, from more recent studies by Segall and Roberts (1980) and by Hadlow and Pitts (1990), that such differences have decreased. Nevertheless, there remain several 'key' medical terms which are not adequately understood by many patients. It is also the case that during a consultation, patients may use some of the medical jargon which they see as appropriate in that context, but it may also be that identical terms are being both used and understood differently by doctor and patient. Many words have both a medical and a 'lay' meaning and when these become confused the patient is even less likely to understand what is being said: psychological expressions such as depression or hysteria would be cases in point. Ley (1988) summarizes a number of studies which examine patients' understanding of the diagnosis of their condition and the medical regimen prescribed. He estimates that the percentage of patients failing to understand their medication varied from 5 per cent to as much as 53 per cent. Most especially, patients are found to have very patchy ideas about dosage and timing of medication. Hermann (1973) asked patients who had been prescribed drugs to be taken either twice, three or four times a day to indicate when they would take them. He found 15 per cent unable to specify a schedule at all and very wide variation between times between doses, from nil to twenty-one hours in some cases.

Again, Alfredsson et al. (1982) asked patients who had been instructed to take medication three times a day to record when they took the medication and found only 2 per cent taking it with such an interval. Kendrick and Bayne (1982) asked patients how many tablets they would take in a day if they had to take one every six hours. Some 22 per cent gave the correct answer. Patients are not infrequently taking a number of different medications, at different times of the day and with different specifications – with food, on an empty stomach, as required and so forth. It is hardly surprising that they become confused and forgetful. Charts and other memory devices are some help, but it is important to remember that these people are ill – and perhaps less able than usual to cope with cognitive demands.

Memory and compliance

Even if patients can understand what they are told during a medical consultation, the amount which they are able to recall after the consultation has repeatedly been shown to be fairly small. Studies have investigated 'real-life' situations where patients are interviewed after a consultation and their recall is measured. Also, 'analogue' studies have been carried out where healthy volunteers are tested for recall of 'dummy' medical information, which does not relate to them personally. There are quite strong similarities between the findings from these two methods of research. Ley and Spelman

(1965, 1967) found that approximately 40 per cent of what had been said during a consultation was immediately forgotten: diagnostic statements were best remembered, followed by information about the illness, with instructions poorest recalled. Other studies have not found this same order but this is probably because there is a strong primacy effect which operates during a consultation. In general, the amount forgotten increases with the amount of information given. Ley suggests that if recall is absolutely essential, then only two statements should be made to the patient.

Ley has developed a 'cognitive' model to describe the relationships between memory, understanding, satisfaction and compliance. He describes it thus:

> Understanding will have direct effects on memory, satisfaction and compliance, and, through its effect on satisfaction, an additional indirect effect on compliance. Similarly, memory will affect compliance directly and also exert an indirect effect through its effect on satisfaction. Finally, satisfaction will have a direct effect on compliance.
>
> (1988: 72)

He supports his suggestion for such relationships by examining the correlation coefficients found in various studies of these factors, and indeed there is some support for each of the variables he incorporates. A criticism of such an approach to explain compliance is, perhaps, that non-cognitive variables are underestimated; the roles of stress, mood and anxiety in memory, for example, are now well documented (Blaney 1986; Bower 1981; Isen et al. 1978). Medical consultations are a prime example of where such effects are likely to be operating.

Patient characteristics and compliance

The search for variables within the patient which will predict which patients will or will not comply has largely been fruitless. The health belief model described in Chapter 1 has been applied somewhat more successfully to the compliance area. A review article by Haynes et al. (1979) which examined a wide number of patient and other characteristics concluded that perceived vulnerability, perceived severity of the illness and costs and barriers to treatment were associated with compliance.

Janz and Becker (1984) considered the success of health beliefs in predicting future as well as concurrent compliance; they found in general that the model was effective in predicting future behaviour. One difficulty is that the amount of variance usually predicted by these factors is small and there is still a large amount of variability in compliance which is unaccounted for.

A rather different aspect might be to consider those patient characteristics which are negatively stereotyped by doctors. Najman et al. (1982) report findings from both Australia and North America which indicate that there is a consensus among doctors about which medical conditions or characteristics of patients they find arouse most negative feelings. Those most frequently mentioned were alcohol abusers, unhygienic patients, angry patients, drug abusers, obese patients and patients with minor mental disorders. They found about half of the responses from 2,421 doctors fell into the category of reactions to individuals who might be seen to be 'culpable' in so far as their problems are the result of their own behaviour; this category which contains alcohol and drug abusers, is also now likely to include people with sexually transmitted diseases and Acquired Immune Deficiency Syndrome.

CONCLUSIONS

The process of medical consultation has by now been extensively studied by social scientists, and much has been learned about patients' and doctors' behaviours. It is important that this knowledge be applied to its setting, both by incorporating it into medical training and reminding ancillary staff of its importance for ensuring successful outcomes for medical consultations.

Chapter 5

The experience of treatment

Marian Pitts

REACTIONS TO HOSPITALIZATION

Most people in industrialized societies will be admitted to hospital at least once in their lives, and for a few hospitalization is a relatively regular occurrence. For almost everyone, though, the first entry into hospital signals major changes in the pattern of their daily routines.

There are a number of social changes which inevitably accompany admission to hospital, obvious ones being the loss of privacy and independence. Most adults do not normally allow themselves to be seen by strangers in a state of undress and do not normally take their meals to order. In most hospitals it is still the case that the person becomes the patient and takes on a patient role. Independence is given up; it is no longer expected that one can choose when and what to eat, when to sleep, when to read, bathe and so forth. All these aspects of a person's individual life-style become subsumed to the hospital regime.

Also lost are the normal social opportunities for distraction or enjoyment. At home, if one feels bored, one can go out, telephone a friend, read the paper, go to the pub, listen to a record or the radio. These distracting activities are only available in a very limited way in hospital; it is therefore probably not surprising that one of the most frequent reactions to hospitalization is to become increasingly preoccupied with the hospital regime itself and with one's own clinical signs and symptoms.

These changes need not always be regarded negatively by all patients. If one has been in great pain or distress, then the yielding up of decision making to powerful and competent others can be reassuring. For an increasing number of people, though, entry into hospital is not because of serious illness but for rather more routine procedures to be carried out on an otherwise healthy individual; giving birth is an example of this, and the change from person to patient may not be entirely welcome.

A number of studies have examined the psychological reactions to hospitalization. Taylor (1979) examined patients' reactions in detail. She suggests that loss of control and depersonalization are common features of hospital experience. She describes the 'good patient' role which staff may reinforce. The good patient is passive, undemanding and co-operative. This patient does not ask questions or make demands on staff time. In contrast, the 'bad patient' may indulge in what Taylor describes as 'petty acts of mutiny' such as wandering around, smoking or drinking, or trying to flirt with staff. These are perceived as acts of defiance and place demands on both time and attention of the staff. 'Bad' patients frequently ask questions or query their treatment. Although hospital staff may reinforce the behaviours of the 'good patient', Taylor lists several ways in which being a good patient can be detrimental to recovery. She suggests such persons are in a state of learned helplessness. Seligman (1975) argued that people learn to be helpless – that is, they learn that their attempts to control will not be successful because response and outcome are independent of each other. Taylor suggests that such a state is not uncommon in hospitals and that hospital regimes often inhibit the patient from taking active steps towards recovery. Patients may fail to report new or changing patterns of symptoms; they may remain relatively uninformed about their condition and may find the process of rehabilitation back to independence particularly difficult to achieve. In Goffman's (1961) terminology the good patient may become 'colonized' within the hospital regime.

The bad patient is not necessarily better off; the demands for attention and the refusal to comply with the hospital regime may result in staff ignoring the 'necessary' complaints along with the 'unnecessary'. There is one area, though, where bad patients do seem to benefit. They retain at least some control over their lives and emotions and the leaving of hospital is welcomed and adjusted to quickly and well. Karmel (1972) reported higher morale and fewer instances of depression among a group of patients he labelled 'intransigent' – those who challenged staff and the hospital routine.

Hospital language is a particular example of the changes brought about for adults in this setting. Often the language used, most especially by senior medical staff, reflects a style of speech more commonly associated with children. Patients are invited to 'pop' in and out of bed, to 'slip off their clothes', women are frequently referred to by terms of endearment – 'dear', 'love', stomachs become tummies, backsides become bottoms, and so on. Older patients are particularly likely to receive such speech – an old man becomes 'a naughty boy who wouldn't eat his tea'. Again, there are aspects of this scenario which can be regarded as reassuring – nursery language carries the implications of safety and care; but it is not always received as well as it is apparently meant.

ANXIETY AND STRESS IN HOSPITALS

There are many aspects of the hospital situation which are likely to induce anxiety or stress in patients; evidence suggests that such negative feelings are common. To what extent such emotions are the inevitable consequence of a novel situation has become the focus of much research. Volicier and Bohannon (1975) devised a hospital stress-rating scale and asked patients to rank order a large number of events related to hospitalization. They concluded that events which could be directly affected by hospital-staff behaviour were ranked high; these included knowledge about the nature and prognosis of the illness, and getting pain medication when it was needed. Wilson-Barnett (1976) found during interviews with hospital patients that issues of separation from family, friends and work were major sources of anxiety and concern. Johnston's (1982) study is one of a number to investigate in detail the areas of concern of hospital patients. Johnston compared patients' worries with those that were estimated by staff to be of major concern to their patients. She found that, on the whole, nursing staff overestimated the concerns about aspects of medical care; the patients, at least in the kinds of wards investigated by Johnston, were still more concerned with aspects of their lives beyond the ward. More recently, however, M. Johnston (1987) reports that worries about the outcome of the operation were most frequently reported as concerns by patients.

Van der Ploeg (1988) investigated a range of medical stressors for their frequency and intensity. He found anaesthetics, operations and hospital admissions were among the most highly stressful medical events; but also that poor communication aspects of the doctor's behaviour could produce equally high levels of stress. In particular, 'doctors not giving proper answers to questions', 'having the feeling that the doctor is not listening', and 'insufficient information about the illness and treatment' were all rated as highly stressful.

There have been various estimates of the degree of depression found among medical patients hospitalized on general wards. Moffic and Paykel (1975) found a 24 per cent prevalence of depression as measured by the Beck Depression Inventory (BDI); Fava et al. (1982), and Cavanagh (1983) both estimate around 33 per cent of medical in-patients to be depressed.

There have been many attempts to link this depression with aspects of the disorders which have resulted in hospital admission. Some studies have reported a relationship between severity of illness and depression (Moffic and Paykel 1975; Schwab et al. 1967), but not all studies have found this (Wise and Rosenthal 1982). Length of illness does not seem directly related to depression, and nor does the experience of pain. It is generally considered to be more fruitful to examine social aspects of the experience as an explanation of these high levels of depression. Taylor, as we have seen, links depression with learned helplessness in patients. A recent study by Rosenberg et al. (1988) employed a multivariate design to try to tease out the major variables influencing incidence of depression among medical in-patients. They focused particularly on the role of social support. Some 38 per cent of their sample of medical in-patients were judged to be clinically depressed. No significant sex, race or age differences were found to be related to level of depression in the sample. The most powerful predictor of in-patient depression was the self-rated index of prehospitalization depression. This is not surprising since current depression could be a continuation of a previous state or could induce a negative set when recalling previous affective states. Other important determinants were the patients' perception of the supportiveness of the doctor and the patients' perceptions of the severity of their illnesses. The *actual* severity of the illness was not related to level of depression; once again it is the perception of the situation which is important.

Other studies, such as that of DiMatteo and DiNicola (1982), have also stressed the importance of the doctor–patient relationship. Rosenberg *et al.* (1988) conclude that 'the physician is uniquely qualified to provide the social support which would mitigate the effects of learned helplessness within the hospital'.

PSYCHOLOGICAL RESPONSES TO SURGERY

Patients about to undergo surgery experience greater disturbance and stress than in almost any other medical situation. It is not entirely clear what it is about surgery which makes it particularly stressful: there are probably at least three important elements – the experience of anaesthetic is in itself frightening; it involves the losing of consciousness and control and there are associated fears of 'not waking up' or of 'being aware and unable to communicate the fact'; another element is the degree of pain anticipated post-operatively, and it would be unrealistic to imagine that any surgical operation could be pain free. The third element involves perhaps the very nature of surgery – the fact of incision, the opening of flesh and the use of needles and knives. It may be that each of these separate elements is stressful, but that their unique combination in surgery is particularly difficult to anticipate and cope with.

There have been numerous studies of reactions to surgery, many of them having focused on the relationship between anxiety, preparation for surgery and recovery. The first studies of pre-operative anxiety and its relationship to successful recovery were carried out by Janis (1958, 1969). He interviewed patients prior to surgery and assessed them for their degree of anticipatory fear; he assigned them to one of three groups – low, moderate or extreme fear. He then assessed them all post-operatively for their recovery. He reported a curvilinear relationship between pre-operative fear and recovery. That is, those who he assigned to the extreme- and low-fear groups recovered less well than those in the moderate-fear group. Janis interpreted these results as indicating the necessity for some of the 'work of worrying' to be carried out before surgery. In other words, he regarded moderate fear as a realistic response to the prospect of surgery and thought that this worry enabled people to prepare themselves for the outcome difficulties. In contrast, those people with extreme fear were unable to use their worry constructively as a preparation, while those with only a low fear were denying the reality of difficulties associated with surgical recovery. This was a very influential study which led to much work on how best to prepare people for the experience of surgery. The most important element was the notion that there was a group of patients whose pre-operative anxiety was too low and who would benefit from increased anxiety. Unfortunately, Janis's findings have not been replicated and the original study is open to the criticism that both assessments were carried out by the same interviewer, who was already aware of the patients' classifications. Two more recent studies by Johnston and Carpenter (1980) and Wallace (1984) have failed to find this curvilinear relationship. Instead, they report a more direct, linear relationship between degree of pre-operative fear and anxiety and success of recovery. The debilitating effect of extreme fear remains, but the idea of the drawbacks associated with denial no longer seems to hold. The benefits of an attitude of denial are increasingly becoming apparent in the health literature (Gentry *et al.* 1972; Hackett and Cassem 1975; Maeland and Havik 1987). The mechanism by which pre-operative anxiety can influence recovery has rarely been spelt out; there is the clear implication that anxiety affects the patient's physiology in a way which endures after the operation.

One of the difficulties in drawing firm conclusions from studies in this area are that they rarely compare like with like. A review article by Mathews and Ridgeway (1984) lists some of the ways in which studies of responses to surgery may differ.

1 *surgical procedure studied:* a wide variety of procedures have been examined, from fairly minor surgery such as dental surgery to major cardiac and abdominal surgery. It seems to be the case, not surprisingly, that the more 'major' the operation, the higher the pre-operative anxiety. This makes comparisons across studies which concern different surgical procedures extremely difficult.

2 *measures of anxiety used:* these also vary greatly from study to study. Some studies use self-ratings, others staff ratings, and physiological indices such as palmar sweating are also sometimes taken. It is not at all certain that each of these anxiety measures would correlate highly with the others and so again cross-study comparisons are made difficult.

3 *recovery measures:* Mathews and Ridgeway identify seven major types of recovery measure: behaviour; clinical ratings; length of time between surgery and discharge from hospital; medication counts, usually of analgesics; mood ratings; pain ratings and physical indices such as blood pressure or medical complications. Once again, there is scant evidence that these different measures correlate with each other at all and so studies incorporating different numbers and types of recovery measures are likely to give different results.

PREPARATION FOR SURGERY

In spite of the difficulties outlined above, there is an increasingly large literature which documents the beneficial effects of preparing people for surgery and other stressful medical procedures. The kind of preparation offered has varied a great deal, but the most common kind has been the provision of information of some kind concerning the surgical experience. Two main types of information provision emerge: the first type, called 'procedural information', describes interventions that employ information about the procedures that the patient is likely to undergo – for example, informing the patient of the timetable of events that will take place on the day of the operation. The second type, termed 'sensory information', gives patients details about the sensations that they can expect to experience, such as the nature and duration of pain associated with the surgical incision site. A further preparation method that is related to information giving actually instructs the patients about the types of behaviour in which they should engage to promote recovery. This method is sometimes referred to as 'behavioural instructions'. One reason for distinguishing between types of information in this way is that it is possible that there may be differences in the power of each of these methods to promote recovery. Obviously, these different procedures are aimed at eliciting different reactions from patients. Procedural and sensory information are generally thought to act through the same mechanism of anxiety reduction. However, Johnson and Leventhal (1974) and Johnson et al. (1978) argue that this may not be the case. They present evidence which suggests that sensory information is the more effective of the two methods; they offer an explanation for why sensory information would be effective, an explanation which, they assert, does not hold for procedural information. It is difficult to evaluate this claim since most researchers have designed interventions with pragmatic considerations in mind so that they often contain mixtures of these three types of information. With the little evidence available as yet it is not possible to establish whether any major differences exist between them.

Other interventions that have been attempted are more varied. These include various forms of preparation which focus on the patient's emotional reactions to hospitalization, training in relaxation skills and the teaching of specific cognitive coping techniques. Reassurance has rarely been examined on its own; more often it is combined with some form of information giving, so again estimates of its efficacy are difficult to give. Cognitive coping methods attempt to train patients to deal with their anxiety-provoking thoughts in ways which are more adaptive. They may be encouraged to summon up distracting images and thoughts when they find themselves dwelling on unpleasant aspects of their hospitalization (Pickett and Clum 1982), or they may be encouraged to re-evaluate their threatening cognitions in a more positive manner (Ridgeway and Mathews 1982).

There have been several major literature reviews which have attempted to evaluate the differential effects of these different preparations, of which probably the most wide ranging has been that of Mathews and Ridgeway (1984). There have also been a number of meta-analyses. These synthesize the quantitative findings of separate studies through formulae for averaging either significance levels or size of effects. The meta-analyses of Devine and Cook, (1983, 1986) and Hathaway (1986), as well as that of Dunbar (1989), all find that psychological and educational interventions reliably facilitate many aspects of the recovery of surgical patients. Reviewers have then tried to establish which of the various preparation techniques is most effective. Different methods of allocating preparation type lead to difficulties in assessing relative effectiveness. Dunbar (1989) concludes that the two preparation types associated with greatest improvement in recovery are behavioural relaxation training and cognitive coping training. This latter method was also found by Mathews and Ridgeway to be the single most effective preparation technique. However, it is increasingly rare that a particular preparation method is used in isolation, and the search for a 'single best one' may in the end prove to be fruitless.

INDIVIDUAL DIFFERENCES AND PREPARATION FOR SURGERY

Many of the effects described above show great variability both between and within studies. Some of this variability may be the result of personality differences. These differences may be particularly important in the area of preferred style of coping with threat. It has been suggested by a number of authors (Byrne 1961; Evans et al. 1984; Miller and Mangan 1983) that individuals can be distinguished by the extent to which they seek information about an impending threatening event. Miller and Mangan (1983) studied patients undergoing colposcopy (a mildly invasive medical procedure) and found interactions between coping style and the amounts of information given on dependent measures of self-reported stress and physiological measures of arousal. Results showed that individuals who prefer to remain ignorant about the details of the impending procedure (blunters), but who, nevertheless, were given large amounts of information, were found to have higher heart rates and reported greater increases in distress than those individuals with the same predisposition who were given only the barest details about the procedure. As yet, possible interactions between personality type and information given in surgical situations have not been fully investigated; but it is likely that the variation found between studies of the effect of information giving may well be due in part to personality differences.

Control and predictability have also been extensively studied. Control means being able to determine what we do, or what others do to us. It is usually the case that we need to be able to predict an event in order to be able to control it; but the reverse does not follow – being able to predict an event does not necessarily mean that we can control it. Accurate expectations have sometimes been found to reduce the stress of surgery (Johnson and Leventhal 1974), but sometimes not. Studies of control for surgical patients have not often been carried out – controlling a ward or theatre environment is often regarded as unrealistic; nonetheless, at least one study (Atwell *et al.* 1984) has reported some beneficial effects from enabling patients to control their own anaesthetic administration. There is some evidence that locus of control may be important, with internals requiring more post-operative analgesia (Johnson *et al.* 1971). Once again, however, not all studies have reported the effect (for example, Levesque and Charlesbois 1977). Mathews and Ridgeway (1981) review the impact of personality differences on responses to surgery. They suggest there is evidence that high levels of neuroticism and trait anxiety are associated with poor recovery.

It is not clear from the research to date whether there is a group of patients who respond particularly poorly to surgery, or whether there are simply individual differences in responses to life stresses in general, surgical stress being one such stress. This distinction is important when designing interventions for surgery. Chapter 3 considers individual differences in styles of coping and reacting to stress in a broader context.

Personality differences may not be the only reason for the finding that information is relatively ineffective as a method of preparation. The evidence from Ley (1988) cited in Chapter 4 shows that patients have difficulty in understanding and remembering information given during medical consultations. If these findings hold for patients receiving information prior to surgery, then whatever effect the provision of information is supposed to have will inevitably be restricted. Few studies have checked to see which aspects of the information or instructions given presurgically were remembered, or whether the information was understood.

There have been two types of explanation advanced concerning the mechanisms by which preparation might promote recovery. Most explanations invoke the suggestion that preparation reduces stress; such stress reduction should be accompanied by a reduction in sympathetic arousal and by improvements in a patient's immunological response. Baker (1987) reviewed the evidence that external stressors could affect a person's immunological status and concluded that such evidence was strongly indicative of such effects. In Chapter 3 Evans considers this evidence in rather more detail.

Mathews and Ridgeway (1984) advance a different explanation. They argue that preparations exert their effects by reducing the frequency and extent of maladaptive behavioural reactions that an unprepared patient might exhibit. These two explanations are not incompatible. Evidence suggests that physiological responses are improved by psychological interventions which may be the result of a chain of events which begins with a reluctance to engage in health-promoting behaviours (such as mobilizing quickly after an operation). Recent studies (Kiecolt-Glaser *et al.* 1985; Linn *et al.* 1988) indicate that the measurement of the effects of preparation on the immunological functioning of surgical patients will in future enable us to examine the mechanisms more directly.

OTHER STRESSFUL MEDICAL PROCEDURES

Weinman and Johnston (1988) point out that inherent in most of the preparation literature is the idea that 'stressful medical procedures' can be considered together and equivalent in terms of their psychological impact. They suggest that a useful way of distinguishing between the various procedures would be by considering the function of the procedure and the time line and nature of stress associated with the procedure. Some stressful procedures can be regarded as having a diagnostic or investigative role, such as amniocentesis or a barium X-ray, whereas others have a treatment function (for example, tonsillectomy, cardiac catheterization). Other surgical procedures incorporate both treatment and investigative functions; for example, treatment surgery which also incorporates further exploratory investigations.

Weinman and Johnston distinguish between 'procedural stress' and 'outcome stress'. Procedural stress refers to the negative aspects of the actual procedure itself, the associated pain or discomfort. Outcome stress describes the longer-term fears and concerns associated with the results of the treatment or procedure. Johnston (1982) examined worries of surgical patients and found most to be concerned with longer-term, outcome concerns; she found that relatively few expressed concerns about the procedure itself. Allan and Armstrong (1984) studied reactions to different radiological procedures. They identified outcome concerns as more prevalent for all except the aged (more than 70 years of age), who were more concerned about the unpleasantness of the procedure itself.

This concern with outcome as well as with procedure may serve to explain the finding by Johnston (1980) that anxiety in surgical patients did not diminish as soon after surgery as would be anticipated if the major source of worry were the operation itself. It also points to the possibility of effective interventions *post-surgery* as well as pre-surgery. Weinman and Johnston suggest that a combination of sensation information and cognitive coping might prove beneficial following an investigative procedure. They suggest that encouraging patients to identify particular sensations and interpret them as normal and to be expected may help to reduce persistent anxiety and misattribution of internal sensations.

SPECIAL-CARE ENVIRONMENTS

Over the last twenty years special-care units for the treatment of acute patients have been developed. These units – intensive-care units (ICUs), coronary-care units (CCUs) and special-care units for babies – are characterized by elaborate and expensive equipment, highly skilled personnel and relatively high levels of activity, light and sound. These environments are thought to give rise to a psychiatric syndrome called 'ICU psychosis'. This can be described as a spectrum from mild confusion to extreme agitation, hallucinations and delirium. The physical setting undoubtedly plays a part in this reaction; but also important is the role of multiple medications and possible withdrawal from alcohol or drugs. Weinman (1981) reports a study of surgical ICU with no windows and limited visiting. Patients who were in neck traction became delirious within six days. The initial confusion is often patients feeling unsure whether they are awake or dreaming; reassurance and regular orientation at this stage can alleviate the distress. Attempts to introduce some form of diurnal routine which again helps patients to orientate themselves in time and place have also been ameliorative. Work by Kornfeld *et al.* (1965) led to changes in the environment; they recommended turning off bright lights at night, introducing clocks and calendars and including windows in the design of new units. These changes are likely to have benefited not just the patients in special-care units, but the medical and nursing staff also.

Recent studies, such as Riggio *et al.* (1982) and Dockter *et al.* (1988) have begun to examine the concerns of patients, their families and the nursing staff in intensive-care units in an effort to discover the match or mismatch between their perceptions of needs. There exists now a recognized need to prepare family members for visiting patients in ICU; they need to know what to expect with regard to the patient's appearance and condition and with regard to the procedures and operations of an ICU. Patients on mechanical respiration will have special communication needs which can be met in part by good nurse preparation and family support.

CHILDREN IN HOSPITAL

There has recently been a great deal of work concerning children in hospital. It is beyond the scope of this chapter to consider the long-term effects of hospitalization during childhood; instead the focus will be on attempts to reduce stress in children undergoing elective surgery. Melamed and her colleagues have carried out a number of studies investigating the beneficial effects of film modelling as preparation for surgery. Melamed (1984) describes the task in terms of answering the following practical questions:

- What does the child need to know in order to co-operate with the physician?
- Given the child's age, previous experience and level of anxiety, which preparatory treatment would be most effective?
- When should preparation take place?
- Should the parents be included in the preparation, and if so, what role should they play?

Melamed's work is within the social-learning tradition and an early study looked at the effects of a short film 'Ethan has an Operation' (Melamed 1974). This film depicted a 6-year-old boy from the time he entered hospital through his tests and operation and his interactions with staff and other children. Ethan is seen as a positive model who, although initially anxious, is able to cope with the medical situation and procedures. It also contained information about the nature of preparation for surgery. Children between the ages of 4 and 12 who saw this film the evening before their operations showed less anxiety both pre- and post-operatively than children who watched a control film about a boy going fishing. Similar results came from studies on preparing children for dental visits. A film showing a child receiving a novocaine injection was more effective in reducing anxiety than a similar film with no peer model. It was important to show the injection within the context of the whole treatment session. In fact, simply showing the injection sequence was found to result in more disruption from the child during the dental procedures (Melamed *et al.* 1978).

Melamed cautions against the assumption that the provision of information is uniformly beneficial for children. In a study of slide-show presentation for children between the ages of 4 and 14 Melamed found that younger children (under 7 years of age) and those with a previous hospital experience, reacted negatively to the presentation and were more disruptive. They argue for the use of a distracting film for these children (Melamed *et al.* 1983) and stressed the need to consider what age the child was and what previous relevant experience s/he had had.

CONCLUSIONS

We can see from trends in recent research that the emphasis of most studies of surgical recovery has moved from simple considerations of 'the best preparation method' to a recognition of the need for differing patient preparations. Ideas of 'tailoring input' and 'targeting information' are now discussed and attempts are made to provide a theoretical framework for the findings. As yet, though, it is not apparent, given hospital procedures, how such individual treatment can be achieved. How will patient preferences be identified? And what of the interactive nature of patient, expectations and treatment? It begins to look as if the doctors have been right when they assert that they tell the patient, 'if s/he asks...'.

Chapter 6

Psychoactive drugs: efficacy and effects

Andrew Parrott

INTRODUCTION

> A willingness to take medicines seems to be one of the most fundamental of human attributes. Of the enormous variety of drugs which doctors prescribe or which we prescribe for ourselves, many have effects on mood or experience.
>
> (Greenshaw *et al.* 1984: 1).

The diverse physiological and psychological effects of medicines are well covered in reference texts such as that of Goodman and Gilman (1985). The comprehensive coverage they provide is beyond the scope of the present chapter, which instead concentrates upon those with 'psychoactive' properties (Table 6.1). Many are taken for their psychoactive effects (for example, mood elevation with antidepressants), while with others their psychoactive properties comprise side-effects of medicines taken for other reasons (for example, sedation following an antihistamine taken to treat hay fever).

Parry *et al.* (1973) reported that each year 22 per cent of the general population took psychoactive medicines. Koenig *et al.* (1987) found that 9 per cent of Munich citizens took a prescribed psychoactive drug in any one week. Both surveys found twice as many women taking them compared to men. The elderly also consume large amounts of all medicines, including psychoactive drugs. Swift (1988) found they consumed 35–40 per cent of all UK medicines, although comprising only 15 per cent of the population. Most of these drugs were prescribed by general practitioners, with the majority of psychological or psychiatric complaints being treated in the general health practice. Tyrer (1988: 588) has stated: 'It is a paradox that most psychotropic (psychoactive) drugs are prescribed in general practice, yet most of the studies showing their value have been carried out in patients seen by psychiatrists.' He concluded that more studies of their effects should be carried out in health centres.

There is concern over the inappropriate use of psychoactive drugs. Avorn *et al.* (1989), for example, noted that for residents on antipsychotic drugs in Californian sheltered-care homes: 'Two-fifths lacked medical supervision and had lower levels of social functioning [than the non-medicated] . . .

Table 6.1 Main classes of psychopharmaceuticals and estimated consumption in western countries

Drug class	Examples	Consumption by value ($USm; 1986 estimate)
Neuroleptic	Chlorpromazine Trifluperazine	800
Antidepressant	Imipramine Amitryptyline	750
Anxiolytic	Diazepam Clobazam	1,450
Sedative–hypnotic	Nitrazepam Amylobarbitone	640
CNS stimulant	Amphetamine Methylphenidate	200
Nootropic	Piracetam Hydergine	1,000
Others (e.g. antihistamine, anticholinergic, steroid).	–	–

After: Julien 1985, Koenig *et al.* 1987, Spiegel 1989 and others.

particularly older people receiving high doses'; in North Carolina: 'Two-thirds of rest home facilities for the elderly lacked any drug-administration records'; in Massachusetts, 56 per cent of rest-home residents were taking psychoactive medications (39 per cent neuroleptics, 9 per cent antidepressants, 8 per cent benzodiazepines); while 'In most cases the prescriptions had been written in the remote past and were refilled automatically.' Many of these residents had been seen for a psychiatric problem, but perhaps most worrying was the 25 per cent of the normal elderly residents with no psychiatric history on antipsychotic (neuroleptic) drugs. The rest-home workers giving out these medications also displayed poor knowledge: 'The neuroleptic chlorpromazine was identified as an anti-depressant by 12 per cent and a minor tranquillizer by 47 per cent of staff respondents, while 19 per cent did not know its purpose.' This US scenario is not untypical of care practices for the elderly in many western countries. The misuse of neuroleptic drugs in political prisoners in the USSR has also been well documented, although their overuse in UK prisons is less widely recognized.

SYNAPTIC NEUROTRANSMISSION

Psychoactive drugs generally achieve their effects by modifying neural transmission. The firing of a nerve cell takes the form of an electrical impulse or action potential, which spreads from the point of impulse to the terminal ends of the neurone. This then stimulates the release of a chemical neurotransmitter, which enters the narrow synapse separating the presynaptic and postsynaptic nerves. This next nerve fires once sufficient neurotransmitter has been taken up within its membrane. These principles of neurotransmission are more fully described in basic psychopharmacological texts (for example, Greenshaw et al. 1984; Julien 1985; Warburton 1975).

Several neurotransmitters have been identified including dopamine (DA), noradrenaline (NA), 5–hydroxytrytamine (5-HT), acetylcholine (ACh), gamma aminobutyric acid (GABA), histamine (H) and others (Julien 1985; Warburton 1975). The recent history of psychopharmacology comprises a mapping of neurotransmitter systems within the brain, describing how they are affected in different disorders, and the influence of drugs upon them (Ashton 1987). Each neurotransmitter has been implicated in various behavioural and affective state disorders: schizophrenia with excess sensitivity of DA receptors; Parkinson's disease with low level of DA; anxiety with GABA; low mood and depression with reduced 5-HT or NA; sleep problems with 5-HT and NA; hyperactivity with DA or NA; allergies with histamine sensitivity; senile dementia with reduced ACh. Psychoactive medicines prescribed for these problems are therefore targeted upon particular neurotransmitter systems: antidepressant drugs to boost NA or 5-HT, neuroleptic drugs to reduce DA, and anxiolytic drugs to enhance GABA. The problem is that each neurotransmitter is involved in a number of central nervous system and bodily functions. Thus, DA is involved with control of movement, arousal and alertness, aspects of information processing and cognition. When a drug affecting DA transmission is given, it affects all of these functions to varying extents. Similarly, all other known neurotransmitters affect a number of different behavioural and cognitive functions. Psychoactive drugs therefore have a range of effects, some of which comprise target changes, while others represent side-effects (Ashton 1987; Julien 1985; Warburton 1975). These are described in the following sections.

NEUROLEPTICS (MAJOR TRANQUILLIZERS)

The discovery of the anti-schizophrenic properties displayed by chlorpromazine has revolutionized the treatment of schizophrenia, yet also illustrates the problems of using medicines with strong psychoactive effects. The development of chlorpromazine followed from studies into surgical shock by the French surgeon Laborit. While other drugs proved superior for the pharmacological control of shock, chlorpromazine led to dramatic improvements in many schizophrenics: auditory hallucinations disappeared or subsided, delusions became less firmly held, socially withdrawn patients became more open, people who had been mute for years began to speak. Placebo-controlled trials have confirmed the clinical utility of neuroleptic drugs (Davies and Casper 1978; NIMH 1964), and superiority over earlier 'therapies' such as insulin coma treatment (Potkin *et al.* 1984). Most schizophrenics are now seen as out-patients in psychiatric clinics or in general health centres. Severe problems occur with the many who fail to adhere to their medications, while many relatives are also left suffering from the problems which follow breakdown in medical supervision.

Neuroleptic drugs have strong side-effects resulting from the profound changes they induce in DA and other neurotransmitters (Ashton 1987; Bradley and Hirsch 1986; Spiegel 1989). These include:

- Parkinsonianism (tremor, altered gait, restricted movements);
- altered myocardial function (orthostatic hypotension);
- anticholinergic effects (dry mouth, sweating, constipation);
- hormonal changes (reduced sex drive, impotence, anorgasmia, amenorrhoea);
- tardive dyskinesia (motor disturbances, rolling the tongue, smacking of lips);
- emotional blunting, slowed thought processes.

Different neuroleptics can be broadly equated in their efficacy (which depends upon their affinity for DA receptors), but differ in side-effects, which reflect changes in both DA and other neurotransmitters. For example, chlorpromazine can induce all the side-effects listed above, thioridazine causes lesser Parkinsonian (extrapyramidical) effects, while haloperidol is less sedative in its action. Perlick *et al.* (1986) assessed chronic schizophrenics on a neuropsychological performance test battery. They found that word-learning decrements occurred that did not correlate with neuroleptic potency (efficacy), but did with anticholinergic (side-effect) potency. Recently introduced drugs such as sulpiride have been designed to retain the desired DA receptor affinity, while having lesser effects upon other neuro-transmitters. Unfortunately, although the side-effects are reduced, neuroleptic efficacy is also weak (Ashton 1987; Bradley and Hirsch 1986; Spiegel 1989). This trade-off of desired actions with undesired side-effects is frequently found when prescribing medicines and it may result in patients being given combinations or a cocktail of drugs. For example a patient given a neuroleptic drug may also be prescribed anticholinergic medication to reduce extrapyramidical (Parkinsonian) motor symptoms, even though anticholinergics may have side-effects of their own.

Recent trends in neuroleptic-drug use include the adoption of long-term depot injections, drug-free periods and dose reductions. Drug depots involve an injection of drug in a vegetable oil base, allowing it to be slowly released over 4–6 weeks. This has improved drug-taking compliance, and reduced the incidence of hospital relapse (Capstick 1980). Several studies have investigated the possibility of dose reductions, or the complete withdrawal of medication. In a review of these studies, Kane and Lieberman (1987) concluded: 'Dosage reduction can lead to a diminution in adverse effects and improvement in some measures of well being, however the risk of psychotic exacerbation increases.'

Following treatment with a neuroleptic, thought processes may be slowed, and emotional reactivity reduced, with social skills remaining impoverished (Spiegel 1989). Schizophrenics typically display a low level of social skills, and this generally remains during drug treatment, unless help and training are given. Despite this May (1968) concluded that the only useful therapy in schizophrenia was neuroleptic medication. In a later review, Schooler and Hogarty (1987) agreed with May (1968) about the importance of neuroleptic medication, but concluded that group therapy, individual psychotherapy, social-skills training and life-skills training could each contribute to behavioural improvement in schizophrenia, but only as long as active drug treatment was being given. Leff *et al.* (1982) also found that training the families of schizophrenics to be less verbally critical led to a significant reduction in hospital relapse for medicated schizophrenics.

A simplified model of pharmacotherapy suggests that the drug reduces the excessive cortical activity (flow of ideas, thought preoccupations, delusions) and high arousal (hyperalertness, distractability, sensory hallucinations) typical of schizophrenia. Therapeutic interventions now become possible. Social-skills training, group discussions and the establishment of new relationships can now take place; these may replace the social impoverishment that has occurred during the pre-psychosis years. There are clear implications for the community treatment of the schizophrenic: the current practice of neuroleptic drug treatment alone is insufficient; community-based social-skills centres and therapeutic clinics are also needed.

ANTIDEPRESSANTS

While the discovery of neuroleptics stemmed from medical research into battle and surgical stress, the use of antidepressant drugs followed from tuberculosis research. Under iproniazid, a monoamine oxidase inhibitor (MAO), several of the tuberculosis patients became exuberant and elated (a remarkable 'side-effect' considering the debilitating nature of the disease). Clinical trials with severely depressed patients confirmed the effectiveness of MAO-inhibitors, and tricyclic antidepressants such as imipramine (Kuhn 1970; Morris and Beck 1974; Spiegel 1989). Antidepressant drugs achieve their effects through an increase in neurotransmitter availability, particularly NA and 5-HT. These biochemical changes can also lead to a spectrum of side-effects (Ashton 1987; Julien 1985; Pinder 1988; Spiegel 1989), including:

– sedation, daytime tiredness, slowed psychomotor performance;
– dry mouth, constipation, impotence;
– visual focusing difficulty (reduced accommodation);
– dizziness, headaches;

- delirium (following over-dosage in the elderly);
- suicide;
- tyramine or 'cheese' effect.

Sedation and decreased alertness are most noticeable on initial prescription. Those prescribed these drugs therefore initially must be warned not to drive, or operate machinery. This restricts many occupations (car/bus/train drivers and industrial tasks), while accidents in the home may also be increased (Parrott 1987). The sedative effect may however be useful for those suffering reduced sleep, in which case each daily dose should be taken an hour before going to bed. Several recently developed antidepressants are less sedative than the original compounds, making them more suitable for ambulatory patients (Pinder 1988). With reference to the tyramine effect, this amino acid is present in many foods (aromatic cheeses, cream, yeast extract), and is normally broken down by MAO in the liver. If tyramine builds up in the body, then headache, cardiovascular stress or fatal cerebral haemorrhage can occur; it is therefore important that these foods are not taken if an MAO inhibitor is prescribed as an antidepressant.

Dry mouth, constipation and difficulty in focusing the eyes follow the alterations in neurotransmission of ACh induced by many tricyclic antidepressant drugs (imipramine, amitriptyline). Visual impairments can lead to increased danger, while all the other anticholinergic effects feel unpleasant. Several recent drugs have been designed to reduce anticholinergic and other side-effects: nomifensine, mianserin, viloxazine. Their reduced side-effects make them better tolerated in general, and more suitable for people undertaking demanding tasks and skilled occupations (Ashton 1987; Pinder 1988). Mianserin has a unique profile of action, including an absence of cardiotoxic or anticholinergic effects, making it safer for elderly patients, although it remains sedative. However, these recently developed drugs have their own severe side-effects: haemolytic anaemia with nomifensine, blood dyscrasias with mianserin, and some have recently been withdrawn for these reasons (Pinder 1988). A further problem with antidepressant drugs is that 15 per cent of all suicide deaths are caused by antidepressant drugs. The traditionally prescribed antidepressants have been used for suicides more frequently than the recently introduced compounds. For instance, amitriptyline accounts for 166 suicide deaths for every million patients treated, whereas mianserin is used for only thirteen suicides per million patients (Montgomery and Pinder 1987). Overall, traditional antidepressants such as amitriptyline and imipramine cause far more deaths through suicide than the rare toxicological reactions of the recently withdrawn drugs such as nomifensine. Pinder (1988: 84) has proposed that more accurate cost–benefit analyses need to be undertaken:

Regulatory authorities tend to deem effects at therapeutic dosage as those most worthy of consideration in an analysis of relative risks and benefits.

Antidepressants are peculiar in that their most important risk occurs not at therapeutic dose but in overdosage.

ANXIOLYTICS AND SEDATIVE-HYPNOTICS

The majority of medicines currently prescribed for sleep disorders and anxiety are benzodiazepine derivatives. Taylor (1987) estimated that around three million people in the UK (6 per cent of the population) took benzodiazepines for three months of each year, while 1.2 million took them for the period of a year or more. Ashton and Golding (1989) independently estimated that 1.2 million people in the UK consumed a benzodiazepine on any one particular day. Koenig et al. (1987) found that 6.6 per cent of their Munich sample had taken a benzodiazepine that week, and that benzodiazepines comprised two-thirds of all psychotropic drugs taken.

Following their introduction in 1958, numerous double-blind trials established the effectiveness of benzodiazepines for reducing tenseness and anxiety. Within six years they were more widely used than the barbiturates they replaced. Barbiturates caused drowsiness, were addictive, used for suicide, and were generally poorly tolerated; their use was a major health concern. Many people were prescribed a barbiturate at night to induce sleep, and an amphetamine in the morning to restore alertness. McKenzie and Elliott (1965) were concerned about the use of these drugs in US Air Force aircrew flying prolonged nuclear bomb missions, since 70 per cent were being prescribed barbiturates, and 64 per cent amphetamines (it may be noted that the problems caused by this poly-drug consumption were resolved within weeks by total drug withdrawal and altered work schedules). It was within this scenario that benzodiazepines achieved their popularity, and by 1970 they had become the most widely prescribed drugs in the world (Skegg et al. 1977). They were regarded as being without major side-effects, and many patients entering the consulting room would be asked whether they felt stressed, and given benzodiazepines if 'anxiety' was considered a factor contributing to their medical problem. Only during the 1980s has their popularity waned, with prescriptions on the decrease (Ashton and Golding 1989), and benzodiazepine dependency is now recognized as a widespread problem.

Benzodiazepines have several actions: muscle relaxation, anticonvulsion, anxiety reduction, sedation and sleep-induction (Ashton 1987; Spiegel 1989), but different drugs display these effects to varying extents. Diazepam, the archetypal benzodiazepine, has clear effects upon all these functions, and is often used for general sleep/worry problems. Nitrazepam and temazepam are more sedative and therefore used for sleep induction (Ashton 1987). Clobazam is largely clear of sedative effects, and is therefore useful for anxiety reduction where daytime drowsiness is to be avoided (Hindmarch 1985), while its anticonvulsant actions make it useful as a co-drug for epilepsy (Gastaut 1981).

The definition of a behavioural change as 'target effect' or 'side-effect' depends upon whether it is wanted or unwanted. For instance, sedation is a target effect in a drug given to induce sleep, but a 'side-effect' when given for anxiety or epilepsy (Gastaut 1981; Hindmarch 1985). Muscle relaxation is beneficial when used for pre-surgical anaesthesia, but a 'side-effect' when driving a car. Daytime sedation is a noticeable side-effect with many benzo-diazepines, together with the ensuing impairments in psychomotor skill and information processing (Hindmarch 1985; O'Hanlon 1988; Parrott 1987). Thus, driving and operating machinery should not be undertaken, especially in the early stages of drug administration. This sedation is increased by alcohol, further increasing the likelihood of an accident. Memory is also impaired, and although Ghoneim et al. (1981) reported partial tolerance to these amnesic effects, Lucki et al. (1986) found that mild amnesia remained with long-term benzodiazepine users. The main side-effects of the benzodiazepines can be summarized as follows:

- sedation, drowsiness;
- impaired psychomotor performance, car-driving skills, reduced attention and memory;
- additive effects with alcohol;
- paradoxical reactions (increased anxiety/aggression);
- benzodiazepine dependency.

Severe side-effects may follow from too high a dose, particularly in the elderly. Their metabolic breakdown systems are generally slowed, so that a given amount of drug will generally remain active for longer. Disorientation and disturbed co-ordination are urgent signals for a dosage reduction. Indeed, dose levels for all psychoactive drugs should be lowered in the elderly (Swift 1988). Paradoxical responses such as increased anxiety, aggressiveness and rage have been noted with all age groups, and may follow from the drug being given to an inappropriate patient. Parrott and Kentridge (1982) used the repertory-grid technique to study detailed feelings of anxiety under a benzodiazepine. As expected the high trait anxiety subjects showed a significant reduction in anxiety; in contrast the low trait anxiety subjects showed a paradoxical increase in anxiety. Non-neurotic patients should therefore probably not be given benzodiazepines (for example, during transient stress situations such as examinations or bereavement), since they may abreact against them (Parrott 1985).

Concern has been raised over the use of benzodiazepines over long periods, both with respect to efficacy and dependency. The Committee on the Review of Medicines (1980) noted that benzodiazepines had not been shown to be effective when prescribed for a continuous period of three months. Following this, however, Rickels et al. (1983) demonstrated that diazepam did maintain its anxiolytic efficacy for twenty-two weeks and probably for longer (twenty-two weeks was the longest period studied). Dependence is, however, a major problem (Lader 1983, 1989). Tolerence to the effects of benzodiazepines can occur, both to its target and side-effects (Aranko *et al.* 1985). Some studies, however, have not confirmed tolerance, and individual differences are undoubtedly important. Rebound reactions also occur on drug withdrawal, where anxiety and tenseness return at levels higher than those initially reported. Rebound depends upon the duration of drug administration, the half-life of the drug involved and the rate of drug withdrawal. Fontaine *et al.* (1984) investigated rebound following long-acting diazepam with short-acting bromazepam, and compared abrupt drug termination with gradual dose reduction. The abrupt withdrawal group reported levels of anxiety significantly higher than those noted before medication had been given, while those in the gradual reduction group returned to their pre-medication anxiety levels. Rebound anxiety was also more severe with the short-acting drug (bromazepam). Rebound is not simply a re-emergence of the original anxiety, since it also occurs in patients undergoing long-term benzodiazepine use for reasons other than initial anxiety (for example, to aid recovery from muscle injury; Lader 1989). A further problem with drug withdrawal/reduction is the induction of previously never-experienced sensations: unexplained pains, perceptual hypersensitivity and feelings of unreality. The most severe and unpleasant experiences again follow the withdrawal of short-acting benzodiazepines such as lozazapam (Fontaine *et al.* 1984). The severity of these effects and the availability of alternative drugs have led to the current practice of not giving new patients these short-acting benzodiazepines.

In view of their side-effects, it is paradoxical that short-acting benzodiazepines were originally developed to overcome the side-effects of traditional longer-acting drugs. Diazepam is metabolized into several active breakdown products (for example, n-desmethyldiazepam), which remain for around one week after a single dose. Most benzodiazepines developed in the 1960s and 1970s had similar long half-lives and active metabolites. The major side-effect at the time was considered to be sedation, and it was expected that a short half-life benzodiazepine without active metabolites would represent a pharmacotherapeutic advance. Although sedation was reduced, the problems of dependence became far greater. In a monograph on benzodiazepine misuse, Marks (1978) summarized the prevailing view that benzodiazepine dependence was not a major problem: they were misused, but dependence was rare, with only single case reports appearing in the literature. Nine years later Ashton (1987) suggested that around half a million people in the UK might be dependent on short- *or* long-acting benzodiazepines. The problems of long-acting compounds have emerged with the realization of the generally more severe problems with the short-acting compounds. Many behaviour-modification techniques, such as relaxation therapy, have been shown to be effective for complaints where anxiety is a central problem. In a general health practice study, Catalan *et al.* (1984) showed that such procedures were just as effective as benzodiazepines, but were of course without associated side-effects.

NOOTROPICS

A degree of memory loss or 'benign senescent forgetfulness' (Spiegel 1989) is common during normal ageing. Senile dementia of the Alzheimer type (SDAT) is said to occur when these memory problems become disabling, and emotional confusion and intellectual decline predominate. The proportion of the population defined as 'senile' depends upon inclusion criteria. Katzman (1986) suggested that around 5 per cent of over 65-year-olds had senile dementia, while with older age groups the estimates vary from 10 to 25 per cent.

Several drugs are marketed as nootropics or cognitive activators, but what is remarkable is the lack of evidence for their effectiveness. Recent reviews (Orogozo and Spiegel 1987; Wittenborn 1981) have concluded that the evidence for the utility of some widely prescribed drugs was almost non-existent; only hydergine and piracetam emerged with any creditable support. Piracetam, the first drug to which the term 'nootropic' was attributed, has been demonstrated to alter brain function in animals, and probably to hasten recovery from anoxia in humans, but there is only slight evidence that it is effective in Alzheimer's disease (McDonald 1982). Hydergine demonstrated slightly stronger evidence for nootropic actions, with cognitive improvement in some studies, although non-significant findings were frequent in many studies (see reviews in Ashton 1987; Hindmarch et al. 1980; Orogozo and Spiegel 1987; Wittenborn 1981).

While the efficacy of these supposed nootropics is in doubt, at least they are largely free from side-effects. This reflects their lack of effects upon central nervous system (CNS) functions. When introduced, piracetam was said to be free from neuronal activity (Giurgea 1976), although subsequent studies have suggested slight effects upon neurotransmission. Similarly, hydergine is suggested to exert its effects through acting as a general cellular activator (possibly similar to caffeine). Hydergine may boost CNS vascular microcirculation, and increase cerebral oxygen consumption, but the evidence is again inconsistent. Whether it is effective or just a placebo, it is well tolerated, and remains one of the most widely used drugs in the world. With the proportion of over 65-year-olds in the population increasing dramatically, the search for an effective nootropic has become the primary target for many psychopharmaceutical research programmes.

CNS STIMULANTS

Central nervous system stimulants such as amphetamine and methyl-phenidate have a range of alerting actions. During the Second World War, studies were undertaken to find a stimulant for soldiers undertaking prolonged military duties. Amphetamine significantly reduced sleepiness and fatigue, and became used by both opposing forces (Davis 1947; Seashore and Ivy 1953). Stimulants lead to increased vivacity, reduced feelings of despondency or depression, and higher mood in general. Athletic performance is also boosted, so they have been banned by athletic organizations (Smith and Beecher 1959). Feelings of hunger are suppressed, and until recently some private UK slimming clinics have been allowed to prescribe them under special licence (Farrell 1989b). Amphetamines are also effective in relieving motion sickness (Hill 1937), and combined scopolamine-amphetamine capsules are used both by astronauts and cosmonauts for space sickness (Lukomskya and Nikolskay 1974; see the Anticholinergics section, below). Further clinical uses for amphetamines include treatment of narcolepsy (suddenly falling asleep), and hyperactivity in children (Ross and Ross 1982).

Despite their range of effects, stimulants are now rarely used. Spiegel (1989) stated: 'Psychostimulants today play hardly any role in medical practice.' The reason for this is their potential addictiveness. While a single dose can increase alertness and feelings of well-being, the after-effects include fatigue and depression. One way to relieve this low mood is to take another capsule, thus initiating a cycle of regular drug taking. Tolerance to amphetamine can develop rapidly (tachphylaxis), with dosage needing to be increased to achieve similar results. Repeated dosing can lead to a state of cortical hyperarousal resembling schizophrenia. The addictiveness of amphetamine and cocaine is well documented (for neurochemical explanations see Ashton 1987). What is less readily explained is why under some conditions it does not develop. Dependency does not seem to be a problem with hyperactive children, nor in the treatment of narcolepsy, nor as a counteracting agent for the sedation produced with some anti-epilepsy drugs. Many potentially addictive drugs induce dependency only under particular situations, or with some people. Phillips, Gossop and Bradley (1986), for instance, showed the severity of heroin withdrawal correlated with neuroticism, but not with length of opioid use. Many of the American soldiers regularly taking heroin in Vietnam simply stopped taking the drug on their return to the USA.

ANTIHISTAMINES

Research into synthetic antihistamines initiated the modern era of pharmacotherapy, so it is surprising that antihistamines hardly figure in contemporary psychopharmacology texts (Ashton 1987; Julien 1985; Spiegel 1989; Warburton 1975). This probably reflects the absence of any major neurochemical model concerning their CNS role, although their influence upon alertness is recognized (Nicholson 1985; Uzan et al. 1979).

Two types of histamine receptor need to be distinguished: the H1-receptor involved in allergies, and the H2-receptor involved in stomach ulcers (Nicholson 1985). Early H1-antihistamines such as promethazine and diphenhydramine affected both peripheral H1 receptors involved in allergic reactions, and H1 receptors in the CNS. These central receptors are involved in arousal and alertness (Uzan *et al.* 1979); thus sedation and impaired psychomotor performance are prominent side-effects, although the degree of sedation does differ between compounds (Hindmarch and Parrott 1978; Nicholson 1985; Parrott and Wesnes, 1987). Some recently developed H1-antagonists which either do not cross the blood-brain barrier (astemizole), or have a greater affinity for peripheral rather than central receptors (terfenadine), display minimal sedative effect. These newer drugs therefore comprise the current treatment of choice for allergic rhinitis (hay fever) and other allergies (Nicholson 1985). The treatment of stomach ulcers has been revolutionized by the development of H2-antagonists such as cimetidine and ranitidine. Being less liposoluble than H1-receptor blockers, they only cross the blood-brain barrier with difficulty. They are therefore generally clear of CNS side-effects (Nicholson 1985), although impaired performance and mental confusion do seem to occur in some patients with renal or hepatic failure (Shentag *et al.* 1979).

ANTICHOLINERGICS

Travellers have suffered from motion sickness ever since the development of artificial aids to movement. Camel, ship, car, aeroplane, train and the space rocket can each engender feelings of nausea when the right motion conditions prevail. The battle scarred Cicero admitted he would 'rather be killed than again suffer the tortures of nausea maris' (Reason and Brand 1975: 14). Studies using the deceptively named 'Slow Rotation Room' have clarified the conditions under which motion sickness can be induced (Wood and Graybiel 1968). They either comprise: sensory mismatch between visual and vestibular (balance) information (for example, inside the cabin on a tossing ship, with the vestibular organs of balance signalling motion, while the eyes signal a static cabin); or conflict within the vestibular organs of balance (for example, during zero gravity space travel, with acceleration indicated by the semi-circular canals, but gravity information unexpectedly not provided by the otolith organs) (Benson 1984; Reason and Brand 1975). Neurochemical models of motion sickness emphasize acetylcholine (ACh) neurotransmission (Kohl and Homick 1983; Reason and Brand 1975), and effective drugs for motion sickness are strongly anticholinergic: scopolamine, atropine and promethazine (Kohl and Homick 1983; Parrott 1989; Parrott and Wesnes 1987; Reason and Brand 1975). Acetylcholine is however also involved in many CNS functions – alertness, information processing, sustained attention, the consolidation of new information into memory – and also in several ANS functions – visual accommodation, salivation, sweating (Goodman and Gilman 1985; Parrott 1986, 1989; Warburton 1975). Because of their sedative properties, anticholinergics are ingredients in many over-the-counter sleeping preparations (Goodman and Gilman 1985). Aircraft crew are prohibited from using them for air sickness, due to their sedating action (Benson 1984). Similarly, car drivers who have taken them on ferry crossings should rest on disembarkation. Overall, the side-effects of anticholinergic drugs comprise:

- sedation, drowsiness;
- reduced information processing (impaired attention and memory);
- dry mouth, difficulty focusing on near objects, impaired sweating.

Various procedures for mitigating against these side-effects have been attempted. Aircrew can be trained to overcome air sickness by teaching relaxation techniques while being exposed to increasingly severe motion conditions; then they no longer need any drug prophylaxis (Benson 1984). Astronauts and cosmonauts use amphetamine–scopolamine drug combinations. The two drugs act synergistically upon different neurochemical pathways, to provide a higher level of protection than either drug can achieve alone, while their effects upon arousal tend to cancel each other out (Lukomskya and Nikolskay 1974; Wood and Graybiel 1968). Scopolamine, the most effective single drug for motion sickness, is now available in a transdermal patch. It is applied to the skin like an elastoplast, and the drug slowly permeates through the skin into the systemic circulation. Although effective over a prolonged time period, the level of side-effects is similar to that found with oral tablets (Parrott 1989).

ANAESTHETIC DRUGS USED DURING DAY SURGERY

Day surgery has increased dramatically in recent years, with new facilities being built in many hospitals. The majority of day-surgery cases comprise straightforward operations: dilatation and curettage, abortion, tonsillectomy and herniorrhaphy, although more difficult and prolonged operations are also performed (see below). Of two million operations in the UK each year, Britton (1987) estimated that a quarter to one-fifth are suitable for day surgery. The Royal College of Surgeons guidelines for day-case surgery (1985) included a recommendation of maximum duration for surgery of thirty minutes. Britton (1987: 3) admitted the general utility of this, but stated: 'Surgery for varicose veins or an inguinal hernia often takes longer and both are still perfectly acceptable.' Moss and Hooper (1987: 18) admitted: 'Because of an insufficient number of in-patient beds at Leeds, it has been necessary to perform certain oral surgical operations requiring tracheal intubation as day cases.'

Medical sequelae from both surgery and the anaesthetic drugs include:

drowsiness, headache, nausea, unsteadiness, sore throat and pain (Moss and Hooper 1987; Ogg 1987), while more severe problems include: complications of pre-existing diseases, and drug interactions (Moss and Hooper 1987). The anaesthetist has a wide range of drugs from which to choose. Anaesthetic agents include inhaled nitrous oxide, or intravenous barbiturates such as thiopentone. Short-acting opioids (fantanyl and alfentanil) are used to suppress autonomic and somatic responses to surgery. Benzodiazepines induce muscle relaxation and reduce anxiety. Analgesics range from minor agents such as aspirin or paracetamol, to more major pain killers. Many different drug combinations have been investigated to find those which are both effective, and allow rapid recovery (Britton 1987; Moss and Hooper 1987; Ogg 1987).

Health psychologists have been requested to devise practical tests to assess patient recovery. These have been used to assess the degree of residual impairment following different anaesthetic cocktails, and in the future may be used to test whether a patient has recovered sufficiently to return home. Current practice is to allow patients home once they feel 'better', or when it is convenient (for example, when facilities are closing at the end of the day). Patients should be asked to arrange for a friend to collect them from the ward, but Ogg (1972) reported that 9 per cent of car owners had driven themselves home following anaesthesia, while 73 per cent had driven within twenty-four hours of surgery. It would be better if each patient were released only when s/he had demonstrated a given level of recovery, but there are several problems in assessing this (Herbert 1987). Many test batteries are lengthy and difficult to administer, while short brief tests may look nice (i.e. have high 'face' validity), but demonstrate neither reliability nor true validity. Even if a brief, reliable and valid test were to be devised, it might be a problem to persuade doctors or patients to use it. Many physicians would be loath to foreswear 'clinical judgement' in favour of a psychological test result; also it would be easier to discharge a patient with the instruction not to do anything, than it would to arrange an unplanned overnight hospital bed.

PLACEBO

The placebo effect has been well documented in experimental psychopharmacology (Shapiro 1978). Frankenhaeuser et al. (1963) demonstrated that responses to physiologically inert (placebo) capsules were dependent upon expectations. When subjects were told that the capsule was a stimulant, heart rate increased, psychomotor responses were speeded, and feelings of alertness increased. When told it was a sedative, their physiological and psychological indices were of decreased alertness. The placebo effect is not just a response to an unknown capsule; it reflects the whole process of being in an uncertain situation, and generating hopes and fears over possible outcomes. Any open undefined event can induce marked psychological and physiological changes. Indeed much of medical healing depends upon generating feelings of confidence, and the expectation of positive outcome in the patient.

In experimental psychopharmacology, the placebo effect is sometimes considered a nuisance variable. Spiegel (1989: 159) stated: 'With clinical trials of new medicines, placebo effects are primarily seen as a distorting element since they blend with the specific effects of the product and make a reliable evaluation difficult.' (This is also true of non-drug treatments such as biofeedback: see Chapter 8.) However, during medical treatment the placebo response should be considered to be of great potential use. The incidence of motion sickness can be reduced by around 70 per cent with placebo. Similarly, with disturbed sleep, anxiety or negative mood state, placebo treatment can have significant beneficial effects. On the negative side, placebos can also induce side-effects, with headache and dizziness being noticeable in many psychopharmacology trials. The difficulty of using placebo for medical treatment is that it is unethical to administer a pharmacologically inactive substance while suggesting it is a medicine. However, a procedure which utilizes the placebo factor is to prescribe a low dose; this practice is already quite widespread with benzodiazepines. Another is to use a drug with weak efficacy and minimal side-effects; nootropics, which comprise some of the most widely prescribed drugs in the world, are an example of this. Many non-western medical approaches use herbal remedies with proven psychoactive efficacy, yet in lower doses than used in the west (De Rios 1989). Their preparation and administration procedures are seen as important in determining positive change, through the induction of expectancies and beliefs. The main lesson for western practices is that medicines should be seen as just one aspect of an overall approach to healing and change.

OVERVIEW

Pharmacotherapy ideally requires an effective medicine with minimal side-effects. This goal is gradually being achieved through advances along several avenues. Pharmacologists are attempting to develop medicines with more specific target effects. The most successful example of this approach comprises the H2-anatagonists, since they are highly effective but largely free from side-effects (see section on antihistamines, above). This degree of specificity is more difficult to achieve with CNS disorders. Improved antidepressants have however been developed, where efficacy levels are maintained, while side-effects are reduced (Pinder 1988). The treatment of allergies such as hay fever has also been improved (Nicholson 1985), but similar advances for schizophrenia have not yet been attained. An alternative strategy is to use existing medicines, but in altered dosing regimens. Long-term depot injections have proved to be an important advance in schizophrenia (Capstick 1980). Transdermal delivery systems are being developed for many more medicines, and are proving particularly useful for drugs that are short acting (Parrott 1989). When prolonged drug treatment is required, drug-free periods, or low doses, can be successful. The deleterious consequences of undesired side-effects may also be reduced by warning patients to expect them. This information should be in the form of written package inserts, since verbal information given during consultation is often forgotten. Gibbs *et al.* (1989) found improved knowledge of side-effects, and greater satisfaction over information received, following the use of simple information leaflets. Finally, many problems currently treated with drugs could be treated without them. This is particularly true for many 'anxiety'-based problems, where self-help groups, simple counselling, advice or changes in life-style may be more beneficial (Catalan 1984). Prescriptions for benzodiazepines in the UK have fallen to 60 per cent of former levels over the past ten years, but they still remain high.

Chapter 7

Pain

Brenda May

INTRODUCTION

There can be no argument with the statement that pain is aversive and that it cannot be ignored. Anyone who has had toothache knows well the over-whelming need to make the pain go away! There are many types of activities that people adopt to achieve the reduction of pain – they take pain-killing tablets, hug a hot-water bottle, bandage the damaged area, go to bed, sit in a dark room, read a book to forget about the pain or visit the doctor.

Pain is thus costly to the individual: a familiar comment is that pain is exhausting. It is also very costly to the economy, studies across various countries show that pain accounts for enormous expenditure – in terms of sick pay, disability pensions and insurance benefits (*Ergonomics* 1985). Absen-teeism owing to musculoskeletal pain accounts for approximately 25 per cent of all sick leave (Hettinger 1985).

There is therefore considerable need for ways of effectively controlling the levels of pain experienced in both acute and chronic cases. Effective management relies upon our understanding of the phenomenon of pain – what it is, which factors affect its perception and which are the most effective ways of controlling it.

DEFINING PAIN

In attempting to define pain, Sternbach (1968) identified three components: sensation, a noxious stimulus and response or behaviour. He defined it as an abstract concept which refers to (a) 'a personal private sensation of hurt'; (b) 'a harmful stimulus which signals current or impending tissue damage'; and (c) 'a pattern of responses which operate to protect the organism from harm'. This definition has face validity and seems to describe quite well the subjective experiences of pain. Imagine someone cutting his/her finger with a sharp piece of glass which is stuck in the flesh. The sensation (pain) is not available for anyone to see although it might be intense, the external harmful stimulus (the glass) is clearly responsible for the tissue damage and signals impending damage if not removed (infection), and during removal! The person is likely to engage in a number of behavioural responses; in the short term, s/he may scream, hold the hand, and in the longer term, sit down, rock to and fro, take a tablet, have a cup of tea and perhaps go to the hospital for anti-tetanus injections and a sick note for the following week.

Sternbach's definition can be seen to be based on a linear model: a harmful stimulus leads to a sensation of pain which leads to a pattern of responses. There are various consequences of adopting such a linear model. First, the assumption is made that 'pain' occurs as a consequence of damage which stimulates transmission and which results in pain. A further consequence is that relief from the pain will be dependent upon removing or repairing the damage. It follows that similar damage should result in similar sensations of pain. The pattern of responses is conceptualized as dependent upon the sensation of pain, as an end-point of the linear progression. This linear model does not seem to be an appropriate one for understanding pain and the consequential assumptions are not supported by clinical experience.

There are a number of clinical findings that invalidate the expectation that a similar harmful stimulus which causes damage will result in similar pain experience. Only one in three of a group of severely wounded combat soldiers returning from battle during the Second World War complained of enough pain to require morphine. These soldiers were lucid and well oriented. Surgical civilians with similar wounds required much higher doses of pain-killing drugs (Beecher 1959). This is an example of the absence of levels of expected pain. Phantom-limb pain exemplifies the reverse – pain in the absence of tissue damage. Most amputees report feeling as if the amputated limb is still there almost immediately after surgery. The phantom limb is felt to be the same size and shape as it was pre-operatively, and it appears to move in response to the individual's wishes. Over time this image alters, it may shrink in size, or parts may disappear altogether. Some individuals report severe pain in areas of the amputated limb which may persist for long periods of time, sometimes for years after surgery (Melzack 1973).

In general, though, tissue damage does result in acute pain, and adaptive behaviour follows. In this situation, we engage in behaviour which fosters rest, care and protection of the damaged area. The injury follows the expected course, and as the damage heals, the pain is perceived to subside and individuals gradually resume their pre-injury life-style; they go back to work, no longer need pain-killers, their pain has gone. On occasions though, this expected outcome is not seen, the injury appears to heal, but the sensation of pain still remains or even increases, and the pre-injury life-style is not resumed. Such individuals are described as suffering from 'chronic pain'.

The absence of pain in the presence of damage, the presence of pain in the absence of damage and chronic pain all call into question the assumption that tissue damage is the cause of pain sensation. Our understanding of pain must be able to account for these unexpected responses and the linear model does not offer such an explanation. The more complex model proposed by Melzack and Wall (1965) goes further in explanation and has stimulated research, particularly psychological research.

Melzack and Wall conceptualized pain as a perceptual experience whose quality and intensity are influenced by the unique past history of the individual, by the meaning s/he gives to the pain-producing situation, and by the individual's state of mind. According to this view, psychological variables play a direct role in the pain experience. This model applied to the example given above would suggest that the amount of pain felt by the cut finger would be influenced by previous experiences with damage to fingers, by the fact that the glass belonged to someone else and there was a sick child crying upstairs, as well as the damage done to the tissue.

Early physiological theories proposed a specificity theory of pain where stimulation of specialized receptors, or free nerve endings at the periphery, would result in pain perception. However, stimulation of free nerve endings elicited a variety of sensations – warmth, cold, touch and itching as well as pain. This lack of support resulted in the pattern theory of pain which hypothesized that pain would be felt following any kind of stimulation that was excessive. The temporal and spatial discharge patterns of peripheral nerve fibres were seen as representing 'codes' which would lead to different sensations (Crue and Carregal 1975).

Recent accumulation of evidence (Bonica and Albe-Fessard 1976; Liebeskind and Paul 1977; Sternbach 1978) supports the concept of specialization rather than specificity and this has been incorporated, along with psychological aspects, into the gate control theory of pain (Melzack and Wall 1965). Two main findings have to be accommodated by any comprehensive theory of pain perception: the physiological basis of neuronal transmission and the lack of correspondence between tissue damage and the perception of pain.

Basically, the gate control theory proposes a gating mechanism in the dorsal horns of the spinal cord. This mechanism modulates sensory input by the balance of the activity of peripheral nerve fibres. Fibres that are maximally responsive to pain stimuli are thought to exist. A-delta fibres, which are the slowest of the myelinated fibres, are thought to mediate immediate or sharp pain, whereas unmyelinated C fibres mediate slow, diffuse or aching pain and A-beta fibres which are large diameter fibres. These sensory fibres enter the spinal cord through the dorsal horns where they are packed into layers. These layers contain cells which are especially responsive to activation of A-delta and C fibres. Activity in the A-beta fibres is assumed to activate the cells of the substantia gelatinosa and thereby inhibit the activity of the central projecting transmission cells, or 'close the gate'. Activity in the A-delta and C fibres inhibits the activity of the substantia gelatinosa, or 'opens the gate' and thus facilitates central projecting transmission cells. Fibres then project via the anterolateral system to various higher CNS areas. Those projecting to the ventrobasal thalamus and the somatosensory cortex are involved in the sensory-discriminatory aspect of pain, those projecting to the reticular formation, the intralamina thalamus and the limbic system are related to the aversive–cognitive–motivational and emotional components. The final component of the theory is the influence of descending fibres from the brain on the 'gate'. Higher cortical areas influence the reactions on the basis of cognitive evaluation and past experience.

What does all this mean in relation to the understanding of the experience of pain? According to Liebeskind and Paul (1977) it means that together, *all* of these mechanisms, but none in isolation, are sufficient to account for the experience of pain. Pain is the outcome of many peripheral and central nervous system structures, with signals from the periphery being evaluated in terms of prior experience, and current attentional and emotional states. Pain perception is the final output of sensation and evaluation.

The lack of correspondence between reported pain and tissue damage can be accommodated by the gate control theory. Failure to perceive pain in certain circumstances is explained by the 'gate-closing' effect of descending neuronal activity – the attention given to the activity, the memory of previous experiences, the anxiety level at the time, the reinforcements for behaviour can all affect pain sensation, making the pain greater or lesser. In 1978 Melzack and Dennis extended the gate control theory. They proposed two mechanisms to explain chronic and phantom-limb pain: first, that low-level abnormal inputs produce self-sustaining neural activity, and these can occur at any level of the nervous system. These 'pattern generation systems' are normally inhibited by central mechanisms. Second, memories of prior pain experiences can act as 'triggers' for abnormal firing patterns. Once pain is established, and damage disrupts normal neural activity, the pattern-generating systems will become self-perpetuating and can only be disrupted by either descending neural activity or imposed normal neural patterns via alternative activities.

Many of the components of the theory remain unsubstantiated, and there have been many criticisms. Dyck *et al.* (1976) presented clinical evidence that sensory fibre size does not facilitate or inhibit pain as proposed by the theory. The gate control theory's explanation of the behavioural dimensions of chronic pain is also somewhat inadequate. The theory presumes that the behavioural response is based on the affective component of the pain itself, the output of the connecting cells in the 'gate' is assumed to activate negative affect and an aversive drive. Put another way, pain behaviour is an outcome of the sensory, motivational and cognitive component. If this is viable, there should be a positive correlation between high pain sensation and high avoidance of pain by not engaging in activities that will cause pain. This positive correlation has not been found. Philips and Jahanshahi (1986) found that chronic-pain patients who did not avoid painful activities did not show significantly lower pain sensation scores than those who did avoid painful activities. As it stands, the gate control theory does not examine the relationships of the dimensions of pain it proposes, but it has provided a conceptual framework for considering the integration of sensory, affective and cognitive dimensions of pain.

The understanding of pain has clearly moved from the simple stimulus–response view. It is agreed that at the very least it involves two basic components – a sensory component, which includes the physiological and pathological events happening to the individual, and an emotional-motivational aspect which is primarily psychological in nature. Lethem *et al.* (1983) argue that the emotional-motivational component is best conceptualized as 'fear of pain' and that it will be subject to the same influences as other fears. The fear is seen as being a function of the individual's response to it; that is, fear will reduce if confronted, and will increase if avoided. This is the same way as the fear of spiders, or anything else, is predicted to develop. Avoidance can be either cognitive or behavioural and both are thought to result in a reduction of physical and social activities. Reduction in physical activities will, in turn, lead to secondary problems such as loss of muscle tone, development of adhesions and, possibly, gain in weight. Such consequences are likely to ensure that future pain will be more severe and it is in this way that an 'avoidance spiral' is set up. The psychological consequences of avoidance will be twofold. First, as the individual adopts an 'invalid status' s/he will be exposed to positive and negative reinforcers which again increase the likelihood of the avoidance spiral. Most importantly, the avoidance will result in fewer opportunities for exposure to painful experiences. Painful experiences need to be encountered as Lethem *et al.* propose that they are the equivalent to testing out the strength of the pain, or 'calibrating' as they term it. Lack of such opportunity does not allow the individual to estimate realistically the pain due to various activities and it is likely that their expectations will be exaggerated in the absence of testing pain levels. This will lead to further avoidance and to the avoidance spiral.

The model, then, assumes that the chronicity of the pain from some organic cause will be a function of the coping style of the individual. If avoidance is the response, de-synchrony between the organic, sensory and emotional components will ensue (Rachman and Hodgson 1974). The perception of pain will remain high due to secondary consequences, reinforcements for illness behaviour and lack of opportunity to test out recovery. If confrontation is the response, the secondary consequences will be minimized, reinforcements will serve to increase well behaviour and the individual will have an opportunity to test out how s/he is recovering; synchrony will result.

An example will help to clarify these two responses. Two persons have similar leg fractures and on removal of their plasters, both are instructed by their doctors and physiotherapists to engage in various exercises and activities. They commence their rehabilitation with some pain when exercising. One of them, called 'A', stops doing the exercises, believing that the pain shows that the fracture has not healed and rest is the best thing. The next week is spent with the leg raised and 'A' is waited on hand and foot. Work colleagues visit and fill in at work, the GP calls and prescribes pain-killers to be taken when the pain is bad (this regimen of tablet taking will be positively reinforced by the reduction in pain after the medication). Neighbours are full of sympathy and help. The outcome is that the leg swells, confirming the belief that all is not well and the positive and negative reinforcement consolidates the illness role, de-synchrony is apparent. The other victim, called 'B', is also worried by the pain on exercising, but telephones the physiotherapist and is reassured that it does not indicate any problems with healing. 'B' continues slowly with the exercises, gradually increasing the amount done and notes that the pain gradually eases. On the fourth day, 'B' decides to try walking across the room without a stick and finds that the pain is less than anticipated. The GP calls, and suggests that a pain-killer taken regularly before bed would be helpful (as this tablet is not contingent on pain, taking it will not be reinforced by pain reduction). 'B' encourages the person who is acting as helper to go back to work for part of the day. The outcome for 'B' is that the swelling reduces, the pain, being less than expected, also reduces, and activities are gradually attempted. Positive reinforcement is contingent on achievement, as the helper is supportive of each new activity. The well role is established, and the components of pain move in synchrony.

CHRONIC PAIN

Lethem *et al.*'s model attempts to explain the process whereby 'pain experience' and 'pain behaviour' become dissociated from 'pain sensation'. Non-adaptive avoidance behaviour is of central importance in the development of chronic pain. The model does not however identify the avoidance behaviours that might be engaged in by chronic-pain patients. Philips and Jahanshahi (1986) addressed this question by factor analysing the responses of 267 chronic headache sufferers to a Pain Behaviour Checklist (PBC). The PBC contained forty-nine items compiled from behavioural items commonly reported by pain sufferers. An exploratory factor analysis with orthogonal Varimax rotation produced thirteen factors which cumulatively accounted for 60.5 per cent of the total variance. The first six factors pertained to types of avoidance, the strongest being 'social withdrawal' (avoids party-going, visiting) followed by 'avoidance of housework' (avoids odd jobs, slows down physical movement), 'avoidance of daily mobility' (avoids lifting objects, public transport), 'activity avoidance' (avoids gardening, time on hobbies), 'daily exercise avoidance' (avoids standing, spending time with co-habiters) and 'stimulation avoidance' (lies down, rests, sleeps, avoids going to work). This suggests that 'avoidance' is complex, with six avoidance factors, the strongest of which is social avoidance accounting for 21.9 per cent of the variance. In the same study, increasing chronicity was associated with increasing avoidance behaviour. By dividing the subjects into high and low avoiders, comparisons were possible between these two groups on estimates of pain sensation. Lethem *et al.*'s 'fear of pain' model would predict that low avoiders would be significantly lower on this measure, but no significant differences were found. Philips and Jahanshahi suggest instead that chronic-pain patients may be either confronters or avoiders: which they are is determined by the individual's beliefs about the power of various situations and stimuli to cause pain. Of course this study needs replication on other types of pain patients as the factors may be particular to headache sufferers.

In his explanation of how chronic pain is sustained, Philips has given a central role to the individual's beliefs about the amount of pain that various activities will produce. Avoidance is seen as being influenced by three sets of cognitions:

1 the balance of expectations about the effects of engaging in events: expectations that there will be an increase of pain on exposure and a decrease with avoidance;
2 self-efficacy beliefs: the beliefs about the individual's capacity to cope with the pain produced;
3 memories of past experiences.

Not only is avoidance behaviour sustained by these three sets of cognitions, but avoidance will itself affect the strength of the cognitions so that in chronic-pain patients, a self-defeating cycle is set up.

Evidence in support of this explanation is limited but encouraging. Linton (1985) found that the activity levels (non-avoidance) of chronic pain sufferers were related to their expectation of pain as a consequence of the activity, and not to present pain levels. Voluntary exposure to a stressful stimulus was significantly related to the memory of the effect of the stimulus on headache pain. Three months after a painful dental experience, anxious dental patients estimated the dental pain as more severe than they had measured it at the time of treatment (Kent 1985). Finally, Dolce *et al.* (1986) found that non-avoidance of chronic-pain sufferers was correlated with their beliefs about their ability to cope with the pain (their self-efficacy beliefs) but not with the level of pain experienced. These studies do tentatively support Philips's proposals that holding an expectation that pain will increase when engaging in events, that the level of one's belief in one's ability to cope with the pain, and memories of past experiences are all important in the willingness to either confront or avoid situations and pain experiences.

Philips's model is in the early stages of development and many aspects remain to be supported. However, it has made an important contribution, as did the gate control theory earlier, in focusing attention on psychological factors; on the attitudes and beliefs of pain sufferers regarding their understanding of their situation, and their own capabilities (Turk and Rudy 1986).

In addition to the transactional relationships, the patients' attitudes and behaviours will elicit responses from others with whom they interact. In the cut-finger example given, both members of the household and the GP were suggested as important sources of reinforcement which would affect future behaviour. Such environmental factors have been proposed for some time, mainly in the operant models of pain experience (Fordyce 1976). This model focuses on the observable communication from the patient, both verbal and non-verbal, and the responses of others which may reinforce their behaviour. Patient behaviours such as complaints (verbal) or lying down (non-verbal) may be positively reinforced by others. Staying away from work may be negatively reinforced by allowing patients to avoid situations which are in some way difficult for them, or positively reinforced by receiving sickness benefit. This operant model may have validity as far as the behavioural component of pain is concerned, but the pain sensation is not directly changed by the reinforcement. Changes in this component will only be explained by the more complex models. However there is evidence that pain behaviours are affected by environmental factors.

A study by Block *et al.* (1980) looked at the amount of exercise performed by chronic-pain patients who were instructed to 'exercise to tolerence'. This means that they were to stop when the pain was as much as they could cope with. The patients had either supportive spouses (who gave positive and/or negative reinforcement for pain behaviours), or non-supportive (reinforcement not given for pain behaviours), each subject was told that his/her spouse would be watching half of a structured interview from behind a one-way screen. The other half of the interview would be watched by a health-care professional. Sequence effects were controlled by balanced presentation. At the mid-point of the two ten-minute blocks, patients were asked to rate their current pain levels. Patients with supportive spouses gave higher ratings when the spouse was observing, whereas those with non-supportive spouses gave higher ratings when the spouse was absent. Similar environmental effects have been shown for exercise levels by Cairns and Pasino (1977) and Fordyce *et al.* (1979).

MEASUREMENT OF PAIN

The attempts to understand 'pain' and construct theoretical models which take account of the empirically identified factors which influence this distressing phenomenon have produced a very complex concept. The real test of the utility of the models lies in the development of interventions and management programmes which can be shown to reduce the distress experienced. Outcome studies of such interventions are only valid if there is some reliable way of measuring 'pain' and it is not surprising that this has not yet been achieved.

Any measurement instrument should have the following properties:

1 it should be reliable: it should yield consistent results over different short testing periods, independently of the person administering and scoring the scale;

2 it should be valid: the measure should measure 'pain' or some clearly operationally defined aspect of pain;

3 it should be versatile: it should be possible to use in a variety of settings and types of pain problems;

4 it should be practical: administration should be accomplished in reasonable time with reasonable resources – a measure which takes three weeks to analyse is of little practical value;

5 it should be sensitive: changes in pain state should be reflected in score changes; and

6 it should have sound psychometric properties.

Many of the attempts to measure pain do not meet these requirements. Efforts to evaluate pain have been allied to the prevailing conceptualizations of the time. Early attempts were unidimensional and later ones multidimensional. Medical assessments were based on the sensory-physiological model where pain is viewed as a sensation directly linked to the extent of the tissue damage. Pain, using this model, is measured for two distinct reasons: as an estimate of the underlying damage – patients are usually asked to describe their pain and categorize it as either 'slight', 'moderate' or 'severe'. This categorization is repeated for the second reason, that of estimating the rate of recovery. The reliability and validity of this method is obviously questionable and the extension of the method into visual analogue scales (VAS) is very little better. A VAS consists of lines of a specific length, frequently 100 mm, with verbal descriptors as anchors, for example 'no pain at all' to 'the worst pain I can imagine'. The psychometric properties of this scale are unknown; it is unlikely to be an interval scale – the size of the difference of intensity of the pain between the least and half-way points is unlikely to be the same as that between the half-way and the most severe point. The reliability is equally difficult to examine as there is no objective criterion against which to validate it. Changes in intensity on the scale may be due to changes in pain perception or the unreliability of the scale itself.

Melzack (1975), applying his sensory/affective/evaluative model to the measurement of pain, devised a questionnaire which attempts to measure the three components (McGill Pain Questionnaire). The questionnaire consists of pain adjectives which are thought to assess the quality as well as the intensity of the pain. These 102 adjectives are categorized into twenty groups, and each group is intended to reflect a specific pain quality. The words within each group are thought to be rank ordered for intensity, the final descriptors in each group representing the most severe intensity. The groups are combined to form the three components of Melzack's model. Examples of the sensory descriptors are 'pounding', 'spreading' and 'crushing', for the affective, 'exhausting', 'awful' and 'nauseating', and for the evaluative, 'agonizing', 'excruciating' and 'miserable'. The patient ticks one descriptor in each group.

The questionnaire has frequently been used as the dependent variable in pain-treatment evaluations. Dubuisson and Melzack (1976) and Fox and Melzack (1976) claim the scale discriminates among patients suffering from different kinds of pain-producing conditions. There are a number of problems with the scale. Some of the descriptors are words not in common usage, for example lancinating, and the verbal ability of the patient may affect the reliability and validity of the measure. Replication studies have found different groupings of descriptors, different loadings on factors, different factors and inconsistency in the order of words for the intensity measure (Reading, Everritt and Sledmore 1982). Turk *et al.* (1985), and Brennan *et al.* (1987), who used clinical patients, found strong correlations among factors, so supporting the existence of one general factor accounting for a large proportion of the variance. This recent research is disappointing because if the three factors were reliable and valid, the score profiles would be useful in deciding the focus of appropriate intervention – for example, low scores on the sensory but high on the evaluative components would indicate that attempts to change the cognitions of the pain patient would be the most effective intervention.

An alternative way in which patients can communicate their levels of pain is by their behaviour. Behaviours are observable and measurements of them should be reliable. According to Fordyce (1976) there are a variety of pain behaviours which include verbal complaints of pain and suffering; non-verbal complaints such as moans and sighs; body posturing and gesturing such as limping, and holding the painful area; displays of functional limitation such as lying down; and the quantity and frequency of medication use. Such behaviours have been measured by three methods:

1 asking the patient to record the frequency of a variety of behaviours in the form of a diary;
2 from information gathered during a structured interview;
3 by direct observation either during an interview or in the natural environment.

All of these methods have limitations, for example the failure to define adequately the behaviour to be recorded (how much of a grimace is to be counted?), difficulties in obtaining contextual information (what was happening at the time the behaviour was emitted?), difficulties in recording multiple behaviours (is 'groan' to be recorded or 'grimace' if they both occur at the same time?). Any observation of behaviour, whether it is self-recorded or recorded by others, is subject to reactivity. Reactivity produces two types of interference to the reliability and validity of the measures. First, the act of self-recording can alter the frequency of the measured behaviour – for example, if the patient is to record the frequency of tablet taking, this may be reduced by the mere act of recording, and changes will thus not be tied to changes in pain levels. Second, the presence of an observer may have an effect, the ward nurse may have a different effect from the patient's spouse. The observed frequency of behaviour from such records may be a reflection of these intervening variables, rather than a direct estimation of the pain behaviour due to the levels of pain.

Assessments of pain behaviours have now become more sophisticated. A multiple-baseline approach has become more frequent, making observations on a range of behaviours, or a predetermined specific behaviour (for example, facial expression) across a range of activities and situations. A study by Cinciripini and Floreen (1983) exemplifies the problems in assessing the behavioural component of pain, and of using this type of measure as an indirect measure of 'pain'. Twenty-five chronic-pain patients suffering from back, leg, neck, shoulder or headache pain were videotaped during an interview. As part of the interview, four questions were asked: two focused on pain and two were of neutral focus. The patient was also asked to do two behavioural tasks, to rise from the chair, walk round the room and pick up an ashtray from the floor, and to pick up and carry an eight to ten pound chair several feet to the other side of the room. The behaviours measured were non-verbal expressions of pain: touching (the subject touched, rubbed, patted, etc. a body part associated with pain), grimacing (frowning, gritting of teeth, biting lip, facial expression of discomfort, displeasure or pain), gesturing (limping, staggering, gross movements used to express discomfort). Other measures taken included eye contact, and the fluency, loudness, affect and duration of speech. The results supported the relationship between environmental factors and the pain behaviours measured. There was a clear differentiation between the frequency of pain behaviours during the occasions when the focus was on their illness and when it was not, and overall, few significant differences were found between pain behaviours during illness topics and the behavioural tasks. This study clearly shows the influence of illness-related topics on pain behaviour and calls into question yet again the validity of using such measures as estimates of pain. Such estimates are made during conversations about the patients' pain and may bear very little relationship to non-pain focused times.

The assessment of the cognitive processes of pain is least developed. Cognitive processes in the study of pain are the thoughts, self-statements or evaluations when in pain, the beliefs, attributions about the pain, and the patients' appraisals about the impact of the pain on their lives. Measures that build on Beck's (1976) cognitive theory of depression have been devised. Lefebvre (1981), using vignettes relating to problems, personal limitations or interpretations of patients with low back pain, found that such individuals made cognitive errors similar to depressed non-pain patients. Kerns et al. (1985) used an initial pool of forty questions to develop the Pain Experience

Questionnaire (PEQ). The aim of the PEQ was to measure the degree of negative cognitive appraisal during episodes of severe pain. Significant pre–post treatment changes on the twenty-five final items were found for thirty pain patients and this suggests that the scale may provide an effective method to assess pain-related self-statements. Rosensteil and Keefe (1983) found that patients frequently reported using cognitive coping self-statements as a help in suppressing the level of pain and that the use of these was related to measures of behavioural and emotional adjustment to chronic pain. Measures of the cognitive processes involved in chronic pain are being used in three areas: those designed to measure the cognitive component of pain; those designed to assess the cognitive consequences of pain and those assessing appraisals of the impact of pain on their lives.

Knowledge about patients' appraisals of their plight and their coping resources, including personal, financial and social support, have become of central importance in both the assessment and management of pain. Assessment instruments specifically designed to evaluate these psychosocial dimensions are now being developed. Kerns et al. (1985) have developed the Multidimensional Pain Inventory (MPI), the first two parts of which assess the patients' appraisal and impact of pain on different domains of their lives and their perceptions of the responses of others to their distress and suffering. The third part assesses the frequency of specific behaviours performed because of their pain. The MPI appears to have satisfactory psychometric properties, and is a welcome move towards attempts to assess the multidimensionality of pain. A number of studies show that assessments of different dimensions do not co-vary (for example, Romano et al. 1988; Fordyce et al. 1984) and it is likely that a pain experience profile rather than a summary measure should be the final form. The danger is that the large quantities of data collected for an individual will be difficult to integrate. The present-day concept of pain, as exemplified by Philips's model, is a complex transactional one, and this necessitates a complex, multidimensional assessment, and an understanding of the ways in which the dimensions transact. Until this understanding has been achieved and assessment tools developed, the management of the pain patient will be eclectic rather than theory based.

TREATMENT OF PAIN

Over the past few years, there has been a rapid increase in the growth of pain clinics. Clinical psychologists as members of the multidisciplinary teams are implementing psychological interventions as part of the management packages aimed at reducing the distress of pain patients. The approach to management of these teams has moved since the early 1960s from a unidimensional focus, concentrating on attempts to change patients' overt behaviours, to comprehensive programmes. The central philosophy of these is perhaps best expressed by Keefe (1982: 903):

Recognition that chronic pain is a complex neurophysiological, behavioural and psychological phenomenon has led to the development of innovative treatment programs. These programs share one common assumption: if chronic pain is complex, then a combination of treatment techniques is needed to successfully treat patients.

This philosophy has of course led to a variety of techniques, based on various theories being used in various combinations, for a variety of pain patients. Some of the most widely used techniques are based on a learning-theory approach. In this approach it is important to distinguish between respondent and operant pain behaviours (Fordyce 1976). Respondent behaviours are those which are controlled by antecedent stimuli – in the case of pain, by the nocioceptive stimuli. Operant behaviours are those which are controlled by events which follow them – in the case of pain this refers to behaviours which are controlled by environmental reinforcement and/or by reductions in pain sensation. Of course operant pain behaviours can also be maintained by the punishment of well behaviours, and/or by the differential reinforcement of other behaviours. Well-meaning friends and relations may prevent the patient from engaging in activities, or 'confronting the pain'. 'You sit down, I know it hurts you to do that, I'll do it for you' may be thought to be a kind offer, but may be a disservice to the pain sufferer!

The goal of any pain-management programme is the reduction (or elimination) of 'pain' behaviours and the restoration of well behaviours, and from the learning-theory viewpoint this is attained by changing the reinforcement contingencies. Positive and negative reinforcement is made contingent on well behaviours and not on pain behaviours. Other behavioural techniques are usually included such as the setting of clearly defined goals, and record keeping is instigated so that achievement of goals is monitored. One of the main areas of concern for any behavioural programme is that of generalization to the natural environment and in order to achieve this it is often necessary to include 'important others', such as family and friends, as partners in the programme. This enables the environmental contingencies to be controlled, and the planning of out-of-clinic events. Training the patient in self-control and self-reinforcement techniques is also common as an aid to increased self-efficacy and perceived control over the pain.

The inclusion of cognitions is an important area of intervention. According to cognitive therapists (for example, Beck 1976; Ellis 1962) the way a person feels and thinks are important determinants of coping, so it follows that these areas are targets for change. Cognitive therapy for pain can be seen as including three aspects (Marlatt and Gordon 1980): patients are taught to re-conceptualize pain by emphasizing how it can be controlled by thoughts, feelings and beliefs: skills, such as relaxation, use of imagery and attention diversion are taught: and the practice and consolidation of these in general situations are required.

One of the problems of using a multicomponent treatment approach is knowing which component is responsible for changing which behaviour. The aim of Philips's (1987) study was to clarify the nature of the changes produced by the components of the programme. The measures were chosen to assess subjective experience of the pain; the pain behaviours – avoidance and complaint; self-efficacy; depression level; and the impact of the pain on various areas of the patient's life. The patients had a variety of pain problems and were either allocated to a waiting-list control group or to the treatment group. Treatment was for nine one-and-a-half-hour sessions, and included the following components: relaxation; graded increase in exercise and physical fitness, graded reduction in medication, increased control over episodes of pain, and training in a number of preventive strategies. There were a number of important findings: overall, the treatment was effective with only 8 per cent of the treatment group feeling it necessary to seek further treatment for their pain. Many of the patients had spent the last eight years searching for help with their pain. The large increase in self-efficacy ratings and expressed control over the pain indicates considerable attitude changes. Examination of the nine separate measures showed that the main effects of the programme were on avoidance behaviour, affective reaction to pain and depression, with little or no change on the other measures. These changes appear to be linked to the specific management techniques of the programme. The aim of these was the development of strategies of control of pain and engagement in activities in spite of pain. The reductions in avoidance behaviour persisted at two months follow-up, and at twelve months follow-up there were significant changes in the other indices of pain showing across the board improvements.

This study is encouraging in its methodology and aims. In a critical review of behavioural treatments for chronic pain, Linton (1982) points out that the general quality of outcome studies is poor. Most investigations lacked appropriate and adequate control groups, outcome measures and/or follow-ups. Overall the literature does suggest that (1) operant methods lead to increased activity levels, decreased pain reports and drug intake; (2) relaxation approaches result in reduced tension; (3) cognitive techniques are still speculative and (4) multimodal programmes produce a variety of improvements, but the diversity of treatments makes general statements impossible. These conclusions by Linton would seem to have face validity: operant and relaxation approaches result in changes in the focus of the approach, and the type of improvement shown in the multimodal programmes will depend on what is included in the programme. All will be dependent on the quality of the measures used and the match between the psychological characteristics of the pain patients and the rationale of the programme. Dolce (1987) points out that patients who fail to display increases in efficacy expectations for coping may constitute a group of patients who are at risk for relapse.

CONCLUSIONS

The present understanding of the problem of chronic pain is far removed from a simple linear model. Rather it is a complex, circular transaction of physical and psychological factors although the relationships and transactions involved are not yet clearly understood. Until this understanding is gained, the assessment and the efficacy of management programmes will be unclear. Which type of intervention is needed for which type of pain experience, and for which individual? These are questions that remain unanswered.

Chapter 8

Biofeedback

Keith Phillips

INTRODUCTION

Biofeedback refers to training procedures used to modify physiological responses or patterns of physiological responses. Biofeedback training has become widely used as a clinical intervention that aims to achieve self-regulation of maladaptive responses and disordered states. It has been defined as 'a set of procedures that enable the individual to control some specified physiological process by providing an external cue or monitor to indicate the activity of that process' (Phillips 1979).

Though now concerned almost exclusively with human clinical studies, biofeedback developed from experimental learning studies that involved training animals to modify physiological responses for negative or positive reinforcement. Those studies implied that, contrary to previous belief, *all* responses, including those governed by the autonomic nervous system, could be brought under voluntary control (Miller 1969). They raised important theoretical issues, including questions about the fundamental nature of the learning process which have still to be resolved. Despite uncertainties about the mechanisms involved in learning to modify responses the use of biofeedback training for the treatment of clinical disorders is firmly established.

Biofeedback represents the prototypical approach of a recently defined discipline called 'behavioural medicine' which was first introduced in 1973 by the appearance of a book by Lee Birk entitled *Biofeedback: Behavioral Medicine*. Behavioural medicine has become established since as 'that broad interdisciplinary field of scientific enquiry, education, and practice which concerns itself with health and illness or related dysfunction' (Matarazzo 1980). Within behavioural medicine, biofeedback is one clinical technique among many others which have been introduced as interventions for health disorders (see Steptoe 1989).

Despite often inflated claims for its efficacy, biofeedback training is in reality one method among many for allowing individuals to achieve changes in physiological responding. In judging its effectiveness as a treatment it can be compared with other interventions, including for example cognitive therapies, relaxation, or drug treatments. This chapter outlines the principles of biofeedback training and considers some of its more popular applications, before concluding with an assessment of its clinical effectiveness and future prospects.

PRINCIPLES OF BIOFEEDBACK TRAINING

Studies of biofeedback began in the late 1960s when it was shown that certain physiological responses which are regulated by the autonomic nervous system and which had been assumed to be outside voluntary control could be modified and brought under instructed control in human subjects, i.e. learned as a result of training that provided information or knowledge of results about the response. Such training became known as the voluntary control paradigm (Figure 8.1).

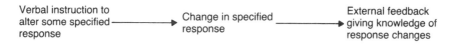

Figure 8.1 Biofeedback – the voluntary control paradigm.

There are four essential elements of biofeedback training.

1 *Instruction.* An appropriate verbal instruction is given that identifies a particular response to be altered, for example 'try to lower your blood pressure' or 'slow the rate at which your heart is beating'. This instruction indicates to the subject both the physiological system to be regulated and a directional requirement (raise/lower, speed/slow, increase/decrease) for the response that is to be modified.

2 *Patient/subject motivation.* For biofeedback to be successful it is necessary that the subject should be motivated to try to achieve the changes in response indicated by the instructions given. Assuming that the patient, or subject in an experimental study, is motivated, then attempts will be made to alter the response.

3 *Some means of recording and monitoring the physiological response specified by the instructions to the subject.* This in fact is fairly straightforward since many of the changes in bodily responses are electrical in nature, involving changes in electrical potential or resistance, for example, and these can be recorded via electrodes attached to the surface of the skin. Other responses may involve physical and non-electrical changes. Blood pressure, for

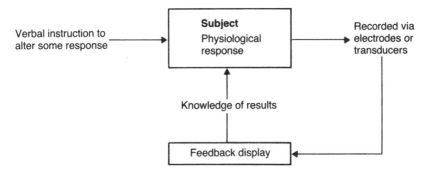

Figure 8.2 The elements of biofeedback training.

example, involves variations in pressure within a closed circulatory system. In instances of this type, however, other devices called transducers are used to convert the physical changes into electrical signals. The techniques for measuring a wide range of physiological responses including responses measured from the skin (electrodermal activity), cardiovascular system such as blood pressure and heart rate, patterns of brain-wave activity, gastro-intestinal responses and patterns of muscular activity (electromyographic responses) are well established (Martin and Venables 1980). There are available commercially many devices for measuring these responses and using the responses to generate external feedback signals.

4 *Feedback signal.* The electrical signals recorded via electrodes or transducers are used to generate an external signal such as a sound that varies in loudness or pitch, or clicks, whose rate fluctuates, or a display of several lights where the number lit alters. Patients or subjects are told to attend to the external signal and informed that the changes indicated by the signal will provide them with the knowledge of whether or not they are successfully controlling the response specifed by the initial instructions.

The elements of biofeedback training are summarized in Figure 8.2.

Early experimental demonstrations of biofeedback used a form of conditioning which gave subjects rewards for successfully controlling the response instructed by the experimenter. Shearn (1962), for example, was able to train volunteer subjects to increase their heart rates by several beats per minute in order to avoid delivery of a mild electric shock. The threat of electric shock and successful avoidance of its delivery by appropriate responding may be considered as both motivating and rewarding and the same technique can be used successfully to train equivalent response changes in animals other than humans using an operant-conditioning procedure which is illustrated in Figure 8.3 (Brener *et al.* 1977).

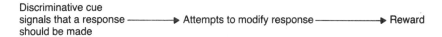

Figure 8.3 Operant conditioning of a physiological response.

Extrinsic rewards including shock avoidance or payment with money may be used successfully for biofeedback training with humans but they are not necessary. Using the voluntary-control paradigm the knowledge of success or failure provided by the feedback display is itself rewarding and is sufficient for successful training. Clinical applications of biofeedback training are based exclusively upon the voluntary-control paradigm.

The desired goal of biofeedback training is voluntary control by which an individual is able to self-regulate some physiological response or state without further needing to rely upon the external feedback signal. In some way the individual has to learn to recognize and achieve the desired goal through his/her own internalized control processes. The mechanisms by which such control becomes realized are still poorly understood, and though several theoretical models have been suggested there is no agreement about how control becomes established. Whatever the mechanisms are, the finding that biofeedback training can be used to train self-regulation is a well-replicated and consistent finding for many different physiological responses. As a consequence, biofeedback has been adopted as a clinical intervention for disorders that involve dis-regulation of physiological activity.

CLINICAL APPLICATIONS OF BIOFEEDBACK

Biofeedback has been used in the treatment of a huge number of clinical disorders. In some instances the rationale is clear but in others, reasons for its use appear to be at best speculative. Further problems exist when examining the literature on the clinical efficacy of biofeedback, including the fact that the training techniques themselves differ considerably between studies on a number of dimensions – for example, number and duration of training sessions, type and amount of feedback given, support by additional exercises and so forth. Moreover, the methods used to assess the effect of training also differ considerably from uncontrolled single case-study designs, single-treatment group studies with before and after designs, to larger-scale controlled group outcome studies (Blanchard and Young 1974). It is the latter that are desirable for making a true assessment of biofeedback's clinical effectiveness. Unfortunately these designs have been rarely used and much of the clinical literature reports studies that have employed weak methodological designs, which limits the conclusions that can be drawn.

Two quite distinct methods of applying biofeedback as a clinical intervention can be identified. The first of these may be called 'direct symptom control'. In this case some clearly identifiable target symptom or response is identified as requiring modification and the biofeedback training is based exclusively upon that single feature. A good example of the direct-symptom-control approach is the treatment of elevated blood pressure in the patient with hypertension by training based upon a feedback signal generated from monitoring of the patient's blood pressure. In this case the response selected for training may be regarded as the pre-eminent symptom of the disorder. Other examples of the direct control approach include feedback of patterns of brain-wave activity (the electroencephalogram, EEG) for treatment of epileptic seizures, feedback of muscle activity (electromyographic activity, EMG) for various neuromuscular disorders including muscle spasticity or paralysis, and feedback of heart rate for cardiac arrhythmias.

The second type of application involves the use of biofeedback for training relaxation to achieve a generalized change in physiological state rather than direct control of a single response. During the last fifteen years it is this approach that has become most widespread and it has been used for the treatment of a bewilderingly diverse range of disorders. For these applications the choice of which physiological response is adopted to provide the external feedback signal is essentially arbitrary. All that is needed is a source of feedback that indicates an individual's generalized state of arousal or relaxation. Any response that varies according to these states would be appropriate. In practice particular responses have been adopted at particular times, including, in early studies, one type of brain-wave activity known as the alpha rhythm, and more recently electrodermal activity and EMG activity.

The existence of these two very different types of application presents something of a puzzle, or what Yates (1980) has referred to as the 'paradox of biofeedback training' as it raises a question about what type of influence the training is having upon the physiological systems involved and the accompanying learning processes. Is biofeedback a means of training specific control where the specificity of the trained response improves with practice? Or is it simply a means of signalling to individuals their general state of activation? If it is the former then applications for relaxation seem inappropriate, but if the latter then applications for specific control of individual responses would be excluded. Insufficient consideration of the nature of the mechanisms involved in biofeedback has undoubtedly hindered the development of successful clinical applications for biofeedback training. This point will be considered further in the section upon judging the clinical effectiveness of biofeedback.

RELAXATION TRAINING

Relaxation training has become one of the central interventions of behavioural medicine (Blumenthal 1985). Its use is predicated upon the assumption that the disorder being treated is stress related and that it is accompanied by a generalized state of sympathetic nervous-system activation which maintains the disorder. That state is argued to represent a dis-regulation of physiological systems (Schwartz 1977) with consequences that threaten the individual's well-being. In these circumstances relaxation training is used to restore normal regulation by eliminating the maladaptive state and replacing it by an antagonistic condition described as 'cultivated low arousal' (Stoyva and Budzynski 1974) in which parasympathetic nervous responses are dominant.

Various relaxation methods, including progressive muscle relaxation, yoga, meditation and autogenic training, as well as biofeedback, have been used to produce changes in autonomic and skeletal responses in the direction of parasympathetic control and reduced muscle tension. It is often assumed that the mechanisms by which they have their effect are the same. Yet this may not be so; it is not clear that meditation, for example, produces reductions of autonomic and endocrine responses, although muscular relaxation training does (see Steptoe 1989). Biofeedback may be used in isolation to train relaxation responses or in combination with other relaxation techniques as part of a treatment package (Phillips 1979).

Biofeedback may be used to train relaxation by self-regulation of physiological responses. The rationale for this approach is based upon the assumption that learned changes in one response system will be accompanied by parallel changes of other response systems. Thus, lowering of heart rate, for example, will be accompanied by similar reductions in other autonomic responses. If this assumption of generalization is appropriate then in principle it does not matter which response system is employed to generate the feedback signal given to the patient. Early clinical studies frequently used feedback derived from a particular frequency of brain-wave activity measured as the electroencephalogram (EEG) called EEG alpha activity. EEG alpha activity is frequently seen during meditational states (Elson et al. 1977) and it was assumed that alpha enhancement would promote the relaxation state. However, while biofeedback can be used effectively to modify EEG activity there is no evidence that alpha activity is associated with any specific therapeutic benefits, nor that, in itself, it produces generalized relaxation. In recent years most studies of biofeedback training for relaxation have adopted EMG feedback as the preferred technique.

Many stress-related disorders are accompanied by muscle tension in specific muscles or throughout the skeletal musculature and at first sight it would seem appropriate to provide EMG-biofeedback training to reduce that activity. However, there exists again an implicit assumption that generalization will occur, and that assumption may be unwarranted. Most EMG-biofeedback treatments generate the feedback signal from electrodes recording the activity of a single muscle, the frontalis muscle of the forehead. Patients are encouraged to learn to decrease tension within this muscle in the belief that the effect will generalize to other muscle groups in the body. Empirical studies have found that this is not so. Alexander (1975) found no evidence of generalization from reduction in frontalis EMG to levels either in forearm or leg. Similarly, Shedivy and Kleinman (1977) found no evidence of generalization from frontalis EMG to muscles of the neck. A further problem is that even where successful reductions of EMG activity are trained these are not inevitably accompanied by subjective sensations of relaxation (Paul 1969; Shedivy and Kleinman 1977). Clearly, unless the patient 'feels' relaxed, then whatever changes in EMG activity have actually occurred, the treatment has little hope of success. Finally, there is no guarantee that relaxation training based on EMG biofeedback will generalize from the clinic to real-life situations where real or potential stressors are encountered. Even after prolonged training such transfer may not occur (Raskin *et al.* 1973). All in all, there is no convincing evidence to support the notion that generalization of effects will occur following EMG training based upon recordings from one specific muscle site such as the frontalis muscle (Carlson *et al.* 1983).

Despite these serious reservations there is evidence that EMG-biofeedback training can be beneficial for some disorders, and particularly in the treatment of various forms of pain, including tension headaches (Budzynski *et al.* 1973) and chronic back pain (Bush *et al.* 1985). The success of biofeedback in these instances, however, may be related not to changes in physiological state *per se*, but rather to changes in the cognitive activity of patients. For example, biofeedback training may alter patients' perceptions of pain and their beliefs in their own efficacy in controlling the pain (Andrasik and Holroyd 1983; Flor *et al.* 1983). These cognitions may be quite independent of measured changes in the response being recorded and monitored during training.

Other forms of biofeedback including thermal and electrodermal biofeedback are also employed for relaxation training. Again the rationale underlying their use is suspect and their effectiveness is doubtful. In general the use of biofeedback to train generalized relaxation does not offer any specific advantage over the more traditional techniques such as cognitive therapy or muscle relaxation. What it does do is to focus attention upon the patients 'doing something for themselves'. This non-specific characteristic of biofeedback training is highly self-motivating and may be helpful for achieving the cognitive changes that are associated with its effectiveness in treating headaches and other types of pain.

BIOFEEDBACK FOR DIRECT SYMPTOM CONTROL

There are several examples of disorders with a clearly identifiable symptom that may be treated using biofeedback training to modify the physiological process associated with that single symptom. Several applications of bio-feedback have been attempted for disorders of this type, including disorders of the gastrointestinal system (peptic ulcer), skeletal muscular system (muscle rehabilitation), cardiovascular system (cardiac arrhythmias) and central nervous system (epileptic seizures). It is impossible to review each of these here but amongst these some of the greatest successes are associated with neuromuscular disorders and cardiovascular disorders, including cardiac arrhythmias and Raynaud's disease. These are considered in detail below.

Muscular disorders

Several different types of muscular disorder have been successfully treated using biofeedback. In some cases specific feedback devices have been developed to treat motor abnormalities. For example, head position trainers sensitive to changes in the position of the head have been used to treat patients with cerebral palsy (Wooldridge and Russell 1976) and weight (load) distribution monitors may be fitted to a patient's shoe to correct an abnormal gait (Flodmark 1986). Essentially these applications are examples of rehabilitation using feedback devices.

Rather different applications involve the use of EMG biofeedback to train patients to modify and gain control over specific muscles that are weakened or even apparently paralysed, for example hemiplegia, or muscles that may be over-active, for example spasticity. Many studies have employed EMG biofeedback for the rehabilitation of patients following cerebrovascular accident (stroke), which frequently results in paralysis or spasticity of the muscles. In these instances EMG biofeedback can be used to train patients with muscle weakness to increase muscle activity, or to reduce muscle activity in the case of spasticity. In either instance control over the affected muscles can be relearned. It is important to appreciate that in this instance the patients are not learning anything new; they are re-establishing control that had existed prior to occurrence of the stroke. Biofeedback training allows the central nervous system to re-establish or re-programme control over the musculature. Patient characteristics such as the length of time that has elapsed since the stroke occurred, and the site of cerebrovascular lesion, are important factors influencing the success of biofeedback training, but even allowing for these it has consistently been found that combined treatment of biofeedback, together with physical therapy, is superior to treatment by physical therapy alone (Wolf 1983). Similar successes have been claimed for EMG-biofeedback-assisted treatment of a wide range of other muscular disorders, including torticollis, tics, Parkinson's disease and myofacial pain.

However, as Jahanshahi and Marsden (1989) have pointed out, its effectiveness is often difficult to assess since interpretation of the clinical studies is bedevilled by their methodological weaknesses. Considerable caution is necessary before claiming that EMG-biofeedback is an effective treatment for all muscular disorders (Health and Public Policy Committee 1985), though it undoubtedly makes a valuable contribution within combined therapies.

Cardiac arrhythmias

A small number of studies have reported that heart-rate biofeedback training can be used successfully to treat patients with abnormal rhythms of heart beat, cardiac arrhythmias, including premature ventricular contractions (PVCs) and sinus tachycardia. In a study where eight patients with PVCs received extensive training both to increase and decrease heart rate and to maintain heart rate within a specified range, Weiss and Engel (1971) reported that five of the eight showed significant reductions in PVCs. These beneficial reductions successfully transferred to the patients' home environments and for four of the five patients reductions were maintained at a twenty-one month follow-up. Subsequent case reports confirmed the effectiveness of heart-rate biofeedback training for reducing PVCs (Engel and Bleecker 1974; Pickering and Gorham 1975; Pickering and Miller 1977). Heart-rate biofeedback training is also reported to be effective for patients who show another form of arrhythmia, sinus tachycardia, which is characterized by an abnormally rapid heart rate. Again, case reports based on single-subject designs have indicated that biofeedback training to reduce heart rate can be used to eliminate the patients' tachycardias (Scott et al. 1973; Blanchard and Abel 1976).

Raynaud's disease

Raynaud's disease is a distressing disorder characterized by episodes of vasoconstriction of the peripheral blood vessels in the fingers or, less commonly, the toes. These episodes can be triggered by either exposure to cold or to stressful experiences. The aetiology of the disorder remains poorly understood but there is good evidence that emotional stress precipitates the onset of digital vasoconstriction. Freedman and Ianni (1985), for example, compared the finger temperature responses of thirty-two patients with Raynaud's disease with twenty-two control subjects in response to three different tape-recordings containing descriptions of a social stress, loss of gloves in a snowstorm and a beach scene. The two groups differed significantly only in their response to the snowstorm tape, with the patients, but not the control subjects, showing vasoconstriction. Raynaud's disease has proved a difficult disorder to treat and no generally successful medical solution has been found. Surgical interventions and drug treatments provide only partial relief for patients. Behavioural treatments using temperature biofeedback offer some more promising solutions.

Studies by Keefe (1975) and Taub (1977) established that normal subjects are able to use temperature feedback training to learn to increase finger temperature to a substantial extent (more than one degree centigrade). On the basis of this finding others have used temperature biofeedback to train patients with Raynaud's disease to increase finger temperature. Freedman *et al.* (1981) found that such training resulted in significant reductions in frequency of symptoms reported by these patients. More significantly, the effect persisted and symptom reductions were still present three years after the original temperature biofeedback training (Freedman *et al.* 1985). Since there are no adverse side-effects associated with biofeedback training, this therapy offers a more acceptable treatment to Raynaud's-disease patients than either surgery or drug treatments.

BIOFEEDBACK AND REACTIONS TO STRESSORS

Though biofeedback training has been used as a clinical treatment primarily to teach individuals to control and regulate the symptoms evident on an enduring basis within some existing disorder it may also be used in anticipation of reactions to stressors. All individuals facing potentially painful experiences and other aversive events show psychophysiological reactions that include autonomic activation. However, some individuals show greater reactivity than others and exaggerated autonomic reactivity has been implicated in the aetiology of certain disorders, including hypertension (see Chapter 12). It is possible that biofeedback training could be used to reduce an individual's reactivity to aversive events or situations, in which case it might be a valuable intervention that offers protection against future disease.

Feedback training is often offered to individuals in a relatively stress-free environment while resting in a quiet clinic, for example. This is entirely appropriate if the patient's condition involves tonic maladjustment of some response that endures and represents a sustained dis-regulation. Some individuals, however, may only experience their maladaptive response as a reaction to, or anticipation of, particular events or situations. For example, fear of pain or anxiety about public speaking might provoke an exaggerated reaction that is so severe that the individual finds it disabling. In these circumstances biofeedback training could be given to allow patients to reduce their symptoms on those specific occasions that they encounter their particular environmental stressor. Used in this way biofeedback is analogous to the use of a beta-blocker such as propranolol to control cardiac reactivity during anxiety, but of course being a behavioural treatment it does not suffer from the adverse side-effects that so often accompany use of these medications.

A number of studies have been reported which indicate that biofeedback may be useful in such circumstances. Studies by Sirota *et al.* (1974, 1976) showed that volunteer subjects given heart-rate feedback were able to acquire control over heart-rate reactions in anticipation of an electric shock applied to the forearm. Significantly, self-ratings of the painfulness of the experienced shocks corresponded to changes in heart rate, i.e. where reductions of heart rate were trained during anticipation of the shock, these were accompanied by lower ratings of the subsequently experienced pain. A further study by Victor, Mainardi and Shapiro (1978) examined the effects of biofeedback training upon subjects' ability to regulate heart rate while experiencing a painful aversive experience in the form of the cold-pressor test. This involves immersing the hand up to the wrist in a freezing mixture of ice and water for thirty seconds. This experience reliably provokes cardiac acceleration and subjective reports of pain. Subjects were given appropriate feedback and asked to control their heart rate during immersion of the hand in the freezing mixture. It was found that even during the painful task, subjects could regulate both increases or decreases of heart rate that were greater than changes shown by subjects not given feedback. In addition, self-reports of pain corresponded to heart-rate changes; those subjects increasing their heart rate reported most pain and those regulating decreases in heart rate reported the least levels of pain.

Biofeedback training is not unique in allowing individuals to reduce reactivity to experimental challenges. Other techniques, including relaxation training and muscle relaxation, are also effective in decreasing reactions to environmental stressors (Connor 1974; Puente and Beiman 1980). However the effects achieved through biofeedback training do not seem to be produced by some non-specific relaxation-type effect since the reductions in reactivity observed are specific to the feedback used. Gatchel *et al.* (1978), for example, trained subjects to use EMG feedback recorded from the frontalis muscle to reduce EMG activity in anticipation of mild electric shock. However, though EMG activity was successfully reduced there were neither similar reductions for heart rate nor electrodermal responses. This is of course consistent with the view that biofeedback training is most effective for training direct symptom control and that it may be less effective for producing generalized relaxation effects.

JUDGING THE CLINICAL EFFECTIVENESS OF BIOFEEDBACK

When first introduced, biofeedback training was hailed as a panacea whose 'uses cover nearly the entire range of human emotional and physical disorders' (Brown 1977). The techniques of biofeedback training were enthusiastically adopted by clinicians with little regard to its underlying mechanisms and applied to what in retrospect seems a bewildering variety of behavioural, psychological and psychiatric disorders as varied as alcoholism, sexual dysfunction or obsessive-compulsive behaviours (for comprehensive coverage of these and other applications see Yates 1980). The rationales for many of these applications were often unclear and the clinical designs used were poorly controlled. Not surprisingly, reports began to emerge of the 'failures' of biofeedback and the question posed was whether biofeedback represents 'a promise unfulfilled' (Blanchard and Young 1973). Almost two decades have passed and that same question is still being asked. This is no longer reasonable since there exists a huge literature on clinical applications of biofeedback and some sort of judgement about its clinical usefulness should be possible. This section will examine some of the issues that have a bearing upon this question, and finally propose an answer to it.

Placebo effect

The point of biofeedback training is that the provision of feedback, an external signal that has meaning and gives knowledge of results, should influence the patient's ability to self-regulate some specified response or state. In addition to this aspect, however, biofeedback training also inevitably involves non-specific effects upon the patient: simply, the fact that the patient is involved in a clinical programme may in itself lead both the patient and the clinician to expect beneficial changes to follow. Those expectancies are not specific to biofeedback and might accompany other quite different types of treatment. Yet they alone could account for any change in the patient's condition quite independently of the specific effects offered by the feedback. It has been suggested that non-specific or 'placebo' effects could account entirely for any beneficial clinical gains that result from biofeedback training (Stroebel and Glueck 1973). The power of placebos in clinical settings is well documented and biofeedback training fulfils many of the criteria that characterize placebos. It is innovative, impressive in its technology, and involves investment of time and effort on the part of both patient and clinician (Miller and Dworkin 1977).

In terms of the outcome for the patient it may not matter whether any clinical improvement results from specific or non-specific effects, but from the point of view of understanding the mechanisms that underlie clinical success it is important to distinguish between them. This can be done by adopting appropriate clinical designs when evaluating biofeedback training. This issue has been well aired by Blanchard and Young (1974). They identify five types of design ranging from, at the weakest level, anecdotal case reports to the most powerful design of controlled group outcome studies. These compare the effects of biofeedback training given to a homogeneous group of patients with the effects of a control condition that gives equal attention but no feedback training to an equivalent group of patients suffering the same disorder. The non-specific effects should be the same for both groups but the experimental group additionally has the benefit of the specific influences of feedback training. Unfortunately, few biofeedback studies have used this powerful design and studies with less adequate designs are often difficult to assess since the specific and non-specific effects of training are confounded.

Clinical relevance and applicability

In addition to design methodology Blanchard (1979) has identified other dimensions which he argues can be used to evaluate clinical applications of biofeedback. Taken together they can be viewed as indicators of the extent to which the outcome of biofeedback training has clinical relevance and applicability for the patient's life. He makes the simple but often overlooked point that the changes in response or symptom can be statistically significant and yet still lack clinical significance. For example, if biofeedback training reliably reduced blood pressure by 1 or 2 mm of mercury then the effect might be statistically significant, though it could hardly be claimed to have altered the patient's condition to any significant degree. Another way of measuring success is in terms of the number of patients treated who show clinical improvement. It may be that biofeedback is effective for some individuals but not others. When assessing its effect over all it is important to know what proportion of patients with a particular disorder might be expected to benefit from this form of treatment.

A further problem concerns the transfer of training. The outcome of biofeedback training is often measured immediately following treatment in a clinic. Beneficial effects of biofeedback training may reliably be found in the clinic but the outcome cannot be considered successful unless the effect transfers to the patient's home and work environments and endures over a substantial period of time. Evaluation of these factors requires testing in real-life settings with follow-up studies to assess the long-term effects of training. Again these procedures have frequently been neglected in clinical biofeedback studies.

Comparison with best alternatives

When judging its clinical effectiveness it should not be forgotten that biofeedback training is often applied to disorders that have proved highly intractable to other forms of treatment. It is unfair to measure the absolute rate of success; a much more appropriate measure is its efficacy relative to alternative treatments. In making this comparison there are several factors apart from the treatment outcome that are relevant, though that is obviously the most important. Other factors that may also be considered include its efficiency, convenience, cost-effectiveness and generality, and the durability of the treatment. Each of these can be assessed though all too frequently they have not been. In a review of the relative benefits of biofeedback compared with relaxation training, Silver and Blanchard (1978) concluded that for those disorders where comparisons have been made, such as hypertension, migraine, tension headaches and pain, 'there is no consistent advantage for one form of treatment over the other'. For certain other disorders the comparison has not been made, and for some of these, including Raynaud's disease, sinus tachycardia and peptic ulcers, biofeedback does seem to offer some promise. Of course to evaluate biofeedback truly one would need to compare it with alternatives other than relaxation, including cognitive therapies, drug treatments and other behavioural interventions. It is disappointing that so few comparative studies exist.

Biofeedback in combined therapies

Much consideration has been given to whether or not biofeedback is effective as a treatment for various disorders. It has been suggested that some applications have been successful, though not all. Evaluations of its clinical efficacy have usually considered biofeedback as an *alternative* to other treatments. A more meaningful approach, however, might be to examine the extent to which biofeedback can be used as an adjunct to other treatments within combined treatment programmes. The nature of biofeedback training suits it very well for combining with other types of treatment such as muscle relaxation or autogenic training (Phillips 1979) or drug treatments to reduce the amount of medication required, for example, in the treatment of anxiety (Lavallee *et al.* 1977), or in more comprehensive treatment packages that contain several different elements such as that developed by Patel and her colleagues (Patel and North 1975) for treating hypertension (see Chapter 12). As a part of combined treatment approaches, biofeedback is assured an enduring role in the treatment of disorders that have a psychophysiological component.

Biofeedback does not represent 'a promise unfulfilled' since the original expectations of what it might achieve were unrealistic. Biofeedback is a valuable weapon within the armoury of behavioural medicine. What is required is consideration of what it can offer before it is applied to particular clinical disorders. It has a contribution to make if applied to well-defined psychophysiological maladaptations. As Yates (1980:499) has pointed out 'the failure of biofeedback training . . . stems from its use as a blunderbuss rather than a rapier or precision instrument'. Where biofeedback has been used to modify clearly defined physiological symptoms, as in Raynaud's disease or some neuromuscular disorders, for example, it has shown considerable success. For other disorders such as hypertension it may be unsuccessful when used in isolation but yet still contribute to combined treatment packages. Biofeedback training is a treatment to be used with circumspection and with considerably greater regard for the nature of the disorder to which it is applied than has previously been the case.

CONCLUSIONS

Biofeedback training offers techniques that allow patients to learn to self-regulate physiological responses or states. It has been widely applied as an intervention for disorders of widely differing origins and with mixed clinical success. Most of its successful applications have arisen from its use as a 'precision instrument' for direct symptom control in disorders that have a clearly identifiable psychophysiological component. It has been less successful in comparison to alternative treatments as a technique for training generalized relaxation. In the past its indiscriminate use has cast doubts upon its clinical efficacy, but its effectiveness for the treatment of a narrowly defined group of disorders including some types of pain, cardiac disorders such as types of arrhythmia and Raynaud's disease, and several neuromuscular disorders, is well documented. Future applications may extend its use within combined treatment packages and its use for the prevention of ill-health by reduction of physiological reactivity to stressors.

Chapter 9

Rehabilitation and coping with chronic disorders

Marian Pitts

INTRODUCTION

Most of the work in the preceding two chapters has dealt with the progression of an acute illness. Much research has focused on the processes of symptom perception, help seeking, diagnosis, treatment and outcome. In contrast, surprisingly little research has examined longer-term recovery or rehabilitation. This chapter will consider certain themes in the processes of recovery and rehabilitation. There is also a group of people who cannot anticipate recovery as they suffer from chronic disorders and we will examine those areas of psychological research concerned with the progression of chronic illness, disability or disease. A comprehensive review of the research into recovery, rehabilitation and coping with chronic disorders will not be attempted: instead, we will search for common threads or themes which might unite these diverse areas. In particular, the concepts of coping and control will be examined.

First, however, we need to examine the issues of recovery and rehabilitation and what they entail. We will consider the areas of recovery from neurological impairment, rehabilitation following myocardial infarction, and the trauma of spinal cord injury; in each area an important theme of the research literature will be discussed. Following this, research from the areas of two chronic disorders, multiple sclerosis and Parkinson's disease, will be evaluated. Finally, a model of coping with illness will be examined. Coping in a broad health context has been discussed in Chapter 3 by Philip Evans. In this chapter we will be concerned specifically with a psychological model which centres on the issue of control as the most important dimension in coping with the stressors of long-term illness.

RECOVERY FROM NEUROLOGICAL IMPAIRMENT

An important aspect of the concept of recovery is that it is a time-related process. Time must pass in order for it to become apparent that recovery has occurred. But the passing of time does not, of itself, cause recovery; something must have occurred during that time. Miller (1984) outlines several types of recovery theory: the first type is referred to as artefact theories. These theories assume that there are two components of the impairment of function which is observed immediately after brain injury. In addition to the primary lesion which results in tissue damage, there is also secondary impairment which may impair or temporarily disrupt some functions. Recovery of some function is then 'artefactual' since nothing has actually been 'lost'; it has simply been suppressed. Oedema, which frequently occurs in tissue surrounding the area damaged by lesion, is an example. As the swelling surrounding a lesion spontaneously reduces over time, so some function will return; this function has not been lost directly as a result of brain injury but simply suppressed by the oedema. Hence, function could be regarded as being 'resumed' rather than 'recovered'. Sometimes, the apparently spontaneous recovery of speech following a stroke (CVA) is the result of the reduction of oedema.

The second type of theory described by Miller involves anatomical reorganization. These theories would imply that other parts of the brain which are undamaged can take over functions normally associated with damaged parts. Some recent attempts at remediation of aphasic difficulties following CVA have focused on training the right hemisphere to 'take over' some of the speech functions usually associated with left-hemisphere functioning.

Finally, Miller refers to theories incorporating the notions of functional adaptation. The basic idea underlying these theories is that a person may be able to relearn a skill which has been lost following brain damage by using novel means, for example by adopting new cognitive or motor strategies. An example is given from Landis *et al.* (1982). They describe a patient who was unable to read words following brain damage from mercury intoxication. Instead he used his fingers to trace the patterns of words to allow their identification by this alternative means.

Miller argues that the search for a single correct explanation of recovery is inappropriate. The types of theory described here are not mutually exclusive and it is most important to identify which explanations are appropriate for which disorders and in which situations. It is particularly important to consider the characteristics of the patient concerned in each case – for example, a young person might benefit more from a functional-adaptation approach than older patients with similar disorders.

The issue of time as an integral part of recovery has been considered in this section. As has been shown, time is not *responsible* for recovery in most instances; other dimensions such as relearning or retraining are also usually involved.

REHABILITATION POST MYOCARDIAL INFARCTION

The concept of rehabilitation is also a complex one; there are many facets to people taking up their lives again after a trauma, accident, injury or disease.

Much of the interest in this area has focused on physical rehabilitation, or on rehabilitation in a social or work setting. Less research has considered the psychological adjustment or readjustment necessary after a major life change. Lip-service is frequently paid to the allied notions of bereavement and loss and to the adjustments necessary to changed situations; but the specifics of what exactly a person experiences and whether there is a characteristic pattern or set of experiences which one can expect to encounter or experience have largely gone unstudied.

Let us take rehabilitation post myocardial infarction (MI) as an example of the area. Cay *et al.* (1976) outlined two main issues in the rehabilitation of patients following a heart attack: the physiological and pathological limitations imposed by the disease itself and the psychological problems of accommodating to a serious illness and holding it in perspective during subsequent life. According to the Mair Report (1972) the aim is 'restoration of patients to their fullest physical, mental and social capability'.

The most extensively studied area of adjustment following MI is return to work (RTW). This is relatively easy to measure and is assumed to be linked with emotional and economic well-being. This assumption is presumably also related to the predominance of middle-aged males as sufferers of MI. Estimates of the number failing to return to work within one year of MI vary greatly, but most fall in the 20–35 per cent range. The most important determinant of RTW is usually found to be social class: white-collar workers consistently have higher return rates. The reasons for this are likely to be complex: their jobs are probably less physically demanding than working-class trades, and they are likely to have skills which are in greater demand from their companies. They may also know the boss rather better than their 'blue-collar' counterparts. In other words, there is a social framework which can accommodate their RTW more easily. Psychological factors are also held to play a part in the likelihood of a successful RTW. Maeland and Havik (1987) found a strong linear relationship between the levels of anxiety and depression reported by patients while in hospital and RTW. They also found that patients' appraisals of future functioning while in hospital were also linearly related to RTW. Patients who anticipated few problems in future work had a three times higher RTW rate than those who anticipated a large reduction in their work loads. Trelawny-Ross and Russell (1987) extended the scope of interest from work alone to include exercise, leisure and physical activity. Six months post MI they found that 55 per cent had returned to work, 77 per cent had satisfactory outcomes in terms of leisure activity, but 23 per cent were taking very little exercise and 45 per cent had not returned to previous levels of sexual activity. They argue convincingly that there is a sub-group of recoverers from MI who would benefit from more psychological and social support during rehabilitation. Garrity (1981) reports that the best predictor of behavioural adjustment (RTW, leisure activities and morale) six months after MI was patients' perception of their health status, which is in itself uncorrelated with their clinical status. Cay *et al.* (1976) target the time of return to work as a particularly important stage in rehabilitation. The greater activity and demands on the person may result in tiredness and weakness. There is a tendency to interpret these symptoms as evidence of deterioration in cardiac functioning, which can lead to an unwillingness to resume more activities.

There have been a number of attempts at psychological interventions in the rehabilitation phase of MI, but as Evans points out in Chapter 13 on coronary heart disease, these have either been poorly controlled, or lacking a sound theoretical basis. Evans also cites recent evidence to suggest that interventions aimed at modifying the Type A Behaviour Pattern are likely to be premature.

Thus, we have seen in this section that rehabilitation is a multifaceted concept, and estimates of recovery or rehabilitation will vary greatly depending on the measure of rehabilitation chosen. Most often, rehabilitation carries with it the notion of complete or partial recovery. However, there are many other possible outcomes. Of interest next are those traumas which result in permanent impairment of function such as amputation or spinal-cord injury. Spinal-cord injury is a trauma which, while resulting in permanent disability, does not now necessarily carry with it implications of a severely limited life-span.

SPINAL-CORD INJURY (SCI) – THE PSYCHOLOGICAL CONSEQUENCES OF TRAUMA

It has been estimated that between 7,000 and 10,000 new spinal injuries occur each year in the USA. Lawes (1986) suggests that an incidence in the UK of 2,000 would be a conservative estimate. Spinal injuries are defined by the level of the spine at which the injury has occurred. Injuries occurring at the cervical (C) level of the vertebral column (neck) will result in quadriplegia (tetraplegia) if complete and quadriparesis if incomplete. Injuries occurring at the thoracic (T), lumbar (L) or sacral (S) regions will result in paraplegia if complete or paraparesis if incomplete. The motor impairment suffered will differ according to the level of the lesion. Lesions at C1 and C2 will result in no function below the neck and breathing will be via a respirator. Independent functioning will be limited to the facial muscles. With lesions at C6 and below there is some chance of independence, there should be some wrist extension and the possibility of transference into and out of a wheelchair. Sensory impairment will roughly approximate to the area of motor loss. Below the level of lesion there will be loss of the sense of touch, temperature, pain and position.

There are a number of complications often associated with spinal-cord injury; pressure sores (decubitus ulcers) are common, as are burns. Bowel and bladder functions have to be relearned and sexual function depends upon the level of lesion. Initially there is frequently pain at the lesion site; there can be hypersensitivity immediately below the lesion level and there can be 'deep root pain'. Muscle spasms can be a great problem, as can rapid changes in blood-pressure levels and temperature.

Who receives a spinal injury? Young *et al.* (1982) collected data via the National Spinal Data Research Centre in the USA and estimated the ratio of paraplegia to quadriplegia at 48–52 per cent. However, the more serious cases are referred to such a centre and this ratio is unlikely to be truly representative. The causes of spinal-cord injuries vary from country to country; in the USA and the UK the main causes are road-traffic accidents and sporting accidents; in other countries there is a higher proportion of industrially related accidents, most especially in the mining industry. In both sets of circumstances it is likely that relatively young active men will be the principal victims. In the USA 50 per cent of persons injured are under the age of 25, and 82 per cent are male.

It is a commonly held belief that people who have experienced trauma such as we are considering here must work through a series of stages of adjustment to their disability. Kerr and Thompson (1972) claim there are three stages of adjustment:

- mental shock, fear and anxiety
- grief and mourning; and
- anger and rebellion.

Hohmann (1966) suggests that there are 'normal reactions to an abnormal situation' such as the trauma of a major disabling incident. He reports:

- denial lasting from two weeks to two months;
- depression – withdrawal and internalized hostility;
- aggression – externalized hostility; and
- reaction against dependence.

The evidence for the existence of such 'stages', however, is not particularly strong or reliable and the number of suggested stages varies from two up to five. Dunn (1969) partially tested the concept of stages by administering a personality test, Cattell's 16PF, twice with a four-week gap to persons becoming rehabilitated post SCI. He found no evidence of change and most of the other evidence is only anecdotal. Silver and Wortman (1980) reviewed stage models of adaptation to a variety of traumatic events and concluded that while these models have an intuitive attraction there is little if any reliable evidence to support them.

A number of studies have looked at the incidence and type of emotional reactions to SCI. Boureston and Howard (1965) compared Minnesota Multiphasic Personality Inventory (MMPI) profiles of three disability groups: persons with rheumatoid arthritis, with multiple sclerosis and with spinal-cord injuries. They found that those with SCI had the most benign profile;

they showed least distress and least concern with somatic problems. The average SCI profile was well within normal limits. The nature and course of the three disorders is very different, and given the varying demographic aspects of the disorders it is difficult to interpret such a finding. Taylor (1967) studied a group of persons with SCI within one month of injury and compared them with a random sample of male university students. There was no evidence of severe depression, anxiety or psychosis amongst patients with SCI; only an increased incidence of mild depression was found. Lawson (1976, 1978) studied ten patients with quadriplegia longitudinally five days a week for their entire hospital stay, a mean duration of 119 days. He took four measures of depressive affect: semantic differential, number of words spoken per minute during taped report, ratings by ward staff and endocrine measure of daily output of urinary tryptamine. He found that there were no clear periods of depressive affect and no patient had an extended period where more than three of the measures were in the depressive range. Scores were very comparable to normal (non-SCI) persons.

Nevertheless, many clinicians have argued that depression is experienced by all persons who acquire SCI (Burnham and Werner 1979; Tucker 1980). Empirically based studies have reported only a significant minority of sufferers from SCI experiencing depressive disorders, between 23 and 38 per cent (Frank et al. 1985; Fullerton et al. 1981). This disparity between estimates may result from staff expectations that depression will occur and from the reactions of rehabilitation staff to those who show negative mood. A recent study by Westbrook and Nordholm (1986) reports that health-care givers perceive patients with paraplegia who are depressed as behaving more typically and appropriately then those patients who are optimistic. Claus-Walker et al. (1972) found that spinal-cord lesions altered the excretory rhythms of catecholamines and could dampen the excretion of 17–hydroxy-corticosteroids; these changes may influence the prevalence of depression, especially when combined with the daily problems experienced by SCI. Dinardo (1971), Lawson (1978) and Malec and Neimeyer (1983) all report that depression is inevitably disruptive to rehabilitation and adjustment to disability. Malec and Neimeyer (1983) administered the Beck Depression Inventory (BDI), a symptom check-list and the short form of the MMPI, to twenty-eight SCI patients on admission to an in-patient reha- bilitation programme. Of the several measures derived from this testing, they found that measures of distress and depression predicted both duration of in-patient rehabilitation and performance of self-care of bladder and skin at discharge.

Frank et al. (1986) conducted a series of studies which investigated the reactions of rehabilitation staff and of college students to a depressed person with spinal injury. Both staff and students reported experiencing dysphoric mood and hostility after listening to a tape of a male depressed SCI. Frank et al. (1987) investigated gender differences in the interpersonal responses of students to persons with SCI. Students listened to tapes which depicted either male or female depressed or undepressed SCIs. Students completed the Multiple Affect Adjective Check-list (MAACL) before and after the tapes and reported their reactions to the target. Results showed that regardless of gender, those targets which simulated both depression and SCI were more rejected than those with no depression. Depressed targets were viewed as less competent and less attractive. Just as there is an expectation in the hospital setting of the 'good patient', so it would seem there are expectations on the part of rehabilitation staff of 'good' SCIs, and those persons who do not appear cheerful and co-operative are likely to arouse negative feelings in staff, which in turn may influence treatment (but see Westbrook and Nordholm 1986).

Another way to measure the degree of distress or depression following SCI would be to examine the incidence of self-neglect or suicide amongst this population. Wilcox and Stauffer (1972) followed 423 consecutive patients with SCI; in this sample there were fifty deaths, of which 94 per cent occurred before the sixth anniversary of the injury. Seventeen deaths (34 per cent) were from avoidable causes, for example suicide, overdose, multiple pressure sores. Nyquist and Bors (1967) studied the records of US war veterans with SCI. Suicide occurred in 85 of 258 deaths. Half of these suicides were in the first five years following SCI. This is likely to be an underestimate since they did not include extreme self-neglect resulting in death. Thus, there is some evidence that a proportion of persons with SCI do not rehabilitate well.

There has also been interest in the emotional experience of persons with SCI from a theoretical viewpoint. Schachter (1971) proposed that emotion is a function of the state of physiological arousal and the cognitive interpretation of this state. This leads to a series of hypotheses of which one is relevant to SCI: 'Given cognitive circumstances, a person will act emotionally, or describe feelings as emotions, only to the extent that there is an experience of physiological arousal.'

It could be argued, then, that persons with SCI do not feel depressed, or indeed anything else much, because they do not experience the associated state of arousal. Hohmann (1966), himself suffering from paraplegia, tried to test this by giving structured interviews to twenty-five SCIs when he asked them to compare their feelings post injury with those prior to injury. He found that persons with lesions at C or high T reported a marked reduction in feelings of sexual stimulation, fear and anger. With lower lesions there was a mild to moderate reduction reported. Almost all reported an increase in sentimentality post injury. Hohmann concluded that the disruption to the ANS causes notable changes in experienced emotional feelings.

Lowe and Carroll (1985) attempted a replication of Hohmann's study. Some 29 SCIs with a median duration of ten years since injury were interviewed and presented with eight common emotional states: affection, anger, enjoyment, excitement, fear, grief, guilt and hate. All were asked to imagine situations in which they had experienced these emotions before and after injury, and to compare the intensity. Relative strength of emotion was measured as greatly decreased through to greatly increased. There were a hundred instances of reports of no change, sixty-eight of increase and forty-six of decrease. No differences were found for six of the emotions. Affection was generally reported to have increased and nothing much else. These findings are very difficult to interpret with the lack of any form of control group. Perhaps everyone, irrespective of physical health, might report such changes, or lack of them, over time. This question of the relationship between physiological arousal and emotion remains unresolved and will need research strategies which are not so reliant on retrospective self-report.

Rehabilitation research has not then supported the notions of stages of adjustment to any great degree. Frank, Elliott, Corcoran and Wonderlich (1987) point out that such approaches have limited psychologists to passive roles. The stage models presuppose that time will, of itself, influence adjustment and that all the patient must do is wait for time to pass. These approaches have been largely superseded by a perspective which allows for individual differences in coping and recovery strategies and which does not regard depression as a necessary and inevitable part of rehabilitation following spinal-cord injury. The patient is increasingly viewed as an active participant in the rehabilitation process, not the passive receiver of change. The issue of depression still lies, though, at the centre of psychological research in the area of rehabilitation following spinal-cord injury, and in this respect it is interesting to compare research from the related area of chronic disease.

CHRONIC DISEASE

Most acute illnesses are self-limiting; the individual suffers from classic symptoms: fever, nausea, pain and so forth, and these are hopefully accurately diagnosed shortly after their onset, treated and the individual recovers. In contrast, most chronic diseases are characterized by vague symptoms, which are relatively mild at onset. Such symptoms initially go unrecognized by people and undiagnosed by doctors. Such diseases, often progressive, are difficult to treat and sometimes impossible to cure. There may be a gradual or rapid deterioration of function. There have been two conflicting tendencies in the literature: the first is to consider 'chronic illness' as a unitary concept irrespective of the nature of the illness, its duration and its prognosis; the other tendency has been to cite the 'psychological effects of. . .' and then examine a specific disorder without regard for literature on other illnesses which might have some bearing. This review will try to steer a course between Scylla and Charybdis by considering two diseases which may have rather different implications for rehabilitation or management.

Multiple sclerosis – a degenerative disease

Multiple sclerosis (MS) is a disease of the central nervous system; it has been the focus of many studies of reactions and adjustment to a chronic illness (Brooks and Matson 1982; Stewart and Sullivan 1982). It is a chronic, progressive and debilitating disease which is neurological in basis. It destroys the myelin sheath which protects and nourishes brain cells and spinal-cord tissues. It can have disabling effects upon vision, speech, co-ordination, intellectual and emotional capacities, muscle strength and bowel and bladder control. It characteristically has periods of exacerbation and remission. It can appear in a variety of degrees of severity and does not respond particularly well to medical treatment. Given these characteristics, a person developing MS is faced with a number of years of self-management and adjustment to an illness which in itself will probably change and progress over time. Hence, the nature of the coping mechanisms employed will also need to be flexible and adaptive to change.

Stewart and Sullivan (1982) focus on the pre-diagnosis phase of MS. Data were gathered through in-depth interviews with sixty individuals with MS and their immediate families. They record that it took an average of five and a half years for an individual to be correctly diagnosed. During this lengthy pre-diagnosis phase they delineate three main phases: the non-serious phase, the serious phase and the diagnosis phase. During the first phase, individuals tended to try to disregard their symptoms and usually took no, or very minimal, medical advice. The serious phase began with the person redefining the symptoms as serious and an 'illness', and seeking medical advice; the diagnosis phase describes the stage during which specific tests are undergone which usually end with the MS diagnosis.

The most common early symptoms experienced were numbness and tingling sensations, co-ordination problems, blurred vision and general fatigue. Given the very general nature of these symptoms, they were frequently ascribed to a variety of causes, the work situation, family stress, 'a bug' and so on. People tended to regard these symptoms as indicators of ailments rather than illness. The change to the view that these represented 'an illness' usually came with increased symptom severity. Medical care was sought and this often resulted in initial misdiagnoses. Patients spent an average of around two-and-a-half years at this stage, before receiving an accurate diagnosis. Stewart and Sullivan report that their sixty patients consulted between them a total of 227 different doctors for a total of 407 diagnostic appointments, not including follow-ups for treatment and tests. Patients underwent a diversity of treatments for this variety of diagnoses.

Individuals' responses to this stage were very similar; they became increasingly critical of their doctors and began to try to 'self-diagnose' by reading medical textbooks. Changes also took place in the social-support networks. These people were in the ambiguous situation of viewing themselves as sick but of not being socially defined as such. They report that their fairly frequent discussions of symptoms with families and friends in the early part of the serious stage gradually tailed off. They assume others are tired of hearing the same complaints without also hearing of some resolution. They found increasing difficulty in convincing others that they *were* sick. More than half the patients described psychological symptoms which accompanied this stage – depression, anxiety, irritability. This phase ends either with the beginnings of a tentative diagnosis of MS or with referral to a hospital for tests which result in the MS diagnosis. This diagnostic phase was, for most of this sample, accompanied by a reduction in stress. Patients on the whole felt fairly positive immediately after the MS diagnosis was confirmed. They gave four main reasons for this uplift in feelings:

1 They finally had a name for their symptoms.
2 They received greater social support from others including their families, friends, doctors.
3 Some patients had become convinced they were terminally ill, often with cancer, and they regarded the MS diagnosis as less final.
4 They were unrealistically optimistic about their prognosis and this was reinforced by their doctors. 'MS didn't frighten me because I thought my condition would never get any worse. My doctor told me a lot of research was being done. . . I was just waiting for the cure to be discovered.'

Stewart and Sullivan conclude: 'surprisingly, the diagnosis of multiple sclerosis often resolves more psychological stress than it creates'.

Progress after initial diagnosis has also been the basis of research. Brooks and Matson (1982) used a longitudinal design to analyse the adjustment process of 103 people diagnosed with MS in their middle and later stages. The average age of the sample was 52 years and the mean duration since diagnosis was seventeen years. They found that more than 48 per cent of their sample sought medical attention once a year or less. Some 13 per cent sought no professional service at all for their MS. They used changes in self-concept as a measure of adjustment to MS and found most changes occurred in the years immediately after diagnosis. After that, self-concept remained fairly stable and fairly positive. They stressed the importance of social and personality aspects in achieving this adjustment. Employment and living arrangements and family income are important determiners of adjustments, as much if not more than the disease *per se*. They endorse the argument put forward by Feldman (1974) that the only management possible of MS is concerned with the components of illness other than the disease itself.

A number of papers have focused on personality, coping and adjustment in MS. An excellent review article by Devins and Seland (1987) outlines the problems associated with such research. Probably the most important criticism is that there is often a confounding of MS symptoms with somatic symptoms of distress measured by such scales as the MMPI and the General

Health Questionnaire (GHQ). This leads to considerable difficulty in interpretation. The most that can be said from studies conducted so far is that there is a general non-specific negative emotional response – which is not really saying very much at all!

An interesting study by Dalos *et al.*(1983) compares MS out-patients with persons with spinal-cord injuries, using the GHQ. They reported that in spite of the fact that the SCI group were more disabled than the MS group, the latter were more distressed, even when their symptoms were in remission. These findings need to be treated with caution, however, because of the methodological problems outlined above. An examination of the psychological literature concerned with MS indicates a continuing search for personality dimensions associated with the disease, either in its etiology, or in the characteristic responses to it. Before we can conclude that such dimensions exist, though, it is important to examine a comparable disorder for similar findings or differences.

Parkinson's disease

Much can be learned from a comparison of MS with another degenerative chronic disease – Parkinsonism. Parkinson's disease affects about one person in a hundred over the age of 50, although there are a number of people who suffer the onset of the disease at an earlier age. It is the result of a failure on the part of a specific area of the brain stem (substantia nigra) to produce a neurotransmitter, dopamine. Symptoms which indicate the lack of dopamine are: tremor, an intermittent and rhythmic tremor when the limbs are at rest; 'cogwheel rigidity' experienced as muscle cramps or soreness and brady-kinesia, a slowness and poverty of movement. There are also numerous secondary symptoms such as spatial and visual disorders, hot or cold flushes and constipation. The history of investigations of the psychological aspects of this disease, as outlined by Dakof and Mendelsohn (1986) is interesting and instructive. They characterize studies as falling into three historical sections: early studies ranging from 1817 when the disease was first described through to 1957; 1957–1967; and post 1967. Early studies tended to stress the psychosomatic nature of the disease; suggesting, in some cases, that psychic conflict was its *cause*. Dakof and Mendelsohn point out that such apparently naive theorizing took place in the absence of any knowledge of the biochemistry of the disorder and point out that, even today, 'assumptions about psychological origins of disease depend on the absence of identifiable biological pathology for their plausibility. Rarely have they been based on positive findings.' Alternative early approaches regarded certain psychological reactions such as depression, apathy or irritability as 'normal reactions' to the disorder, an approach which mirrors the arguments put forward by Hohmann with regard to spinal injury. Machover (1957) argued that since each chronic disease had a unique configuration of physical symptoms, then its effect on people's emotions should equally be different. This presupposes that each individual will respond to the disability in the same way, a supposition with little support.

The middle years of research into Parkinsonism (1957–1967) were marked by the use of stereotaxic surgery and the consequent investigations pre and post surgery. The contributions and the conclusions drawn from these studies are characterized by Dakof and Mendelsohn as 'slight'. More recent studies have examined Parkinsonism in the light of Sinemet and other drug treatments which, to some extent, alleviate the severity of at least some of the symptoms. The clinical research has been dominated by the study of depression. There is the customary debate about the prevalence of depression with a range of 12–52 per cent between studies, and the consistent finding of elevated levels of depression when Parkinson patients are compared with healthy controls (Horn 1974; Marsh and Markham 1973). Comparisons of patients with Parkinsonism with patients suffering from other diseases also consistently give higher depression scores for the former group. This has lead to the hypothesis that there is a direct biochemical or neuroanatomical basis for the depression. If this were to be the case, then some predictions could be made: that disease duration and severity of depression should be positively related. This has not been found – indeed, frequently the opposite is recorded, i.e. that depression is more commonly linked with the disease in its early stages. This is not so surprising: Cassileth et al. (1984) and others have reported increased psychological disturbance in the early stages of a large number of illnesses. Singer (1974) reports that the longer patients had Parkinson's disease, the more stoical they were about the symptoms. This argument also seems to conflict with the discussion of the diagnosis of MS by Stewart and Sullivan reported above. Other reasons for not accepting the suggested simple biochemical link are that there is no clear relationship between severity of neurological symptoms and depression, and that placebos decrease levels of depression (Andersen et al. 1980, cited by Dakof and Mendelsohn 1986). Knight et al. (1988) review the psychological deficits associated with Parkinson's disease and conclude that no cognitive deficits exclusive to the disease have been identified. They also consider the increased risk of depression and suggest that this might be indicative of the problems such patients face in adjusting to the effects of this chronic and irreversible disease.

Yet again, the search for a characteristic response to a particular physical disease has not been very fruitful. It is still not clear whether there are unique aspects to the psychological disorders associated with Parkinson's disease, or indeed, any other chronic disorder, rheumatoid arthritis, MS or diabetes. Antonovsky (1979), and others since, have argued that the search for a reason for the depression experienced by some proportion of persons suffering from a chronic illness is less useful than the search for explanations for the ability of the majority of persons to remain effective and psychologically intact in the face of the enormous difficulties and stresses which accompany illness and disease.

The study by Cassileth *et al.* (1984), referred to earlier, compared the emotional impact of six different disorders: cancer, diabetes, renal disease, arthritis, dermatologic conditions and depression. Their conclusions are that the emotional impact of chronic illness may be quite uniform across the range of disorders, and across a variety of populations. No group, with the exception of the depressed patients, differed from the general population on measures of anxiety, depression, positive affect, emotional ties, control and global mental health. They conclude: 'our results. . .cast doubt on the notion that emotional traits are unique – either in cause or effect to a particular illness.' We have shown in this chapter that the reactions to disorders as different as myocardial infarction, spinal-cord injury, multiple sclerosis and Parkinson's disease share many similarities. In particular, the theme of depression as a response is shared by research into all these disorders. How to cope or combat the psychological effects of illness and disease will be considered in the next section.

COPING AND CONTROL

Ben-Sira (1984) stresses the issue of resources as the fulcrum of coping with chronic illness. These resources will clearly include medical and other health-professional care, but also support from other areas – family, work, friends, self-support groups and the Church. These 'other' agencies may be especially important at times when the doctor's inability to cure, and perhaps a past history of misdiagnoses of symptoms, may lead to a breakdown in the primary medical relationship. Schradle and Dougher (1985) confirm a positive association between social support and health. They caution, however, that tangible forms of support such as money and other material aid are frequently confounded with psychological support. The latter can be divided into emotional support and problem-solving support. Schradle and Dougher describe emotional support as interacting in an intimate non-directive manner in such a way that feelings and concerns can be expressed; while problem-solving support offers advice and information, and can provide feedback on a person's coping efforts.

An alternative approach to coping looks for concepts which might link the diversity of research findings outlined above. Such variety as there is in psychological responses to different disorders can possibly be explained by considering the concept of control as at the centre of rehabilitation and adjustment. Devins and Seland (1987) point out that it has been applied to healthy people (Garber and Seligman 1980), and to a small number of disorders including epilepsy, endstage renal failure, SCI and MS. They suggest that, prior to the onset of an illness, control derives from physical strengths and abilities and from a variety of social, economic and environmental resources. Following the onset of a chronic disease or disorder, however, the person's ability to control can become severely compromised. Barriers to control can be both *general* and applicable to all illnesses and *specific* to the particular illness suffered. Hence, the degree to which symptoms or progress of the disease are predictable can be important in determining how well a person can mobilize resources to cope. The distinction made by Lazarus and Folkman (1984) is probably useful here; they suggest there are at least two types of coping: *problem-focused* coping which is directed at changing the troubled relationship between the person and the environment; and *emotion-focused* coping which is aimed at managing the distressing emotions themselves. They claim that the former is most often employed when people are suffering from an acute physical illness, while the latter is probably the more important for those suffering from an unpredictable and chronic condition like MS or Parkinson's disease. Emotion-focused coping can take a number of forms: denial, avoidance, relaxation therapy, turning to others for support or the use of humour.

The importance of these ways of coping with the stresses associated with long-term illness is becoming increasingly recognized. Taylor (1983) studied the adjustment to breast cancer and postulates a theory of cognitive adaptation. She argues that the adjustment process centres around three themes: a search for meaning in the experience, an attempt to gain mastery over the event and one's life, and an effort to enhance self esteem. Attribution theory suggests that people will make attributions in order to understand, predict and control their lives and their environment. Faced with an event which threatens this process, Taylor found that the women in her study spontaneously offered explanations as to why they had developed cancer. No single explanation seemed more functional than the others, but the need to explain was almost universal. Meaning was also found for the experience in terms of what life now meant to these women: 'it puts things into perspective'; 'I feel as if I were for the first time really conscious.' Mastery over the event is achieved by beliefs about personal control, especially over the progression or recurrence of the disease. Control over the treatment also enhances a sense of mastery. The third theme identified by Taylor was an effort to restore self-esteem. This is achieved via comparisons, especially downward comparisons with others who have been less fortunate. Hence, women with lumpectomies compared themselves favourably with women with mastectomies, but never vice versa. Taylor says: 'the need to come out of the comparison process appearing better off drives the process itself; the process does not determine the outcome.' These cognitions are largely based on illusions; causes for cancer are not easily determined, the degree of personal control over the development of the disease is limited, and it is always possible to find people who are better or worse off than oneself. Nevertheless, such illusions can be beneficial in providing coping strategies which allow people to be adaptable to threatening situations such as chronic or long-term illness.

CONCLUSIONS

The research described in the areas of recovery and rehabilitation is often confused and this limits the conclusions that can be drawn. Many suppositions, such as those concerning stages of recovery, have been largely unsubstantiated. Similarly, the search for personality profiles associated with certain chronic conditions such as multiple sclerosis and Parkinson's disease has also proved fruitless. Future research will move beyond these considerations, hopefully, to a more concerted approach to aid the lives of people coping, often successfully, with disease and disability. Psychologists have much to offer in this regard, and a more 'interventionist' approach which seeks to develop individuals' coping skills should offer considerable scope for their contributions to the areas of recovery, rehabilitation and living with chronic disorders.

Part III

Health issues

Part III examines interventions by psychologists directed towards specific illnesses and diseases and the application of theories and methods described in Part I and Part II. It begins with the topic of AIDS – the most recent and arguably most pressing health issue facing health psychologists. The chapter outlines the need for effective behavioural strategies to be implemented as part of health-education programmes. Chapter 11 considers the controversial topics of contraception and abortion. It examines the application of psychological models to decision making for contraception and abortion and considers the impact of legislation on those decisions. The following two chapters concern the related issues of essential hypertension and coronary heart disease. The management of essential hypertension by behavioural methods is evaluated in Chapter 12 and the problems of adherence to behavioural management programmes are discussed. Chapter 13 critically reviews the evidence that the Type A Behaviour Pattern is a psychological risk factor for coronary heart disease and questions whether behavioural interventions can be recommended.

The health consequences that follow ingestion of drugs that are socially acceptable in many cultures including the UK are reviewed in Chapter 14. The actions of nicotine, alcohol and caffeine are described and their effects upon health discussed. Chapter 15 examines diabetes mellitus, a disorder which has been extensively studied by health psychologists. The self-management of diabetes is discussed and the effects of age and family factors upon such management are evaluated. The final chapter broadens the perspective upon health. Chapter 16 looks at child health and considers the influences of styles of parenting and family functioning upon the child's health. It argues that health in its broadest sense is dependent upon a child's social environment and that health professionals can play an important role in promoting beneficial health practices for parents and their children.

Taken together, these chapters give an indication of the diversity of health issues with which psychologists are concerned and the approaches which are increasing our understanding of the psychology of health.

Chapter 10

The primary prevention of AIDS

Keith Phillips

INTRODUCTION

The human immunodeficiency virus (HIV) destroys the Helper T-cells of the immune system which normally provide resistance to disease. Infection with HIV makes the body vulnerable to several opportunistic infections such as Pneumocystis carinii pneumonia, protozoal and fungal infections, and tumours, including a rare form of skin cancer named Kaposi's sarcoma, and lymphomas. Acquired Immune Deficiency Syndrome (AIDS) is diagnosed by the presence of such specific diseases in the absence of any other known cause of immune system deficiency. HIV may give rise to a range of symptoms such as fevers, fatigue, sore throat which may be diagnosed as AIDS related complex (ARC) and persistent swollen lymph nodes. Many people with HIV infection show no symptoms at all for several years and the epidemiological statistics indicate that the progression from infection with the virus to the development of AIDS is between five and eight years. Also, it is generally accepted that several co-factors such as poor nutrition and stress assist the progression to AIDS (Siegel 1988). The presence of these and other co-factors may account for the differences that exist for epidemiological patterns and risk factors in different countries.

AIDS was first reported among young homosexual men in USA in 1981 (CDC 1981). Since then it has been reported in countries world-wide in heterosexuals as well as homo- or bisexuals, and among injecting drug users, prostitutes and recipients of untreated blood products including haemophiliacs. It is estimated that at the time of writing (June 1989) there may be 100,000 cases of AIDS world-wide and a further 5–10 million people infected with HIV. Because of the progression from HIV infection to the development of AIDS the full impact of deaths attributable to AIDS has yet to be felt. In the UK, 2,192 cases of AIDS were reported in March 1989 with 1,149 deaths attributable to AIDS. It is predicted that over the next ten years in England and Wales 100,000 men and an unknown number of women will die of AIDS (OPCS 1989).

The medical facts concerning HIV infection and AIDS have become well known (Hersh and Petersen 1988) and yet the prevalence of AIDS continues to grow and it is generally agreed that the peak of HIV infection has yet to be reached. A major problem is that no vaccine for HIV is available and nor is it likely that one will be available within the next five years (Zuckerman 1989). Though some drugs, combined with a programme for self-management of infection by attention to diet, exercise and relaxation, may be effective against some of the opportunistic infections, they are not a 'cure' as they cannot eliminate HIV infection itself.

In the absence of any medical solution the best strategy against AIDS is its primary prevention through elimination of those behaviours that allow transmission of the HIV virus (Phillips 1988). Unfortunately the research on AIDS prevention shows that thus far the strategy has had only limited success. This is not surprising when one examines the literature on other areas of health psychology in which behaviour change is required to avoid illness, or more significantly, the risk of future illness in individuals who are currently well, as the statistics on smoking or drinking show (see Chapter 14).

This chapter will examine the behaviours associated with the transmission of HIV, consider interventions that may be used to persuade people to adopt behaviours that will limit the spread of HIV, and assess their prospects of success in the future.

BEHAVIOURAL TRANSMISSION OF HIV

Despite rumours and myths to the contrary there is no evidence that social contacts can transmit the virus from an infected to a non-infected individual (Fischl et al. 1987). The virus is easily destroyed outside the body and mere exposure does not result in infection. There are only three effective routes of transmission of the virus from an infected to a non-infected individual; by transfer of either blood or sexual fluids, or by perinatal transfer from mother to foetus. The virus has been identified in other fluids including saliva and tears but there is no evidence that infection has occurred from contact with these fluids (CDC 1985). There is some risk of infection for breast-feeding infants from the milk of an infected mother (Ziegler et al. 1985) and though recent estimates suggest that this risk is low, HIV seropositive women are advised to bottle-feed their infants (Mok 1988).

Efforts to prevent AIDS have concentrated attention upon those behaviours that allow transfer of blood and sexual fluids between individuals. The particular behaviours that are significant vary from country to country. The patterns of transmission are not the same and it is important that primary prevention programmes recognize this fully (Piot et al. 1988). In some countries the greatest risk of transfer via blood may come from untreated blood products used in surgery, or from unsterilized injecting equipment used in hospitals. In the USSR, for example, there was reported an instance of seventy Russian children and their mothers becoming infected with the virus via contaminated syringes where the source could be traced to a single child born with HIV (*Guardian*, 5 June 1989). In western countries, that risk no longer exists though of course in the early days of the AIDS era many haemophiliacs were infected with HIV via untreated blood extracts. In western countries the greatest risk of transfer of HIV via blood is by intravenous drug users sharing inadequately sterilized injecting equipment.

Intravenous drug use

Intravenous drug users (ivdus) are seen as key individuals in the fight against AIDS as through their drug practices they expose themselves to risk of HIV infection and their sexual habits may present further risks to their sexual partners and their unborn children.

The initial spread of HIV infection among homosexual males in the USA has slowed as several homosexual communities have altered their behaviours to reduce high-risk sexual activities (Winkelstein *et al.* 1987). But HIV infection continues to increase among intravenous drug users, their partners and increasingly their children. In the USA 17 per cent of AIDS cases are attributable to heterosexual ivdus. In Western Europe the problem is equally large – the proportion of AIDS cases accounted for by heterosexual ivdus has risen from 1 per cent at the end of 1984, to 7 per cent at the end of 1985, and to 15 per cent at the end of 1986 (Conviser and Rutledge 1989).

Ivdus and the subculture that supports their behaviours present a major challenge for those involved in AIDS prevention (Mulleady 1987). Innovative policies are called for that decriminalize drug use in favour of public-health education for safer drug use. The potential impact of this approach can be seen by comparing the seroprevalence in Glasgow and Edinburgh (Conviser and Rutledge 1989). In both Scottish cities it is legal for pharmacists to sell syringes and needles to ivdus, but in Edinburgh police pursued a policy of arrests for those found carrying injecting equipment, whereas in Glasgow no such policy existed. Sharing of equipment occurs in both cities but because of this difference in policing, sharing occurs in small local groups in Glasgow, whereas in Edinburgh sharing exists between many more drug users in so-called 'shooting galleries' (these are places where drugs are sold and buyers share or rent the injecting equipment with several others). In Glasgow the rate of HIV infection among ivdus at the end of 1986 was around 5 per cent while in Edinburgh the rate grew from 3 per cent in 1983 to 50 per cent in 1984 and is now endemic among the city's ivdus (Robertson *et al.* 1986).

One approach to reduce the spread of HIV infection among ivdus is to encourage safer drug-injection practices by policies operating at a national level, for example through needle-exchange schemes. These schemes were pioneered in Amsterdam and are being evaluated in the UK (Stimson *et al.* 1988) and other European countries. They legally allow ivdus to exchange used needles and syringes for sterile ones. In addition, however, they bring ivdus into contact with counselling and advice services which allows the opportunity for health education messages to be conveyed. These include messages for 'harm minimization' (Landrey and Smith 1988) which involve a hierarchy of behavioural changes for ivdus to reduce the risk of HIV infection:

- do not use drugs;
- if you must use drugs, do not inject;
- if you must inject, do not share injecting equipment;
- if you must share, sterilize the injecting equipment before each injection.

Though this strategy has been criticized for condoning drug use, there is no evidence that further drug use is encouraged, and it does recognize the realities of factors in the ivdus' lives that increase personal and public risks of HIV infection (Mulleady and Sher 1989). Currently the USA does not have needle-exchange schemes but evidence from community-based 'outreach' programmes, where ivdus are taught how to sterilize injecting equipment using a bleaching agent, indicates that ivdus can reduce the risks of HIV infection within their local community (Watters 1988, 1989). This style of approach for ivdus involves a shift from treating their chemical dependency upon drugs by trying to achieve abstinence to educating users about safe practices they can adopt to minimize the risks to themselves and others. To be successful national policies must necessarily reflect that shift to decriminalize drug use in favour of health-education programmes.

The dangers associated with injecting drugs also threaten the sexual partners of ivdus and their unborn children. It is a fact that most women diagnosed with AIDS here and in USA are either ivdus or the sexual partners of male ivdus. It is becoming increasingly recognized that women ivdus and women sharing relationships with ivdus require specific policies to protect themselves and their children against AIDS, including advice on safer drug use *and* advice on safer sex, but also advice on contraception, pregnancy and childcare (Mulleady *et al.* 1989). It is vitally important that women in these circumstances are not regarded as 'transmitters' of HIV either to men by prostitution or by pregnancy to infants, but as a special group that needs protection against their own drug-using behaviours or the behaviours of their sexual partners (Cohen *et al.* 1989).

Paediatric AIDS

Paediatric AIDS was first identified in 1982 in the USA in cases of children less than 13 years old showing signs of cellular immunodeficiency without obvious cause (CDC 1982). Since then an elaborate and comprehensive classification system has been developed to identify HIV infection in children (CDC 1987). Infants may become infected with HIV perinatally, during the birth itself, or possibly postnatally through mothers' breast milk (Rogers

1985). The true risk of perinatal transmission from a mother infected with HIV is unknown but has been estimated to be between 20 per cent and 65 per cent (Schwartz and Rutherford 1989). The prognosis for children with AIDS is poor. Women who are HIV positive should receive specialist counselling concerning the effect of their pregnancy upon their own health as well as the health implications for their infant and its future health care. As women account progressively for a greater proportion of individuals with HIV the instances of paediatric AIDS will increase. This tragic consequence requires urgent consideration of policies for women and their infants. It is a particular problem in parts of Africa where a high proportion of AIDS cases result from heterosexual transmission and a much higher percentage of women are represented among the HIV-positive population.

Sexual behaviours and AIDS

The risks from sexual activities have been well publicised. Some degree of risk is associated with any practice that transfers bodily fluids: the greatest risks are associated with penetrative sex including anal intercourse (particularly for the receptive partner), and transfer from man to woman or, to a lesser extent, woman to man during vaginal intercourse. The risks can be substantially reduced by the precaution of using a condom as a barrier to the transfer of HIV, particularly if used in association with the spermicide nonoxynol-9, which is claimed to be effective against the virus. The risks are not eliminated totally, however, as condoms may fail, or may be used inappropriately, and they do not present the complete answer since a couple may wish to avoid their contraceptive effect if trying to achieve conception. Others may have firmly held religious objections to their use. Monogamy for non-infected partners or celibacy offers complete protection, of course, but their costs are clearly unacceptable for many individuals. This illustrates the dilemma facing health educators; preventive behaviours have value in protecting an individual against future illness but they also have costs associated with them. Decisions to adopt healthy behaviours will depend in part upon the individual's perception of the reward–cost payoff. Effective health education must maximize that payoff.

Since sexual transmission is a common cause of HIV infection it is important that health-education messages provide accurate and appropriate information about the risks associated with unprotected sex and the opportunities for safer sex practices among individuals of different sexual preferences. In this context safer sex can be interpreted as minimizing the risk of HIV transmission, which in most cases means avoiding the exchange of body fluids from one individual to another (Aggleton *et al.* 1989).

The difficulties of persuading people to alter their sexual behaviours are enormous, but changes are possible (Becker and Joseph 1988). Statistics from some American cities show that local groups of homosexual males have reduced high-risk sexual activities and adopted safer sex practices (Winkelstein *et al.* 1987). They have recognized the risks and adjusted their behaviour accordingly. This does not however mean that high-risk behaviours have been abandoned by *all* individuals. For example, a postal survey conducted in the UK found that while many homosexual males had adopted a policy of safer sex, those who continue to engage in high-risk activities such as anal sex without a condom may be particularly sexually active (Golombok *et al.* 1989).

Public education campaigns to persuade heterosexuals to alter their behaviours have not been obviously effective. There may be many reasons for this. One is undoubtedly the fact that a myth has developed that AIDS is a disease associated with minority groups – homosexuals and drug users – rather than the reality that it is associated with particular risk behaviours and there are no 'risk groups'. The existence of this myth allows people who do not regard themselves as belonging to those minorities to deny any risk to themselves. A damaging side-effect of the myth is that it encourages blaming of those groups and stigmatization of individuals with AIDS. People's perceptions of AIDS are determined by a complexity of beliefs, attitudes and values that may be shared with others and which collectively form a social representation of the disease (Phillips 1989b). The social representation of AIDS needs to be shifted if individuals are to make realistic decisions about their own behaviours (Markova and Wilkie 1987).

A further obstacle to change is that individuals are unrealistically optimistic about their own health and see themselves as being at less risk than others in a similar situation (Weinstein 1987). This 'illusion of invulnerability' prevents people from making realistic estimates of personal risk, which in turn acts against the adoption of preventive behaviours. This is a fundamental problem for preventive health programmes and though not unique to AIDS its impact can be seen in studies of sexual behaviours and contraceptive use (see Chapter 11). A recent study of Oxford University undergraduates (Turner *et al.* 1988) found that these students estimated their own personal risk of AIDS to be less than that for others of their age and sex. This was true even for individuals who were engaging in activities associated with greater risk for AIDS such as unprotected intercourse with bisexual partners, ivdus, and prostitutes.

It is not only estimates of personal risk that are important, however. Even when the risks are recognized, individuals may not take appropriate precautions to reduce the risks. Our studies with students and young people have found that the precautions against AIDS that are favoured by many are mandatory screening for HIV, and vetting of partner's past sexual history. The obvious unreliability of both of these measures is seemingly denied by these young well-informed people (Boyle *et al.* 1989; White *et al.* 1989). A number of studies have found little evidence of changes in behaviour by adoption by young heterosexuals of the simple preventive measure of condom use for penetrative sex (Baldwin and Baldwin 1988; Kegeles *et al.* 1988). This may reflect the difficulty in persuading people to alter attitudes to practices that are perceived as having excessive costs, for example loss of pleasurability (Chapman and Hodgson 1988).

Adolescents are a particularly important group for future AIDS education campaigns (Melton 1988). A recent American report on AIDS (NRC 1989) recognizes the special importance of effective health-education messages for adolescents, recommending that all teenagers should receive sex education in school including information about prevention of HIV infection. The report states that 'young people are not particularly skilled in managing their sexual lives: inevitably this places them at risk of HIV infection and health educators need to recognize this as being so.' It must be acknowledged, however, that they need more than information alone: they additionally require opportunities for learning about relationships and the social skills required to manage the dynamics of relationships. It is self-evident that intimacy involves social interactions between partners and negotiations about sex may not be equitable (Byers and Lewis 1988). For example, coercion or compliance may cause an individual to disregard his or her intention to allow sexual intercourse or to use a condom during intercourse. Information encouraging safer sex must be accompanied by education about adhering to intentions for preventive health. Much more research on this aspect of adolescents' behaviour is necessary.

CHANGING RISK BEHAVIOURS

Epidemiological studies of AIDS have clearly identified the particular behaviours that present to the individual risks of contracting HIV infection. The success or otherwise of behavioural approaches to the prevention of AIDS depends upon persuading people to take responsibility for actions they may regard as private, personal, and which they do not perceive as a threat to either their own health or that of others. Interventions to promote changes in behaviour for reducing the risk of future illness should be based upon theoretical models that identify the determinants of behaviour change. Unfortunately, modelling preventive health behaviour has proved to be an enormously difficult task. Several models focus upon the importance of socio-cognitive variables in preventive health. Among these are the health belief model (Becker 1974; Rosenstock 1974) and the theory of reasoned action (Fishbein and Ajzen 1975; Ajzen and Fishbein 1980), both of which emphasize the importance of volitional decisions by individuals about the perceived utility of their actions. (See Chapter 1 for detailed explanations of these models.)

According to the health belief model the significant variables that influence the adoption of precautions against a perceived threat to health are a person's perceived vulnerability to the threat, the perceived severity of the threat and the cost–benefit payoff that is associated with adopting preventive behaviours. Consideration of these variables in relation to AIDS indicates the difficulties faced by health educators. Despite public education campaigns there is little evidence that the bulk of the population see themselves as personally vulnerable to HIV infection. Furthermore, in the absence of perceived personal risk, individuals may estimate that the costs of safer sex such as using a condom are greater than the benefits which would mitigate against the adoption of effective preventive measures.

The theory of reasoned action identifies intention as the most immediate determinant of behaviour. Intentions are themselves a function of privately held attitudes towards the particular behaviour and socially determined subjective norms that represent a person's belief that others think s/he should behave in a certain way. The model attaches values to each of these factors. The particular values attached to each of these factors will depend upon the individual's beliefs and thus in many ways this model is similar to the health belief model.

One difficulty with this model is that it identifies a direct link between intentions and behaviours, but intentions are not always translated into actions. Even when an individual holds an intention towards some behaviour, action does not necessarily result. When considering sexual behaviours and safer-sex practices there may be one or several reasons for individuals' failures to carry out intentions to act in ways that are perceived as beneficial. An action may not be possible in a particular situation or at a particular time, it may be difficult or time consuming or it may simply be suppressed, for example if the use of intoxicant drugs accompanies the behaviour (Stall *et al.* 1986). Much greater consideration needs to be given to the impact of situational influences of this kind upon adherence to intentions to act in accordance with prevention. As pointed out elsewhere (Phillips 1989b), adherence to intentions for safer sex may be particularly vulnerable since sexual relationships involve a partner. What happens when one partner's intentions for sex do not coincide with those of their partner? Inevitably social processes will occur which may involve one partner abandoning his/her intentions in deference to the wishes of the other.

There is a clear need for empirical studies that test these and similar models for the adoption of preventive health behaviours since interventions have implicitly accepted the assumptions contained within them. If the determinants of precautionary behaviours could be identified, this would be a significant step forward in campaigns against AIDS and other behavioural diseases. There is little doubt that the principal variables identified by these models – perceived risk, perceived severity of the disease, perceived effectiveness of precautions and cost–benefit payoff – are important predictors of preventive health behaviours of many kinds (Janz and Becker 1984). However, these models have their limitations and a more recent approach emphasizes the dynamic aspects of preventive behaviours.

The precaution-adoption process

Weinstein suggests that the precaution adoption process involves a progression through distinct stages which differ qualitatively from each other. The factors that are important at any particular time therefore depend upon which stage of the adoption process an individual has reached (Weinstein 1988). One of the advantages of this model is that it recognizes that as people move through qualitatively different stages towards adoption of preventive behaviours, the interventions that are appropriate also change. In Weinstein's words 'The idea of matching the communication to the audience follows naturally from a stage model' (p. 380).

Though this model remains to be tested, it offers a wider perspective on the adoption of preventive behaviours and may be more compatible with the fact that target behaviours do not exist in isolation. Attempts to modify an individual's sexual or drug-using behaviours will inevitably impinge upon other significant aspects of that person's life. The process of precaution adoption will reflect this interdependence of behaviours.

Interventions that are planned on the basis of theoretical models of behaviour change must also be prepared to provide the resources required for those changes in behaviour to be realized. Interventions that encourage safer sex, for example, might require that condoms be widely available and at an affordable price. Similarly, harm-minimization programmes for safer drug use will involve making sterile needles and syringes available for those who wish to use them. Psychologists and educators promoting interventions must be prepared to address the social and political implications of their interventions (Ingham 1988).

POLICIES FOR PROTECTING AGAINST AIDS

World-wide, many different policies to prevent the spread of AIDS have been adopted, including programmes for international co-operation and collaboration, national measures including legal restrictions upon all or some citizens or mass health-education campaigns, local and community-based projects for selected groups of individuals. Each of these policies is concerned with altering people's behaviour in some desired direction: each may have several impacts upon individuals' behaviours and their perceptions and the social representation of AIDS. Some of the policies also raise significant questions, including those of the relationship between individual rights and public welfare, and the objectives and policies for health education. The following section considers the value of some of the measures adopted as precautions against AIDS.

HIV testing

Governments' reactions to the AIDS health crisis have varied. Some have adopted mass education campaigns designed to alert the public to the existence of HIV infection and to encourage changes in behaviour that would reduce individuals' personal risk of exposure to the virus. Others have adopted authoritarian measures that seek to legislate against individuals with HIV, against groups who are perceived as presenting a risk for transmission of the virus, or against behaviours that might transmit the virus. Legislation against particular individuals or against groups is discriminatory and may abuse individuals' rights as well as presenting a threat to civil liberties; measures against particular behaviours will inevitably be ineffective since the behaviours concerned, sexual and drug practices, are private and beyond effective control by the authorities. In the midst of these various measures there has been great debate about the merits of screening and testing for HIV, or rather, antibodies to the virus since their presence is indicative of infection.

A number of countries including Cuba and Bulgaria have expressed a wish or intention to have mandatory screening for HIV of their entire population. Others require testing of citizens returning from abroad, for example Iraq, or of some visitors to the country, for example the USSR, or immigrants, for example the USA. Many more countries have introduced legislation that allows mandatory testing of selected individuals including prostitutes (Austria, Israel, South Korea and others), injecting drug users (Hungary, Bavaria), or in some instances individuals suspected of these activities (Hungary). Some countries have introduced mandatory notification of HIV infection (Japan). In all of these instances the authorities have dismissed the danger inherent in all such measures, namely that the problem is not eliminated but simply driven underground, causing the emergence of marginal groups outside the reach of health services and beyond the scope of educational programmes. Appeals for mass screening also ignore the prohibitive financial cost that would be involved, particularly as to be effective, screening would need to be repeated at regular intervals. Long-term reliance upon screening or testing for HIV is a recipe for the continuing increase in the prevalence of HIV infection.

Anonymous HIV testing has also become a contentious issue. In the UK there has been considerable debate amongst doctors and politicians as to whether blood taken from a patient for other tests should be tested anonymously for HIV. Anonymous testing would mean, of course, that the donors could not be informed of the outcome of the test and could not be advised of their own health status. However, anonymous testing would allow statistics to be gathered to show the true incidence of HIV infection in the population, something that is otherwise difficult to establish. These statistics are needed to allow accurate projections of health provision for AIDS patients and their likely health costs. Critics, however, argue that anonymous testing would be an abuse of individual rights. Even though it might establish the prevalence of HIV, anonymous testing would be of extremely limited value for planning policies for prevention since it provides no information at all about the way in which the virus is being transmitted within a population. This information is critical for planning measures that may be effective against further transmission in that population. As discussed below it cannot be assumed that modes of transmission will be identical for all populations; preventive measures must take account of different patterns of transmission and the ecology of AIDS.

Voluntary testing with informed consent of the client is offered by health services in several countries and may be regarded as a compassionate measure that should be available on demand to individuals who see themselves at risk. Even in this instance, however, there may be costs for the individual: someone whose test is negative on one occasion may continue to engage in behaviours that place him/her at risk for the future. There must be guarantees of confidentiality if discrimination against individuals is to be avoided and counselling must be provided for all volunteers, not only after their test results are known, but also beforehand to explore the meaning of the test and the possible social, health and employment consequences for someone following the test outcome (Acton 1989). In some instances, of course, voluntary testing may be of considerable value. For example, pregnant women may wish to know their HIV status if they consider themselves at risk and would wish to consider therapeutic abortion if they found themselves to be infected. Similarly, women injecting drugs may wish to know their HIV status in consideration of contraception and planned pregnancies.

Adults (for example, see Moatti et al. 1988) and young people (White et al. 1989) have identified screening for HIV as an effective preventive measure against AIDS without apparently recognizing the difficulties and uncertainties outlined above, and many express the opinion that they would be prepared to take a test themselves. This may simply reflect anxieties about their own behaviours. It certainly indicates a failure to recognize effective precautions against HIV and suggests the need for further education about prevention of HIV transmission.

Public education campaigns – awareness, knowledge and attitudes

Several countries, including the UK, have introduced national AIDS campaigns providing public education by means of messages distributed via delivery of leaflets to individual homes, television, radio and print media. Evaluations of these campaigns clearly show that they have been highly effective in increasing awareness of AIDS among the general populations of the UK (DHSS and Welsh Office, 1987), Sweden (Brorsson and Herlitz 1988), and the USA (Singer et al. 1987). Of course, awareness of an issue is far removed from action by individuals in respect of that issue; knowing that

AIDS may be life threatening will not have any impact upon the behaviour of people who do not consider themselves at any risk of having AIDS. There is little evidence that mass campaigns have been effective in bringing about changes in behaviour that are effective precautions against HIV infection (see Phillips 1989b). This is not surprising when one considers the psychological processes that underlie behaviour change and the precaution-adoption process discussed earlier.

The assumption underlying mass education campaigns has been that knowledge about AIDS will cause people's attitudes to change which in turn will lead to changes in behaviour. This simple sequential process, in which knowledge leads to a rational decision to alter behaviours in favour of prevention without any regard to costs that may be incurred as a result of those changes, is clearly inadequate. It fails to take account of both the interacting complexities of variables that determine people's behaviours and the fact that behaviours do not exist in isolation; change in one behaviour has implications for other aspects of an individual's life that may be unacceptable (Hunt and MacLeod 1987). Moreover, there is no compelling evidence that mass education campaigns have altogether been effective in communicating accurate information and increasing knowledge about HIV and AIDS. One difficulty is that the audience is not made up of passive receivers of information. They have 'lay beliefs' that will influence their attention to the messages and their willingness to accept or reject the 'truth' of those messages (Aggleton et al. 1989). In part, individuals' lay beliefs may be determined by information received from other sources, including media messages that distort the facts or confirm myths and stereotypes associated with AIDS or persons with AIDS (Wellings 1988). Furthermore, they do not share equal amounts of knowledge about AIDS, and messages that contain no new information for some may be beyond the comprehension of others. This is a particular problem when trying to present material that is appropriate for young people who may, for example, have limited experience of sexual practices. Lay beliefs may further interfere with accurate perceptions of risk and provide obstacles to the adoption of preventive behaviours. Education involving personalized learning experiences which is beyond the scope of mass campaigns is necessary to bring about changes in behaviour. For young people greater opportunities could be made of learning within its traditional context, i.e. schools.

If increasing knowledge is difficult, then altering attitudes may be yet more problematic. Several survey studies in different countries have examined people's knowledge and attitudes towards AIDS before and after particular education campaigns (for example, Mills et al. 1986; Sher 1987) or as trends over time following cumulative exposure to educational messages about AIDS (for example, Singer et al. 1987). They find that though the general level of knowledge has increased, particular gaps in knowledge may remain. For example, there remains uncertainty about the risks of transmission of HIV associated with casual contacts or by oral sex. However, attitudes have changed much less. In particular there is little indication that the population as a whole recognizes the need to change behaviour. Many studies have shown that individuals, and particularly heterosexuals, are not adopting effective preventive measures and do not intend to alter their sexual behaviours. Further interventions are required to bring out the desired alterations.

School-based education

There are opportunities for many different kinds of learning experiences for young people within school settings. Effective health education could easily be included in the school curriculum. The advantage of using schools for health education is that young people's beliefs, values and attitudes may be malleable, unlike the more firmly held attitudes of older groups. If so, appropriate attitudes towards social responsibility can be encouraged that enable appropriate precautions to be taken against AIDS. Learning experiences of this type could make use of person-centred approaches rather than simple exposure to information. This would allow youngsters to develop their own knowledge structures, at their own rate and within the context of experiences within their own lives. It is quite clear that adolescents do require more information about HIV and AIDS (White *et al.* 1988, 1989), but information is not enough: they also need the opportunity to make use of that information for risk assessment and decision making, and most importantly they need to acquire social skills that allow them to adhere to their decisions even in social contexts that exert pressures against those decisions. AIDS education in schools should be a major aspect of policies for preventing HIV infection.

Community programmes

Just as schools are an appropriate context for encouraging preventive behaviours in young people, so community groups and local social networks are appropriate for other groups. Rather than aiming for educational messages suitable for all, which will inevitably be unsuccessful, a social-marketing approach can stratify groups and develop messages that are tailored to the needs, interests and existing knowledge and beliefs of specific groups and communities (Lefebvre and Flora 1988). Within a community there is then the possibility of adoption of new ideas or practices that can spread by social diffusion. A model derived from communication studies (Rogers 1987) predicts that the adoption of new ideas such as 'safer sex' takes time. Following introduction of the innovation, the time course of its adoption is influenced by the way in which it is perceived and the means available for its transmission – can it be advertised by media or does its spread depend upon interpersonal communication? Is there sufficient time available to allow its effectiveness to become confirmed or will it be rejected? And is the innovation compatible with the social norms that exist within that community? The characteristics of the community, its social structures and social norms, will determine the response to the innovation and whether it becomes adopted by the majority within the community. Each community will differ, and advocates of innovations should take account of this and present their messages accordingly. It may be that particular communities require special initiatives, for example prisons, and it may be that aspects of a community could become more involved in promoting educational messages, for example the work-place, trade unions, health clinics and Church organizations.

THE ECOLOGY OF AIDS

It is important to appreciate that though some groups are overrepresented in the statistics on AIDS, there are no high-risk groups, only high-risk behaviours. The key to preventing AIDS is changing behaviours. Many of the research studies on AIDS have focused on investigating individuals' attitudes, knowledge and beliefs, but though these are important variables in models of behaviour change, they do not act in isolation. Perceptions of risk, the illusion of invulnerability can be significant obstacles to change. In addition, decision making does not occur in isolation – it involves social influences and social comparisons also, and these will affect behaviour. It must also be appreciated that patterns of transmission of HIV are not identical across different countries (Piot *et al.* 1988) and interventions to limit the spread of HIV should reflect this fact. Unfortunately, because much of the research upon HIV/AIDS has come from the USA and Western Europe, health-promotion messages often reflect the patterns of transmission seen in those countries, even when as for some African countries those messages may be incorrect or inappropriate (Hubley 1988; Pitts and Jackson 1989). International programmes that are sensitive to cross-cultural differences and similarities and the ecologies of different countries are needed for effective world-wide strategies against AIDS.

Several studies have reported that, despite awareness about AIDS and knowledge of the transmission of HIV, the behaviours associated with risk of HIV infection are not changing. For example, a telephone survey of teenagers in Massachusetts found that only 15 per cent of sexually active respondents had changed their sexual behaviour as a result of AIDS and most of these reported being more selective in their choice of partner as the preventive change adopted. Only 10 per cent reported using condoms (Strunin and Hingson 1987). Other studies of young heterosexuals have found similar lack of intent amongst this group to alter behaviour by adopting precautions against HIV (Baldwin and Baldwin 1988; Turner *et al.* 1988). Despite this there is cause for some optimism since other studies do indicate that risk behaviours can be changed, but to be successful, interventions must become more sensitive to the characteristics of target groups and their own particular social conditions. Because of the nature of HIV transmission, by sexual intercourse or by injecting drugs, interventions clearly cannot expect to eliminate all transmission. They can only work to reduce the risk of transmission as far as possible.

In considering the risks associated with injecting drug use, it is not enough just to consider the drug habits of ivdus. Interventions for risk reduction must also understand the sociology of their drug use and provide counselling advice on sexual practices. This will depend on the user's gender, status, whether single or in a relationship, his/her source of money to finance the drug habit and so on (Mulleady and Sher 1989). Ivdus are not a homogeneous group. Different users will require differing assistance to reduce their personal risks of HIV infection. It must not be assumed that there is, or can be, a single solution or set of guidelines that will be effective for all ivdus.

Once HIV exists within a community, then, the local conditions within the social and environmental parameters of that community will determine the spread and prevalence within the community. As discussed earlier, ecological factors can account for the situation in the UK where there is a much higher seroprevalence of HIV in some Scottish cities than others. Similar factors may explain why, in 1987, two American cities both experiencing drug use show very different patterns of HIV infection. In New York City seroprevalence is more than 50 per cent among the clinical population of ivdus; yet in San Francisco the equivalent figure is around 15 per cent (Watters 1989). Watters suggests that although needle sharing occurs in both cities, there are particular ecological factors in New York City that encourage the use of 'shooting galleries' which present such extreme risks that their use is predictive of HIV infection. The social conditions that encourage use of shooting galleries do not exist in San Francisco and needle sharing occurs within more localized and stable social networks.

A further ecological factor is indicated by the differences in HIV prevalence that exist between different ethnic groups in the USA. Studies suggest that Hispanic and black ivdus are at greater risk than white counterparts (Peterson and Bakeman 1989). Why should this be so? It has been suggested that it might depend upon some genetic susceptibility to the virus but it is more likely that it reflects the isolation of these ethnic communities and their associated relative social and economic deprivations, for example in health resources and educational attainment. In addition, the particular social representations that exist within these communities, including the perception that AIDS is a homosexual problem and the associated homophobia within black and Hispanic communities, act as obstacles to the adoption of precautions by heterosexuals (Friedman *et al.* 1987).

More culturally sensitive intervention programmes are needed which recognize the differences and seek to devise appropriate educational strategies and messages that are compatible with the social representations that exist within those communities (Schilling *et al.* 1989).

There are indications that local community-based interventions can be effective in reducing risk. Watters (1989) reports that in San Francisco there have been changes in behaviour that are attributable to community-based initiatives such as use of 'outreach' workers to distribute condoms, bleach for sterilizing works, and as agents to disseminate information about the risks for AIDS and effective precautions that can be taken without abstinence from drugs. They are likely to be more sensitive to local ecological factors that exist for a given community. He argues that effective interventions of this type must be preceded by ethnographic techniques to understand 'the social organization of drug use'. Higher-order policies that may include decriminalization of aspects of drug use such as the possession of syringes and needles, in order to eliminate the existence of shooting galleries, will assist the work of local interventions.

There are also indications that sexual behaviours can be changed. Several reports have noted that homosexual groups have altered their sexual behaviours towards safer sex by reducing (though it must be admitted not eliminating) high-risk activities such as receptive anal intercourse and by increased use of condoms during sexual activity, and by reducing the number of sexual partners (Becker and Joseph 1988; Golombok *et al.* 1989). Such changes within gay communities appear to have arisen as innovations that have been adopted through social diffusion as a result of the well-organized social structure of those communities. In many instances the changes had begun to occur before public education campaigns had begun through education within communities. There remain problems, however, since risk reduction is not practised by all: some individuals continue to engage in high-risk activities (Golombok *et al.* 1989) and further research is required to identify why some individuals comply with messages for risk reduction while others do not. In addition, risk reduction must be maintained over time, but some individuals who generally practise safer sex will on occasions fail to adhere to those guidelines and increase their personal risks. Such recidivism is commonly encountered in other types of health behaviours and the reasons underlying it must also be investigated further in longitudinal studies. Once achieved, risk reduction must be maintained and interventions must aim not only at modifying behaviour but also at supporting and maintaining desirable behaviours once adopted.

CONCLUSIONS

The emergence of AIDS has crystallized for health psychology the central issues of the precaution-adoption process. In the absence of any effective medical solution, behavioural strategies must be devised that promote modification of behaviours for risk reduction and maintain those behaviours once adopted. It has become apparent that little is known about the determinants of risk reduction, but what is clear is that educational messages must be sensitive to the ecological balance of specific communities and groups and to the particular patterns of transmission of HIV that exist in different countries. Studies of gay communities and ivdus have shown that behaviour change is possible though its long-term stability has yet to be demonstrated. To persuade others in the population that they too must change their behaviours for risk reduction will require innovative programmes, beginning with education for young people and the establishment of new patterns of social responsibility. The success of the venture will depend upon the concerted efforts of behavioural scientists, health educators and politicians too.

Chapter 11

Decision making for contraception and abortion

Mary Boyle

for something like three-quarters of that part of the professional abortion-ist's business that derives from urban American married women, he can thank the birth controllers and the current imperfections in the technique of their art.

(Pearl 1939)

it appears to be common practice that women will resort to abortion (whether legal or illegal) if the contraceptive method they are using fails.

(Potts *et al.* 1977)

If these statements conveyed a full picture of the relationship between contraceptive use and unwanted pregnancy, psychologists would have little to contribute to the area. For the statements imply that, if an unwanted pregnancy occurs, attention should be directed to the method of contra-ception and not to the method of use. There is, however, abundant evidence that this picture is incomplete. In spite of the availability of reliable contraception, often at little or no financial cost, the rate of legal termination of pregnancy amongst women aged 15–44 in England and Wales has risen each year since 1983 (OPCS 1987). Ryan and Sweeney (1980) reported that 63 per cent of a sample of pregnant teenagers claimed to have made a conscious decision not to use contraceptives, although less than a third of the sample intended to become pregnant. Similarly, Braken *et al.* (1978) found that 68 per cent of young, unmarried women having abortions had not used any contraceptive around the time of conception. Using a wider age range, Allen (1981) found that 39 per cent of a sample of women granted terminations reported either never having used contraception or not having used it at the time of conception. There are, moreover, several reasons for supposing that these figures may overestimate the relationship between the desire to avoid pregnancy and efficient contraceptive use. First, some of the figures are based on the self-reports of women seeking or granted abortions. If abortion is not available on demand, then it would be surprising if some women did not report using contraception when they had not, in the hope that this might increase their chances of obtaining a termination. They might then maintain this report if questioned afterwards by researchers. Second, figures for use or non-use of contraceptives tell us little about the *pattern* of use: was the pill taken every day? Was the cap used with a spermicide? Was the condom put on before any contact was made? And, third, Ryan and Sweeney's report that around 30 per cent of pregnant teenagers wished to become pregnant seems rather high in comparison with a figure of 10 per cent from a national sample of sexually active teenagers (Zelnick and Kantner 1977). It is possible that some of Ryan and Sweeney's sample, having not used contraception and then found themselves pregnant, decided in retrospect that the pregnancy was intended.

What is clear from these figures is that the relationship between contraceptive use and the desire to achieve or avoid pregnancy is not straight-forward. This chapter will consider some of the factors which are related to the decision to use, or not use, contraception. It will also examine the processes surrounding decisions about the termination of pregnancy. Finally, the chapter will look at patterns of contraceptive use following abortion.

Before this is done, however, there is a feature of the literature which is worth noting, and that is that the majority of research subjects are female. Indeed, an alien reading some of the research would have to conclude that men had nothing to do with either contraception or conception. One possible reason for this bias is that women are more likely than men to form a 'captive' subject pool at family-planning clinics, pregnancy advisory services and termination clinics, or at mother and baby homes. As Chilman (1985) has pointed out, however, another plausible reason is that contraception and the avoidance of pregnancy are, in our society, seen as the responsibility of women and that the structure of research is a reflection of this view. She suggests that this selective attention to women places an unfair burden on them and makes it more difficult for men to share the responsibility for contraception, even if they wished to do so. Similarly, Schinke (1984) has suggested that, because males are less victimized by pregnancy, they are forgotten in most research directed at the prevention of unwanted pregnancy. It is perhaps not quite as bad as this, but of fourteen studies aimed at encouraging teenagers to use contraception, and reviewed by Beck and Davies (1987), seven were aimed exclusively at females and only one exclusively at males.

DECISION MAKING AND CONTRACEPTION

Much of the research into contraceptive decision making has proceeded outside any particular theoretical framework. This is not necessarily a disadvantage, as valuable descriptive data may be gathered and can form the basis of theoretical models. Some of the models which have been suggested have not been subjected to rigorous evaluation. Some, too, such as the health belief model (Becker 1974; Rosenstock 1974), were developed in other health areas, and their applicability to contraceptive decision making is debatable

(Fisher 1977; Herold 1983). The models which have been suggested range from those which emphasize individual factors, such as emotional state or personality characteristics, to those which stress situational and social variables (for brief reviews see Morrison 1985, and Beck and Davies 1987). No attempt will be made here to repeat these reviews. Rather, one of the models, the Subjective Expected Utility Model suggested by Luker (1975, 1977) and Beach *et al.* (1979), will be used as a framework for the presentation of research findings.

This model suggests that whether people will perform a particular behaviour depends on their evaluation of the outcomes and on their expectation of the likelihood of any particular outcome. The behaviour chosen will be that which has the greatest subjective expected utility. As applied by Luker to contraceptive decision making, the model has four elements: the assignment of costs and benefits to contraceptive use; the assignment of costs and benefits to pregnancy; the assignment of probabilities to becoming pregnant and, finally, the assignment of probabilities to the termination of pregnancy. The model emphasizes the social and environmental factors which may influence the decision to use contraceptives. This fits well with the idea of contraceptive use as self-regulation, i.e. an example of behaviour which may involve short-term costs for the sake of long-term gains. As Mischel (1974) has demonstrated, there is considerable evidence that situational factors can strongly influence self-regulatory behaviour. In line with this, Luker explicitly rejects the idea that certain types of people consistently do or do not use contraceptives and the model suggests that, for any one person, usage may vary considerably in different situations or at different stages in life. The factors suggested as having significance by Luker do repeatedly appear as elements in people's accounts of their contraceptive decision making and manipulation of some of them appears to alter the likelihood of contraceptive use. Finally, the model is comprehensive and incorporates many elements of other models, particularly the health belief model and Fishbein's attitude model (Jaccard and Davidson 1972; Pagel and Davidson 1984). The same framework can usefully be used to examine both female and male contraceptive use, although, of course, the values assigned to the elements in the decision-making process may differ considerably for the two groups.

The costs and benefits of using contraceptives

Luker (1975) has suggested that many researchers assume that the benefits of using contraception outweigh the costs and that the costs of non-use outweigh the benefits. The probable benefits of use are obvious: the avoidance of unwanted pregnancy and, for some methods, the avoidance of sexually transmitted diseases. The costs, however, may be less obvious and will vary with people, situations and methods. The costs which appear to contribute to non-use, or the use of unreliable methods, can be divided into a number of types.

Side-effects

Cobliner *et al.* (1975) and Washington *et al.* (1983) found that complaints about side-effects were frequently associated with young women's failure to adhere to a contraceptive regime. These women had been prescribed oral contraceptives and it is these, and also intra-uterine devices, which are most strongly associated with negative side-effects. The apparent relationship between worry over side-effects and non-use of contraception is of particular concern when considered alongside Allen's (1981) finding that many women who obtain birth-control services from their general practitioners are offered only oral contraceptives. Allen noted, too, that a number of the younger women in her sample of those seeking terminations reported that they did not want to use the pill because of possible health risks. They saw other methods as unreliable, however, and therefore used no method at all.

It is not clear from these studies where the women obtained information about side-effects, or how accurate it was. Information about risks, however, may be given in a form which is extremely difficult to apply to individuals. A statement such as, for example, 'the pill increases risk of breast cancer by 50 per cent', may entirely misinform women of the risk for any individual. Women may therefore rely on their own experience, the experience of friends, or on media reports of individual cases of the assumed consequences of contraceptive use.

It appears that women may be expected to endure more side-effects from contraceptives than men. Reading, Cox and Sledmere (1982) have commented on the far greater concern surrounding the effect of a male chemical contraceptive on sexual functioning than was apparent during the development of female oral contraceptives, in spite of indications that they could affect women's sex drive.

Problems in obtaining contraceptives

It is now relatively easy to obtain condoms and spermicides. Obtaining other contraceptives, however, can involve considerable time, effort and anxiety for women. In a study of women who had attended family-planning clinics, Allen (1981) found that a substantial proportion said that they had been nervous or even terrified before their first visit. Some were pleasantly surprised and found the staff friendly and sympathetic; others were dismayed by long waiting times, complicated appointments systems, examinations and lack of privacy. Some found the experience so negative that they never returned, although it is not known whether this led them to abandon contraception entirely or to use less reliable methods. It is perhaps not surprising that it is young, single women who appear to be most vulnerable to these negative experiences, although the mothers of young children were most critical of the lengthy waiting times. These results are particularly dismaying when it is considered that it is only at these clinics that women – and men – are routinely offered the whole range of contraceptive methods, and can discuss problems in using them.

Social sanctions

Morrison (1985) has suggested that part of young people's negative attitudes towards contraception involves the anticipation of guilt feelings and fears of others, particularly one's family, knowing about contraceptive use. Allen's (1981) findings strongly support this. It was single women under 20 who were most likely to report high levels of anxiety before their first clinic visit, and who were most likely to mention anonymity as a reason for obtaining supplies from a family-planning clinic rather than from their general practitioner. Similarly, Allen's sample of those aged under 20 who were seeking abortions had made far less use of family-planning clinics than had the older women. These young women reported that they were too shy, afraid of being turned away or lectured at or of the lack of privacy, to use these services. Sanctions for using contraceptives may also be anticipated from peers and partners. Finkel and Finkel (1975), for example, found that over a third of their male teenage sample would not want their friends to know that they had used condoms, while two-thirds of teenage subjects in a study by Freeman *et al.* (1980) agreed that a girl would feel 'used' if her partner knew she used contraception. It is difficult to know what this figure means, however, because a similar proportion also agreed that 'A boy respects a girl who uses birth control.' The strength and extent of these sanctions will vary in different cultures. Contraception use is, for example, explicitly forbidden or, at least, regarded as sinful, by the Roman Catholic Church, although the rhythm method may be excepted. In other cultures, multiple pregnancies may be valued for economic reasons, because of a high infant and child mortality rate, or as a sign of a man's virility.

The anticipation of sanctions for using contraception may be related to the finding that unwanted pregnancy and unplanned sexual activity are often associated. Zelnick and Shah (1983), for example, found that both male and female teenagers were more likely to use a reliable method of contraception if their first intercourse was planned. It seems, however, that many young people prefer not to plan sexual encounters and give as a reason for negative attitudes to contraception that it makes sex seem pre-planned and less natural and spontaneous. (Morrison 1985; Schinke 1984). It may be that some people derive more enjoyment from unplanned sexual activity and do not arrange contraception for this reason, but this is unlikely to be the whole story. Certainly it does not fit with the often given advice in agony columns to revive a flagging sex life by planning and anticipating sexual encounters! It seems more likely that people who do not belong to groups in which regular sexual activity is sanctioned may be reluctant to be *seen* to be anticipating sexual encounters by carrying or using contraception. In other words, for many people it is not so much that sanctions operate against contraception, but against the sexual activity which its use implies.

Finally, recent legal discussions ('Fighting it in the Streets', Channel 4 Television, 27 June 1989) have highlighted an additional sanction which may operate against women who carry condoms: the possession of condoms may apparently be used as corroborating evidence in support of a charge of soliciting.

Interpersonal anxiety

Schinke (1984) has suggested that one cost associated with contraceptive use is having to discuss the matter with a partner, health professional or even just mention it to a shop assistant. The problem of discussion with partners is particularly severe with methods such as the condom, withdrawal and, possibly, the cap, which are likely at the very least to be commented on during sexual activity. It is perhaps not surprising, then, that anxiety about heterosexual relationships should have been found to correlate negatively with use of effective contraception at first intercourse (Bruch and Haynes 1987), or that embarrassment about birth control should be related to less reliable use (Herold 1981).

In an attempt to deal with this problem, Schinke designed a number of programmes to teach young people the interpersonal skills needed to discuss contraception. The subjects were asked to provide information about the specific problems they had encountered, and the skills were taught in those contexts. At follow-up these subjects, in comparison with a control group, were more consistently using contraceptives and were more likely to have used a reliable method at last intercourse.

Costs, benefits and the AIDS campaigns

In theory at least, the cost–benefit equation for one type of contraceptive has altered considerably with the risk of HIV infection. An analysis of people's response to this risk may help to clarify some of the processes underlying contraceptive use in general.

In a study of 234 male and 91 female teenagers living in the San Francisco area, Kegeles *et al.* (1988) found that the large majority of subjects agreed that using a method which prevents both pregnancy and sexually transmitted diseases was of great value and importance. In spite of these perceived benefits, however, only 2.1 per cent of females and 8.2 per cent of males reported using condoms each time they had intercourse during the study year.

In addition, males' intentions to use condoms decreased during the study, while females remained at the very low level. Unfortunately, the authors did not collect data on the use of other contraceptives, so it is not clear what benefits would have accrued to this sample had they used condoms. What may be the case, however, is that the sample saw themselves as at low risk of HIV infection and saw condom use as having costs which outweighed the perceived benefits. One cost, of course, is interpersonal anxiety and condoms are probably the least likely of any contraceptive method to be used without discussion. Interviews with women (*Independent*, 14 February 1989) who had attempted to persuade their partners to use condoms, usually without success, highlight sexual sensation. The women's accounts, however, also suggest that some men do not know how to use condoms, so that they may have had no direct experience of their effect on sensation and may have been trying to avoid embarrassment. The accounts also emphasize the importance of interpersonal skills in discussing contraceptive use. Some of the women reported feeling unable to assert themselves or to resist their partners' implications that they would be responsible for reducing the men's pleasure. Thus, many social processes may be involved in sexual intimacy, including negotiation, bargaining coercion and compliance. Each will have implications for the willingness of one or both partners to adopt an effective contraceptive method.

The costs of practising contraception may be immediate and concrete. The benefits are in the future (when it is clear that pregnancy has not happened) and uncertain (pregnancy might not have happened even without contraception, or might happen even with it). Under these conditions we should expect inconsistent self-regulation. Given the potentially high costs of using contraception, the values assigned to the remaining factors in the equation become extremely important.

Costs and benefits of pregnancy

There have been few detailed studies of the relationship between the perception of pregnancy and contraceptive decision making, although, as might be expected, a positive relationship has been found between young women's educational and career aspirations and the consistent use of contraception (Herold 1983; Morrison 1985).

Smith *et al.* (1984) compared pregnant teenagers who claimed that their pregnancies were desired with a group whose pregnancies were unwanted. The first group had more positive expectations for improved relationships with their families and friends after delivery. But the relationship between perception of pregnancy and contraceptive use is not clear, because the patterns of non-use were similar in the two groups. This raises the question of whether the first group's failure to use contraceptives was for quite other reasons than the desire to become pregnant, and whether they only later anticipated or experienced benefits to make the pregnancy desirable. Ryan and Sweeney (1980) studied a sample of pregnant teenagers, most of whom had not used contraceptives. Some 47 per cent of them claimed to feel 'happy' or 'OK' about their pregnancy. Only 10 per cent claimed that their parents were 'sorry' or 'upset' about the pregnancy. Some 88 per cent expected to complete their high-school education, although 38 per cent claimed that either they alone, or they and the father, were going to look after the child. As with the previous study, however, it is difficult to know what was the relationship between contraceptive use and these rather positive views of pregnancy.

In both these studies, subjects had not yet given birth and, had not had the opportunity to match the anticipated benefits of having a child with the reality. But it is, presumably, the anticipated costs and benefits which operate at the time of contraceptive decision making and it is not difficult to see how these might differ from reality. But even if the anticipated costs are high, contraception might still not be used in some situations. For example, the costs of obtaining and using contraception might be seen as even higher or cues signalling the likely outcome of unprotected sex may be absent. The influence of the anticipated costs and benefits of pregnancy will also be modified by the values placed on the final two aspects of Luker's equation.

The probability of becoming pregnant

A number of researchers have noted that the belief that pregnancy will not happen is frequently offered as a reason for not using contraception. (Goldsmith et al. 1972; Morrison 1985; Washington et al. 1983). In fact, it is estimated that although the overall probability of pregnancy resulting from any one act of intercourse is about 0.04 (Bongaarts 1976), the probability of a woman becoming pregnant during a year of unprotected intercourse is 0.8 (Potter 1963). Morrison (1985) has noted the interesting finding that adolescents often overestimate the overall probability of pregnancy from a single act of intercourse, giving figures ranging from 0.17 to 0.50. Cvetkovich and Grote (1981) have suggested that any estimate which is less than one may be seen as low or uncertain or may encourage women to see themselves as sub-fertile if they do not become pregnant. For any particular couple, estimates of the likelihood of pregnancy may depend on their prior experience of the outcome of unprotected intercourse and their beliefs about the timing of and circumstances surrounding their sexual activity.

Morrison (1985) has reviewed studies of teenagers' knowledge of the risk periods for conception and found that fewer than half the subjects in these studies were able to answer correctly. Knowledge was related to age, social class, race and sexual experience, with attendance at sex-education classes appearing only as a weak predictor. In addition, many young people appear to hold beliefs which encourage the idea that pregnancy is unlikely. Kantner and Zelnick (1972), for example, reported that 40 per cent of their national sample of 15 to 19 year olds believed that fertility does not begin at the menarche. About a third of Sorensen's (1973) sample agreed with the statement that 'If a girl truly doesn't want a baby, she won't get pregnant, even though she may have sex without taking any birth control precautions.' Some 10 per cent of a sample studied by Cvetkovich and Grote (1983) did not believe that pregnancy was possible the first time a woman had intercourse, while Allen (1981) noted that a number of her sample of women seeking abortions claimed that they had not thought they would become pregnant so soon after starting to have sex.

It would be easy to conclude from these findings that young people have unprotected sex because they lack knowledge of the risks. But there is no logical reason why lack of knowledge should lead to underestimates of risks, and unprotected sex, rather than overestimates and overprotected sex. The beliefs are, in fact, notably self-serving in that they allow the performance of a wanted activity without incurring any immediate costs. There is no reason to suppose that if these beliefs were challenged, another equally self-serving set would not emerge to replace them as long as, for some people, the costs of using contraception remain high.

The probability of the reversal of pregnancy

There has been little research into how women, or men, perceive the likelihood of an unwanted pregnancy's being terminated, or how this might affect the decision to use contraception. The likelihood of being offered a National Health Service termination appears to vary considerably across health regions (OPCS 1987) and it is difficult to know how an individual woman would be able to predict whether she would be successful. Allen (1981) noted that the women in her sample had been unable to judge how their general practitioner or consultant was going to react to their request, and that the women knew very little about the abortion services beforehand. Hamill and Ingram (1974: 232), however, concluded that 'the bulk of women seeking an abortion achieve their end if not in one centre, then in another; if not under the NHS, then privately'.

Conclusions

It is notoriously difficult to collect information from any group about their sexual behaviour and the data on contraceptive use must be interpreted with some caution. Much of the data, for example, consists of self-reports given after contraception has or has not been used. It is therefore difficult to know how accurate usage figures are or, indeed, what 'usage' might mean to different people. It is also possible that some of the reasons given for non-use are *post hoc* rationalizations which had little to do with the actual decision not to use contraception, or are given as the more socially acceptable reasons.

Nevertheless, the results do suggest that, for some people, using contraception may involve considerable costs and that the mere availability of reliable methods, or knowledge of their benefits, will not be sufficient to reduce the rates of unwanted pregnancy.

DECISION MAKING AND THE TERMINATION OF PREGNANCY

As Adler (1982) has pointed out, abortion is unusual among medical procedures in that it involves legal, political, economic, theological and moral as well as psychological issues which impinge on the woman undergoing the procedure. That this is indeed the case is made clear by an analysis of the decision-making processes surrounding abortion. This section will briefly examine these from the point of view of social policy, of the woman seeking a termination and of the professionals who decide whether she should have one. Finally, the section will return to contraception, to look at its use after abortion.

Abortion and social policy

In England and Wales, under the terms of the Abortion Act of 1967, a woman may be granted an abortion if, in the opinion of two registered medical practitioners, either of two conditions is fulfilled. The first is that the continuation of pregnancy would involve a risk to the life of the pregnant woman or injury to her physical or mental health or to that of any existing children, greater than if the pregnancy were terminated. The second condition is that there is a substantial risk that if the child were born, it would suffer such physical or mental abnormality as to be seriously handicapped. The Act also stipulates that in determining whether the continuation of pregnancy would involve such risks to health, account may be taken of the woman's actual or reasonably foreseeable environment.

Radcliffe Richards (1982) and Watters (1980) have examined some of the problems of this form of legislation and of the assumptions which appear to underlie it. Watters, for example, has pointed out that mortality and morbidity rates following a first or second trimester termination are lower than those following childbirth. He also points out that those few studies which have followed up women who were refused abortion suggest that this group fares worse on a variety of psychological and behavioural measures, than do those granted abortions. These two sets of evidence, Watters suggests, mean that anyone who prevents a woman having a safe, legal abortion, if that is what she wishes, is placing her in a situation where, statistically, her physical and mental health are at greater risk than if she is allowed to have an abortion. But what would be effectively abortion on demand is, presumably, not the intention of the legislation and, apparently, is not the way in which it operates.

It might be objected that although the population risk of refusing termination is greater than granting it, the risk to an individual woman might not be. This argument, however, is problematic because there are no rules which allow us accurately to predict, early in pregnancy, what complications might arise in childbirth or how happy or unhappy any particular woman might be with her situation in a few years' time, as compared to her state had the termination decision been different.

Radcliffe Richards has pointed out a further complication of this form of legislation: it is that it conflates two types of decision which ought to be clearly separated. The first is a *descriptive* statement that, if abortion is granted or refused, certain consequences are likely. The second is a *prescriptive* statement as to whether these consequences justify the sacrifice of a child. Radcliffe Richards suggests that, even if we assume that the first type of decision lies within the competence of a medical practitioner, there is no good reason to suppose that the second type does also.

It is not clear to what extent beliefs about the harmful effects of abortion have been influential in framing this legislation. Adler (1982) suggests that research on abortion, or, at least, the conclusions drawn from it, have mirrored historical and social trends in attitudes and legislation. From the 1940s to the 1960s, when legislation was generally restrictive, it was often concluded that abortion was likely to result in psychological disturbance. It may be, however, that some subjects in this research had undergone illegal abortions in sub-standard facilities and that their reactions to the termination were confounded by this. More recently, it has proved extremely difficult to find data to support the idea of abortion as a harmful experience (Adler 1982; Brewer 1977; Greer *et al.* 1976; Lask 1975; WHO 1978). This is not to suggest that some women do not suffer afterwards. It has, however, been found that a negative outcome tends to be associated with, among other variables, lack of social support and negative attitudes of family, and also with terminations carried out for medical reasons. These negative consequences, however, must be considered in relation to the possible negative results of having the termination refused.

Decision making by the woman

Allen (1981) reported that 73 per cent of her sample of women who had had abortions had visited their general practitioners before the eighth week of pregnancy, and over 90 per cent before the eleventh week. The majority of these women had already made a definite decision before the consultation. Both Allen (1981) and Braken *et al.* (1978) emphasize the importance of discussions with friends, relatives and partners, rather than with medical professionals, in the decision to have an abortion. Braken *et al.* suggest that, having reached a tentative decision, the woman then seeks support by discussing the decision with people who might agree with her. Particular importance may be attached to role models – for example, to other women who have had abortions without apparent ill-effect. Although a decision may be reached early in the pregnancy, the woman may still be ambivalent. Braken *et al.* found that about 40 per cent of each of their samples of young women who terminated or continued their pregnancies, changed their minds at least once in the early stages. Allen reported that, although more than half of her sample never had any doubts about wanting a termination, there was greater ambivalence among very young women and divorced and separated women. Among the young women, this seemed to be associated with what Allen calls 'romantic notions' of what it would be like to have a child. The ambivalence may also be reflected in the greater contraceptive risk-taking which Allen noted in both of these groups. This could, however, be related to unplanned sexual activity.

Smetana and Adler (1979) studied the decision-making process using Fishbein's model of behavioural intention (Fishbein 1972). This model predicts that the intention to perform an act, and its actual performance, are a multiplicative function of the attitude towards performing the behaviour in a particular situation, of beliefs about what others expect to be done and of the person's motivation to comply with these expectations. Smetana and Adler found that the intention to have, or not to have, an abortion, stated before the results of a pregnancy test were available, correlated very highly with actual behaviour. In line with the model's predictions, the intention to have an abortion was significantly related to beliefs about the expectations of significant others (mother, partner, clergyman) and to beliefs about the consequences of having a child. Thus, women choosing either action claimed that others wanted them to follow their chosen alternative. The women choosing or rejecting abortion, however, did not differ in their stated motivation to comply with these expectations, with the exception that women choosing an abortion claimed to be more strongly motivated to comply with the expectations of female friends. The two groups also saw the consequences of having a child in very different terms: those who chose abortion stressed the burden and long-term commitment of child rearing, while those who continued their pregnancies stressed their emotional well-being and fulfilment. The groups did not differ in their moral attitudes to abortion.

These results support Allen's finding that the decision to have an abortion is made relatively quickly; indeed, in Smetana and Adler's study, the women did not yet know for certain if they were pregnant. The results also emphasize the perceived role of partners, family and friends in the decision-making process. The results do not, however, offer direct evidence about the nature of this role, as no data were collected from these people.

Decision making by professionals

The majority of abortions in England and Wales are carried out because it is claimed that continuation of the pregnancy would involve risk of injury to the physical or mental health of the pregnant woman greater than if the pregnancy were terminated. It appears that it is the mental health of the mother which is thought to be at risk in the vast majority of these cases, because 'neurotic disorders' or 'personality disorders' are the conditions most frequently given as justification for the termination (OPCS 1987). This means that the majority of abortions (and, presumably, the majority of refusals) involve doctors' judgements about the woman's likely psychological state, taking into account her 'actual or foreseeable environment'. It was pointed out earlier, however, that there is no set of rules by which these judgements might be made, nor have representative data been provided on their reliability. This places those who must make the judgements in a very difficult position. As Radcliffe Richards (1982) has pointed out, it also leaves the way open for the operation of personal beliefs.

Qualitative data presented by Allen (1981) emphasize this problem. Although she found that many of the general practitioners in her sample referred for consultation all women who requested a termination, some did not. One commented that:

> They're entitled to the benefit of the law. I've given up moral judgement. If it's for a reason like they have a heavy mortgage etc., I forget to write sometimes. I say, 'Too late, love, sorry. It's the hospital appointment system. You'll have to have the baby.'
>
> (Allen 1981: 71)

Most of the consultants interviewed claimed that they very rarely refused to perform abortions, but it was clear from Allen's interviews with general practitioners that certain consultants were avoided when referrals were made, presumably because they were less likely to agree to perform abortions.

In a more systematic study of the variables which influence the decision to allow or refuse termination, Hamill and Ingram (1974) examined the decisions reached in 132 referrals for psychiatric opinion on termination. A questionnaire covering general information, clinical and social findings, and contraceptive history was completed by each consultant at the time of examination. Some 64 per cent of the women were granted a termination and 36 per cent were refused. The questionnaire data for these two groups were then compared. Members of the group granted terminations were significantly more likely to be older, married, already to have children, to have claimed to use contraception regularly, and to be rated as showing psychiatric symptoms. There was no significant difference in the overall number of social problems rated in the two groups, but the women refused terminations were significantly more likely to have been deserted by their partners. Some 52 per cent of the women who were granted abortions agreed to be sterilized. The finding here that women who claimed to use contraception regularly were more likely to be granted an abortion is in line with Allen's (1981) report that women who had been 'unlucky' because of contraceptive failure were usually granted a termination without difficulty, and were sympathetically treated by their doctors.

In introducing their research, Hamill and Ingram (1974: 119) noted that

The assessing doctor tends to show bias by labelling psychiatric disorder in those he recommends and vice versa. We hoped to diminish this by avoiding formal diagnoses on the questionnaire and asking instead about the presence or absence of specific symptoms.

There is, however, no reason to suppose that any biases in psychiatric diagnoses would not equally apply to judgements about the presence of the 'specific symptoms' rated on the questionnaire which included 'emotional immaturity' and 'personality disorder'. Hamill and Ingram's results do raise the question of whether those women who were granted termination were somehow seen as more 'deserving' and of whether this judgement might have biased judgements of symptoms. It is, however, very difficult to research this question because the details of doctors' decision making are not officially recorded, nor are the numbers or characteristics of those refused terminations. The high proportion of women who had terminations and were also sterilized is particularly striking. This figure can be compared with the report of the Lane Committee (1974) which found that almost half of all married women granted National Health Service abortions had also been sterilized, although the overall figure for all women granted terminations was 15 per cent. This proportion is now considerably lower: in 1986, for example, it was 4.5 per cent for all women granted termination. A higher proportion of National Health Service abortions, however, were accompanied by sterilization than were non-NHS abortions: 7.8 per cent versus 1.9 per cent (OPCS 1986). It is not clear whether this reflects a different population structure for the two sectors, or a different professional decision-making process.

Contraception following abortion

It seems reasonable to suppose that the values assigned to various elements in contraceptive decision making would alter following the termination of a pregnancy, although we cannot assume that this will always lead to efficient use of contraception. A number of studies have examined the extent of women's use of contraception after abortion. Beard *et al.* (1974) found that 81 per cent of their sample reported using some form of contraception one to two years after a termination, and that some of the remainder wished to become pregnant. This figure compares favourably with that of 41 per cent who claimed to be using contraception previously. Using a sample of 10–18 year olds, Abrams (1985) reported that 79 per cent of those followed up for two years after a termination were using reliable methods of contraception. Lask's (1975) figures are much lower: of a sample of forty-one women followed up six months after the abortions, sixteen were regularly using some form of contraception and five had been sterilized. It is not clear, however, how many of the women were sexually active, nor whether any were trying to become pregnant.

These figures present similar problems of interpretation as those mentioned earlier: they are based on self-reports and give little indication of the pattern of use. Some researchers, however, have reported figures for requests for subsequent abortions. In Abrams's study, these were 7 per cent in the first year of follow-up and 11 per cent in the second. Rovinsky (1972) reported a rate of 5 per cent even with intensive advice about contraception though some requests for repeat abortions would be expected simply from rates of contraceptive failure.

Allen (1981) has noted that advice about contraception has apparently become standard practice following, or even prior to, abortion. As she points out, promises to use contraception may be used as part of a 'bargaining procedure' before the termination is carried out. There is, however, little evidence that this advice is based on an analysis of the factors which may influence a woman's – or her partner's – decision to use contraception. Rather, some of Allen's professional respondents appeared not to acknowledge the difficulties women might experience in obtaining and using contraception. One gynaecologist claimed that it was necessary to 'put the squeeze' on women before the termination because afterwards they 'don't give a damn'. One general practitioner spoke of a 'hard core' who 'like to live with the risk', while another claimed that women didn't experience two unwanted pregnancies 'unless they're hopeless'. This last comment was said by Allen to sum up the feelings of many respondents.

CONCLUSIONS

Psychological research on abortion has tended to emphasize the outcome of the procedure, in terms of 'psychiatric complications', or the psychological characteristics of women seeking abortions. It is, of course, important to know about the outcome of abortion and about the factors which influence it, provided that this research is matched by research on the outcome of refusals to grant terminations. But this implicitly pathological bias could lead to a relative neglect of other important aspects of the subject, particularly of the relationship between social attitudes and abortion legislation, of professional decision making and of the application of research on contraception use to post-abortion counselling. And the neglect of male subjects is notable: their attitudes and reactions to their partners' experiences are often unknown, while they do not appear to be expected to take any responsibility for contraception immediately after a termination. Future research needs to redress the balance and to place abortion in the wider social context in which it belongs.

Chapter 12

Essential hypertension

Keith Phillips

INTRODUCTION

Hypertension is a chronic disorder characterized by sustained elevation of blood pressure level (BPL). It may result from a specific physical cause such as renal failure, adrenal tumour or aortic disease, in which case the disorder is termed secondary hypertension. The treatment of secondary hypertension involves purely medical interventions. Temporary BPL elevations may be caused by the actions of some drugs or may occur during pregnancy. Chronic elevation of BPL is commonly not associated with any identifiable physical cause and in this instance the condition is termed primary or essential (meaning 'of unknown origin') hypertension. This chapter will be concerned solely with essential hypertension, whose treatment may involve pharmacological or behavioural methods, or both. (Further references to 'hypertension' should be understood as meaning essential hypertension.)

Hypertension is said to be asymptomatic, and although a variety of symptoms are reported by hypertensive patients such as headache, dizziness, fatigue and breathlessness, these are neither consistently reported nor exclusive to hypertension. It is reported that 20–25 per cent of the adult populations of the UK and USA exhibit hypertension to some degree. It represents a major threat to health since although itself asymptomatic, hypertension is a risk factor for other diseases including kidney failure and cardiovascular disorders such as myocardial infarction, congestive heart failure and cerebrovascular stroke (see Chapter 13). The objective of treating hypertension is to reduce the morbidity and mortality associated with renal and cardiovascular diseases of these types.

Definition of hypertension

The diagnosis of hypertension depends upon measurement of BPL within the arterial blood system. Blood circulates within a closed circulatory system and has to be forced around the system under pressure. Its movement within this system is determined by several haemodynamic factors, and the BPL within the arteries is a product of the cardiac output from the heart and the resistance to flow presented by peripheral blood vessels. Pressure varies according to the cycle of activity of the heart: peak pressure, which coincides with the contraction of the heart, is called systolic blood pressure and pressure reaches its minimum level in the arteries, the diastolic blood pressure, as the heart relaxes before its next contraction. Within populations, BPL shows a normal distribution and varies according to demographic factors including age, sex and ethnic origin. Within many populations, BPL shows a systematic increase with age, but this is not true of all populations, which suggests that age-related increases are not a direct function of ageing but reflect other, perhaps psychosocial, factors (Steptoe 1981).

Clinically hypertensive individuals are categorized according to the severity of their illness on the basis of either diastolic or systolic blood pressure (measured by the physical pressure unit of millimetres of mercury – mmHg). The precise cut-off points are arbitrary and vary between different classification systems but generally, individuals with systolic BPL greater than 140 mmHg or diastolic BPL greater than 90 mmHg are diagnosed as mild hypertensive. A systolic level greater than 160 mmHg or a diastolic level greater than 115 mmHg is classified as severe hypertension.

Elevation of either systolic or diastolic pressure is associated with greatly increased risk of cardiovascular and renal diseases (Kannel and Schatzkin 1983). Moreover, the association between pressure and risk is continuous, i.e. the higher the pressure the greater the risk (Kaplan 1982); thus, any reduction of BPL is beneficial in reducing the risk.

FACTORS ASSOCIATED WITH HYPERTENSION

Several factors have been identified as being involved in the aetiology of hypertension. They include genetic factors (individuals whose parents are hypertensive have a greatly increased risk), dietary factors such as total caloric intake and intake of particular substances including salt and alcohol, behavioural factors such as exercise, situational factors that collectively may be regarded as stressors, and perhaps also personality styles or traits. There are undoubtedly complex interactions between these various factors (see Steptoe 1981).

Genetic factors

There is considerable evidence from population studies and studies of families that genetic factors are involved in the development of hypertension (WHO 1983). Within families it has been found that there is a significant resemblance between the BPL of first-degree adult relatives and between the BPL of mothers and their infants. Studies of twins indicate that monozygotic twins have BPLs that are more highly correlated than are those of dizygotic twins. Further evidence comes from the finding that there is not a significant correlation between BPLs of adopted children and either their adoptive parents or their adoptive siblings, despite the fact that they share the same environment, diet and so forth. Within populations it is found that BPL shows a continuous distribution, which is indicative of multifactorial determination. It is generally accepted that though BPL cannot be inherited through transmission by a single gene, some form of polygenic inheritance is likely though the exact mode of inheritance has yet to be identified.

Though genetic factors may account for some of the variance in arterial pressure it does not account for all, and the remaining variation must be determined by other factors in the environment.

Dietary factors

Obesity has been established as an independent risk factor for hypertension and obese individuals are between three and six times more likely to be hypertensive than non-obese individuals. It has been suggested that the physiological mechanisms involved in producing this increased risk concern either excessive activity of the sympathetic nervous system or increased insulin secretion and other disturbances of the endocrine system (Sims 1982).

An obvious treatment intervention for hypertensives who are overweight is to lose weight by changing diet, reducing caloric intake, and increasing exercise as weight loss is reliably associated with blood pressure reduction (Rosenfeld and Shohat 1983). Unfortunately, there are problems in achieving adherence to weight-reduction programmes and in maintaining weight loss over time, and there is a need to investigate behavioural strategies to improve compliance.

Sodium levels in the body are influenced by dietary intake of salt and there are indications that high salt intake may contribute to increased BPL. Experimental studies with rats have shown that feeding with a high salt content diet does lead to increases in BPL (Dahl 1961). In addition, it is possible to produce a strain of rats with hereditary sensitivity to the pressor effect of salt through selective breeding, and it may be that it is salt tolerance rather than salt intake that is the critical factor.

Research has not provided conclusive evidence for a role of sodium in the pathogenesis of hypertension. For example, there are differences in salt intake between different populations, and cross-cultural studies find a positive relationship between salt intake and incidence of hypertension (Dahl and Love 1957). Yet other studies have failed to find any clear difference between the salt intake of normotensive and hypertensive individuals within a particular population (Laragh and Pecker 1983). However, despite such inconsistencies, recommendations for treatment of hypertension do include restriction of dietary intake of salt. Belief in the effectiveness of sodium-intake restriction has existed since the studies of Kempner (1948) showed that severe dietary restriction based upon a diet of low sodium foods such as rice and fruit could reduce blood pressure. Unfortunately, this conclusion may be too simple since diets of this kind additionally produce weight loss which is itself associated with blood-pressure reduction, and they also affect the intake of other nutrients and minerals such as potassium and calcium. In a review of studies of salt restriction Laragh and Pecker (1983) question the assumption that salt restriction is of benefit to all hypertensives: it does seem to benefit some but may actually increase BPL in some severe hypertensives. The issue is not yet resolved.

Population studies have shown a direct linear relationship between alcohol consumption and BPL, and high consumption of alcohol is also associated with hypertension (Larbi *et al.* 1983). Heavy alcohol consumption is also associated with increased incidence of coronary heart disease. The effect of alcohol on BPL is reversible: that is to say, when alcohol intake is reduced, then BPL decreases (Potter and Beevers 1984).

Clearly, diet can influence BPL and may be causally implicated in the development of hypertension. If so, individuals' risk could be modified by behavioural interventions that allow self-management of dietary factors.

Exercise

There is evidence that regular exercise has some slightly beneficial effect for lowering BPL in adults though the changes are generally small. However, there are additional benefits in that regular exercise is generally accompanied by lower body weight, less smoking, and lower blood cholesterol levels (Epstein and Oster 1984). Beneficial effects of exercise upon BPL may reflect these changes or may be related to psychological effects since regular exercise is also associated with increased self-efficacy and positive mood states, as well as providing an escape from the experience of daily stressors. It has been demonstrated in animal studies that exercise is beneficial as a coping mechanism to buffer the reaction to stress (Mills and Ward 1986). This was independent of fitness effects associated with exercise and it may be that only very moderate levels of exercise are required for beneficial reductions of BPL in humans (Jennings *et al.* 1986). In addition to altering mean BPL, aerobic exercise has been found in experimental studies to be effective in reducing hypertensives' cardiovascular reactivity to external stressors such as a mental-arithmetic task and playing a video-game (Perkins *et al.* 1986). Since excessive cardiovascular reactivity has been implicated in the aetiology of hypertension it is possible that aerobic exercise may be of value in preventing the onset of hypertension.

Personality traits

There have been many studies that have looked to find associations between individuals' personality characteristics or traits and hypertension following

Alexander's (1939) hypothesis that suppression of hostile feelings leads to elevated BPL. One approach has been to investigate the personality profiles of diagnosed hypertensives. Unfortunately, this approach suffers from the methodological flaw that any factors exhibited by hypertensives may reflect and be a reaction to their diagnosis rather than a characteristic that is causally related to development of the disease. Robinson (1964), for example, found that hypertensive patients attending a clinic had higher neuroticism scores than individuals participating in a programme simply screening BPL, but their neuroticism scores were no higher than those of other out-patients attending a psychiatric clinic. It would seem that it is attendance at a clinic that is the critical feature and that 'any excess of psychiatric morbidity. . . is not part of the hypertensive state but follows upon diagnosis' (Mann 1986: 534).

A superior methodology involves screening a population and identifying the characteristics of those individuals who emerge as the hypertensive subgroup. Using this approach there have been few findings of consistent associations between personality measures and high BPL. For example, Waal-Manning et al. (1986) found that among 1,173 citizens of a New Zealand town, neither neuroticism nor affective factors such as anxiety or depression were associated with high BPL. In another study of this type Mann (1977) did find that hostility was a feature of people with high diastolic BPL. This is of interest as hostility and anger are components of the Type A behaviour pattern which is associated with risk of cardiovascular disease (see Chapter 13 in this volume). Several studies have indicated that anger may be associated with elevated BPL in high-stress urban environments (Gentry et al. 1981; Harburg et al. 1979), but this finding is not universal and was not found in a rural setting (Waal-Manning et al. 1986). A direct link between Type A behaviour pattern and hypertension has not been established (Shapiro and Goldstein 1982).

In order to demonstrate a causal relationship between personality and hypertension it is necessary to conduct prospective and long-term longitudinal studies and it would be interesting to examine further the role of some of these constitutional factors in hypertension; for example the relationships between BPL and styles of expressed anger and hostility. Unfortunately, studies of this type are lacking. In their absence there is no evidence for a clear link between personality traits and hypertension and certainly no evidence that there exists a certain 'hypertensive personality' (Mann 1986).

Psychological risk factors: stress

External and environmental factors are assumed to operate through psychological processes that have an impact upon physiological responses including elevation of BPL. Factors that have been implicated include migration, rapid modernization, and the experience of major life events.

Epidemiological studies and laboratory studies have been conducted to investigate the impact of these factors.

Epidemiological studies have looked at the changes involving migration to a new environment or rapid changes within a local static population. In general these studies have shown that the experience of rapid cultural change, or change from rural to urban environments, are associated with increased BPL (Cassel 1975). However, in at least one instance involving Japanese migrants to the USA, Marmot (1984) has shown that the expected increases in BPL did not occur, and though there was an increased prevalence in coronary heart disease among the migrants, this probably reflects changes in diet and exercise pattern rather than the process of urbanization *per se*. It may also be the case that migrants from any population are a self-selecting group with particular characteristics that predispose them both to migrate and also to develop increased BPL.

Other studies have concentrated upon environmental factors within non-migrant communities and again factors have been found that are apparently associated with elevation of BPL. Animal studies for example, have shown that environmental crowding causes elevated blood pressure in rat communities (Henry and Stephens 1977). Similarly, D'Atri and Ostfield (1975) found that crowding of humans within prisons elevates BPL. Occupational factors may also have a significant effect upon BPL. These may be caused either by direct effects of the work environment or by the demands imposed upon the individual by the nature of the work itself. In the former instance, for example, it has been found that chronic exposure to noise at work is associated with elevated BPL (Johnsson and Hansen 1977). Environments, including work, have great potential for influencing individuals' health, and the impact of environmental factors upon workers' health, including hypertension, deserves greater consideration. More attention has been given to the influence of work-task characteristics upon morbidity and mortality, and it is recognized that many factors can influence health such as work overload or underload, occupational change, responsibility, social support and many others (Fletcher 1988). It is likely that factors of these types interact with the internal characteristics of particular workers to produce effects that have consequences for individuals' BPLs (Theorell 1976).

Laboratory studies have looked at the responses to physical and psychological stressors of normal, borderline and hypertensive subjects. These studies indicate that in many different situations, particularly those involving challenging or provoking demands that require active coping responses, hypertensives exhibit greater blood-pressure responses than do normotensives (Obrist 1981; Steptoe 1981). Exaggerated cardiovascular responses to challenging tasks may depend upon excessive sympathetic reactivity, which has been implicated as a mediator in the pathogenesis of hypertension. This issue is discussed more fully later.

It is difficult to investigate psychosocial variables in isolation. They inevitably interact with individual and environmental factors, and as Steptoe (1981: 153) points out, 'psychosocial influences on essential hypertension can best be understood in an interactional framework'. Much more research is needed on the dynamic interactions between these factors over time in the development and maintenance of hypertension. In a study of this type, for example, DeFrank et al. (1987) found that among 415 air-traffic controllers monitored over a three-year period, obesity was initially the best predictor of BPL, and that alcohol consumption was second-best predictor. However, alcohol consumption rose during the period of study for those subjects who developed high BPL and this was linked with psychosocial variables of low social support and high level of experienced stress. The combined influence of alcohol consumption (linked with psychosocial variables) and obesity together presented the greatest risk for hypertension, and obesity by itself became a less important predictor of BPL at higher levels of alcohol consumption. Only longitudinal studies of this type can reveal the developmental patterns of association between significant variables.

CARDIOVASCULAR REACTIVITY AND THE AETIOLOGY OF HYPERTENSION

Exposure to stressors of many kinds provokes physiological changes in animals including humans. One aspect of those changes is cardiovascular activation indicated by increased heart rate and elevation of BPL. The extent of such activation and its duration of effect varies from individual to individual, and one hypothesis is that exaggerated cardiac reactivity is implicated in the pathogenesis of hypertension (Obrist 1981).

Elevated blood pressure is a symptom. By itself it simply indicates that the usual regulatory mechanisms that maintain homeostasis within the cardiovascular system are not functioning appropriately. Psychophysiological studies have sought to identify the mechanisms by which behavioural factors can affect the control mechanisms that regulate blood pressure. In a healthy organism, when blood pressure rises the cardiovascular system compensates to reduce pressure to normal levels. In hypertension, complex physiological changes involving renal, autonomic and cardiovascular systems occur and become fixed as a response to idiopathic states involving high cardiac output. The result is sustained high BPL (Guyton et al. 1970). In established hypertensives cardiac output can return to normal levels but in this case the process is accompanied by increased peripheral resistance of the vasculature, and this again operates to maintain the pressure within the circulatory system at a high level. In this case, although the symptom, namely high blood pressure, has remained the same, the physiological mechanisms sustaining it are different from those that initially gave rise to it. The key to understanding the disorder is to understand how behavioural factors can influence these various regulatory mechanisms.

One mechanism involved in controlling variability of blood pressure is the baroreceptor reflex arc. The sensitivity of this reflex is suppressed in hypertension. This reflex also influences the central nervous system and individuals' pain thresholds. It has been proposed that the stress of exposure to chronic pain or anticipation of pain causes the sensitivity of the baroreceptors to become reset, and as this learned response becomes established there is a consequent rise in blood pressure which eventuates in hypertension (Dworkin 1988). A recent study has found that baroreceptor reflex sensitivity increased for normotensive subjects during relaxation and was reduced during performance of a stressful task demanding active engagement by subjects, namely mental arithmetic, though not during exposure to a passive stressor, the cold-pressor test (Steptoe and Sawada 1989). Thus, a link has been established between behavioural demands of a particular kind known as active coping, and changes in circulatory regulation that are mediated by the baroreceptor reflex arc and which are associated with hypertension. It remains to be confirmed whether baroreceptor reflex sensitivity is selectively suppressed in individuals at risk for the development of hypertension.

Changes in BPL are a ubiquitous feature of everyone's daily lives. Why is it, then, that some individuals develop hypertension but others do not? It may be that those who are predisposed to develop hypertension are, in certain situations, prone to excessive cardiac reactions mediated by sympathetic-nervous-system actions upon the heart. Young adults who show exaggerated cardiac reactivity experience the high cardiac output state that precedes development of hypertension. The exact processes involved remain unclear but are believed to involve central and autonomic-nervous-system mechanisms, though renal and endocrine systems may also be involved (Guyton 1977). What is clear is that excessive sympathetic influence upon the heart is at least one of the factors that is involved in the aetiology of hypertension.

Many studies have demonstrated that hypertensives do show cardiac responses, including BPL responses, of greater magnitude than normotensives during performance on a variety of tasks including a ball-sorting task, mental arithmetic, competitive games and reaction-time shock avoidance. These tasks and others that provoke this hyper-reactive effect involve active behavioural involvement by the subject. Passive tasks, such as the cold-pressor task where the subject plunges a limb into a mixture of freezing ice and water and passively endures the pain, do not reliably distinguish the cardiac reactions of hypertensives and normotensives (Steptoe 1983). This suggests that it is the active engagement in a task that may be the critical component for hyper-reactivity. It is not the case that hypertensive individuals are over-reactive in all situations but only with respect to certain environmental challenges which provoke excessive sympathetic activation of the heart (Steptoe 1981). In summary it seems that it is those individuals who respond to challenging tasks with exaggerated increases in heart rate and blood pressure that are at risk of progressing from a state with normal blood-pressure regulation to one with maladaptive physiological changes that underlie sustained elevation of blood pressure. Consistent with this hypothesis is the finding that the normotensive children of hypertensive parents have a greatly increased risk of themselves becoming hypertensive as adults and they show excessive cardiac reactions to psychological challenges that require active coping even during their normotensive state (Carroll *et al.* 1985; Manuck and Proietti 1982).

BEHAVIOURAL TREATMENTS FOR PRIMARY HYPERTENSION

Drug therapy with one of the many available antihypertensive agents is currently the major form of treatment for hypertensive patients. However, the effectiveness of these drugs is uncertain. Some patients prescribed antihypertensive drugs do not show BPL reduction (MRC 1985) and compliance with medication may be poor, particularly as many of the drugs have side-effects that can be both distressing and harmful. Adverse symptoms reported by patients taking antihypertensive medication include, for example, insomnia, fatigue, lethargy, impotence and reduced glucose tolerance (MRC trial 1981). In recent years there has been increased interest in non-pharmacological treatments for hypertension involving self-management through behavioural methods. These non-pharmacological methods are most appropriate for the mild hypertensive patient and those who are severely hypertensive will almost certainly remain on medication for treatment of their condition. Even in these cases, however, behavioural measures may provide useful adjuncts to drug treatment.

It will be clear from the earlier section on factors associated with hypertension that there is considerable scope for behavioural management of this disorder. Recommendations for treatment by modification of physical factors include taking regular aerobic exercise, reducing weight, restricting salt intake and reducing alcohol consumption. In addition to these direct interventions there has developed in recent years considerable interest in self-management of hypertension based upon stress reduction techniques which include various forms of relaxation and biofeedback training.

Biofeedback

Biofeedback training is used to allow an individual to gain control over some specified physiological response (see Chapter 8 in this volume). Training can be used either to modify some particular symptom (direct symptom-control approach) or to produce generalized relaxation. Since hypertension is defined by reference to one particular and easily identifiable symptom, namely BPL, it would seem ideally suited as a candidate for biofeedback treatment using the direct symptom-control approach. Experimental studies using normotensive volunteer subjects have shown that biofeedback can be used effectively to train both increases and decreases in BPL (Shapiro *et al.* 1972). The results of blood-pressure biofeedback from clinical studies, however, have been disappointing. Though some applications of biofeedback training to reduce high blood pressure have been successful (see for example, Kristt and Engel 1975), in general the reductions achieved in hypertensive patients have been modest and of little clinical value. Many of the clinical studies have included relatively few subjects and have been poorly controlled. Furthermore, the effects of training do not easily transfer from the clinic to home or work environments and nor do they endure over time. Having reviewed clinical studies that have used biofeedback training, Johnston (1984) concludes that there is no evidence that cardiovascular biofeedback has any specific effect upon BPL in hypertensive patients.

Biofeedback training for generalized relaxation using feedback based upon responses other than blood pressure has also been applied to the treatment of hypertension. Green *et al.* (1979), for example, gave subjects biofeedback training based on temperature feedback measured from the fingertip. Subjects were trained to increase finger temperature and it was found that thermal control was associated with reduction of blood pressure. At least one controlled comparison study has found thermal biofeedback to be superior to relaxation training for the reduction of blood pressure in hypertensive patients (Blanchard *et al.* 1986). The mechanisms underlying the blood-pressure reductions achieved by this method are not obvious but since peripheral temperature regulation involves sympathetic-nervous-system control it may be that thermal biofeedback training is acting as a relaxation technique that acts to reduce sympathetic activation. Biofeedback has also been used within combined treatments for relaxation and these are discussed in the next section.

Stress management

As has already been described, epidemiological studies and experimental laboratory studies have implicated hyper-reactivity to acute or chronic stressors in the development of hypertension. As a consequence several studies have investigated the effectiveness of stress-management programmes for the treatment of hypertension. The precise methods involved differ considerably but the majority include some form of relaxation training such as meditation, yoga, muscle relaxation and biofeedback. In an excellent review of this topic, D.W. Johnston (1987: 100) has identified twenty studies carried out since 1975 which have used stress-reduction methods within clinics and he states that 'in the majority of studies stress reduction techniques are associated with reductions of blood pressure and that these persist for as long as four years'. He argues that the effects are specific to stress management and are significantly greater than for control procedures. Extending this analysis Johnston (1989) has pooled data from twenty-five randomized controlled trials of relaxation-based stress-reduction studies. In total 834 patients received some form of stress-management procedure and achieved substantially greater reductions in both systolic and diastolic BPL than the 561 equivalent subjects represented within control conditions. A similar analysis of other groups of patients whose BPLs were measured outside the clinic in home or work environments again found significantly greater BPL reductions in patients given stress management rather than control procedures (see Table 12.1).

Table 12.1 Comparison of blood-pressure reductions following stress management versus control procedures in clinic and non-clinic studies

	Clinic			Non-clinic		
	Number of patients			*Number of patients*		
		SBP	DBP		SBP	DBP
Stress						
management	834	–8.4	–6.1	313	–6.3	– 4.5
Control	561	–2.7	–2.1	142	–2.1	– 1.9

Note: The figures are adapted from Johnston (1989) and show mean reductions of systolic blood pressure (SBP) and diastolic blood pressure (DBP) measured as mmHg for subjects pooled from twenty-five separate studies.

It seems that stress management is effective in producing long-term reductions in blood pressure, though the mechanisms involved are poorly understood. Some studies have however suggested that the effects of relaxation are mediated by the patients' expectations of benefit and that the BPL reductions achieved are attributable solely to this non-specific effect (Agras *et al.* 1982; Wadden 1984). In a direct test of this hypothesis, Irvine *et al.* (1986) compared for hypertensive patients the effects on BPL of stress management involving relaxation with a control procedure involving physical exercise in which similar expectations of benefit were encouraged. Patients' responses to an expectancy questionnaire showed no difference between the two conditions prior to treatment. Following ten weeks of treatment they found that the relaxation condition was superior to the control procedure immediately post treatment and also at three months follow-up, indicating some specific advantage for the relaxation condition. Whether caused by specific or non-specific effects, or both, what is impressive about relaxation training is that reductions in BPL achieved in the clinic do generalize to patients' home and working environments, and the beneficial effects have persisted when measured at fifteen-month follow-up (Agras *et al.* 1983;

Southam *et al.* 1982). Clinicians using relaxation therapy for blood-pressure reduction frequently complement clinic-based training with the addition of home relaxation tapes to be used by the patient. However, a controlled comparison study found no evidence that their use offers any additional benefit for BPL reduction over and above that achieved in the clinic training (Hoelscher *et al.* 1987). Considerably more research is needed to identify the presentation and components of relaxation training for optimal effectiveness for reducing BPL in hypertensive patients.

By far the most impressive and systematic research on the value of relaxation therapy for hypertension has been carried out by two groups of workers led respectively by Patel, and Agras and Taylor. Agras and colleagues have developed a self-management programme based on progressive muscle relaxation trained in the clinic, together with home exercises and instruction on the application of relaxation for stress reduction in patients' everyday lives. In controlled comparison studies they have found that this relaxation programme is more effective for reducing BPL than control procedures such as no treatment, psychotherapy and self-monitoring of blood pressure and follow-up studies have shown that the effect of lowering BPL persists for at least a year after training (Agras *et al.* 1983). Other studies by this group have demonstrated that relaxation training can be applied effectively in the worksites of newly diagnosed untreated hypertensives (Chesney *et al.* 1987) and also established hypertensives who were responding poorly to anti-hypertensive drug medication (Agras *et al.* 1987).

Patel and her colleagues have developed a highly successful approach to treating hypertension using an eclectic stress-management programme that includes relaxation, breathing exercises, meditation and both EMG and skin-resistance biofeedback. Patients are also given instruction on applying relaxation for managing stressful situations within their everyday lives (Patel and North 1975). Comparison of eighty-nine patients trained in this way with eighty-two matched controls showed that those in the relaxation condition achieved significant reductions in both systolic and diastolic blood pressure which were evident after training for only eight weeks. Follow-ups conducted at eight months and four years found that the substantial BPL reductions were maintained over time. The importance of the relaxation training itself is indicated by the fact that those patients who reported using relaxation to self-manage their condition on a regular basis showed greater reductions in blood pressure (10.9 systolic, 7.0 diastolic) than did those whose adherence was poorer (6.3 systolic, 1.7 diastolic). Even more significant is the fact that on the basis of changes in standard risk factors (smoking, blood cholesterol level, blood pressure) the risk of developing coronary heart disease for the patients receiving relaxation training was substantially reduced by around by 12 per cent (Patel *et al.* 1981, 1985). At the four-year follow-up, patients were also questioned about the effect of the treatment on other aspects of their lives including social life, sexual life, work relationships, general health and enjoyment of life. The results showed that compared to controls, the treatment group showed beneficial changes in many aspects of their lives, and significantly so for general health, enjoyment of life, personal and family relationships, and work relationships. These non-specific improvements may be additional health benefits that result from the relaxation training received by these patients or it could be that the improvements have themselves contributed to the reductions in BPL achieved (Steptoe *et al.* 1987).

CHOICE OF TREATMENT

Though the immediate goal of treatment for hypertension is to reduce BPL by as much as possible and ideally to within the normotensive range, the longer-term objective is to reduce the incidence of renal and cardiovascular disease for hypertensive patients. Appel (1986) suggests that the objectives of self-management programmes can best be met by considering hypertensives as a heterogeneous group whose treatment package should adopt a 'stepped-care approach' starting with procedures that are least costly and best suited to each particular patient, for example weight loss for an overweight patient or alcohol reduction for someone with high alcohol intake, and more costly or effortful procedures introduced only as necessary. Using this approach Glasgow *et al.* (1989) carried out a controlled study of a stepped-care approach that compared fifty-one patients given a stepped-care treatment involving, first, blood-pressure monitoring, followed by blood-pressure biofeedback training and, finally, relaxation training as required with fifty-one control patients. Both groups received medication to keep their BPLs within normal limits. However, the medication of those patients in the stepped-care condition receiving behavioural treatments was reduced as far as allowable to maintain their BPL within the normotensive range. Comparisons between controls and stepped-care patients were made over nineteen months and it was found that the stepped-care-group patients required less medication to control their blood pressure than did the control patients, and their cost of care was also significantly lower. This study shows that patients with moderate hypertension are able to reduce substantially their antihypertensive medications without any increase in BPL by introduction of behavioural treatments to complement the drug therapy. Combined behavioural and drug treatments using the stepped-care approach may offer the most cost-effective therapy for hypertensive patients.

Primary prevention of hypertension

Thus far behavioural treatments have been used for diagnosed hypertensives. However, it could be the case that it is also appropriate to use self-management for individuals who are judged to be 'at risk' for hypertension on some criterion, for example family history of hypertension to prevent the development of the disorder. It should not be forgotten that though hypertension affects adults, the conditions that give rise to it are associated with factors that may well be established in infancy or adolescence, i.e. lack of exercise, diet and drinking alcohol. Future research should examine the possibilities for behavioural interventions introduced during adolescence for the primary prevention of hypertension in adulthood (Coates 1982). Those interventions would probably be based upon modification of physical factors but might also include stress management programmes. For example, the package of treatment for stress management introduced by Patel is estimated to require only one hour per patient, which is highly cost-effective since its beneficial effects persist for at least four years. The difficulty, of course, is identifying those individuals who are at risk and who should be recruited to treatments for preventive care. This can only be done by large-scale community screening of BPL, but given the prevalence of hypertension in the adult population and the associated mortalities by renal and cardiovascular diseases, primary prevention could be more beneficial than trying to treat the disorder (Hart 1987).

PROBLEMS OF ADHERENCE TO TREATMENTS

Chapter 4 has discussed the issue of compliance in medical settings. Non-compliance is a problem for behavioural as well as pharmacological treatments, and particularly so for hypertension. One of the difficulties encountered with hypertension is that being a symptomless disorder, patients may ignore or deny their condition and fail to comply with the treatments advised. This is particularly so when the medication itself causes distressing symptoms, and Sackett and Snow (1979) reported that as many as 50 per cent of hypertensive patients do not comply with their medication regimens. There may also be intolerable costs for the patient associated with behavioural treatments. For example, patients may be unwilling to reduce their alcohol consumption or to change their diet to treat their disorder. Behavioural methods may be used not only as direct interventions to alter individuals' behaviours but also indirectly to improve adherence to either pharmacological or non-pharmacological therapies.

Several strategies have been adopted to improve hypertensive patients' compliance, including self-monitoring of blood pressure and education about the disorder. Self-monitoring of blood pressure is often recommended as a useful component of self-management programmes though the evidence that it is useful is inconsistent and some studies have found that self-monitoring by hypertensive patients did not lead to BPL reduction (for example, Goldstein et al. 1982).

Similarly, it has been believed that education about hypertension and its management will increase patients' adherence to treatment, but again this may not be so. Kirscht et al.(1981) developed an educational programme for hypertensive patients, but although it increased their knowledge about the disorder it did not improve their adherence to treatment. Similarly, Haynes (1979) has found that education increased knowledge but not adherence to medication.

Other strategies that may be used to improve adherence include verbal and written contracts between patient and doctor, social support and individualized treatment programmes that allow the patient maximum flexibility in managing their disorder. Haynes (1979) found that combinations of several such strategies together are necessary to improve compliance, and any one alone is insufficient.

Although there is little evidence that either mood states or particular symptoms are consistently associated with hypertension, hypertensives themselves often believe that they can tell when their BP is elevated and take medication accordingly (Meyer 1985). Unfortunately, this can be effective only when hypertensives' beliefs about their illness are correct and these are not always so (Pennebaker and Watson 1988). However, it may be possible to encourage correct beliefs and to train hypertensives to detect changes in their BPL more accurately by using blood pressure feedback (Barr et al. 1988). Certainly accurate blood-pressure discrimination has been shown to be possible with feedback training (Greenstadt et al. 1986). Accurate detection of changes in BPL, if it could be achieved, might assist patients to adhere to treatments and to employ behavioural and pharmacological treatments to self-manage their disorder more effectively.

CONCLUSIONS

Several factors have been identified as being associated with hypertension but it is by no means certain which of these are responsible for causing the disorder and which are simply maintaining it once established. In addition, the physiological mechanisms by which their effects become realized are poorly understood. Not surprisingly, therefore, there remains considerable uncertainty about the pathogenesis of hypertension. Future research should employ prospective methodologies both for population studies and for clinical and laboratory studies to distinguish factors that are antecedents of hypertension and those that may simply be maintaining the disorder once it has developed. It may be particularly useful to concentrate on 'at risk' normotensives, for example children with hypertensive parents, to compare the personal characteristics and environmental factors associated with those that subsequently become hypertensive with those of individuals who do not.

In terms of treatment there is now good evidence that behavioural methods can provide a valuable adjunct to pharmacological treatments, and in the case of the borderline patient they may provide effective treatment on their own as an alternative to antihypertensive drugs. Though more research is needed to identify the optimal treatment by behavioural methods it is clear that exercise, control of diet and reduction of alcohol intake are all beneficial. More attention should be paid to the psychological factors involved in achieving compliance with these recommended practices. In view of the high prevalence of hypertension in the adult population, community screening programmes to detect elevated blood pressure in its early stages of development could play a valuable role in the primary prevention of hypertension.

Chapter 13

Coronary heart disease

Philip Evans

INTRODUCTION

Coronary heart disease (CHD) is one of the major causes of death in modern industrialized societies. It is also a disease which often kills prematurely or leaves its middle-aged victims with a reduced quality of life. Not surprisingly therefore much research has concentrated on knowing more about the risk factors for CHD.

As a disease concept CHD embraces two major types of coronary disorder: angina pectoris and myocardial infarction. In order to understand both of these, however, we need first to understand the term 'atherosclerosis'. This is the technical way of referring to the process whereby arteries become narrowed as a result of fatty material being deposited on their walls. In some people the coronary artery, which is responsible for feeding blood to the heart muscle itself, becomes so narrowed that the heart can be temporarily starved of oxygen, giving rise to ischaemic pain. This is usually noticed following a period of exertion and constitutes an attack of angina. Atherosclerosis, however, can also lead to a more serious eventuality. A narrowed artery is more easily blocked by an obstructing deposit or blood clot. Such an event is called 'coronary occlusion', and it can cut off the supply of oxygen sufficiently for parts of the heart muscle (the myocardium) to die. Such an acute emergency is called a myocardial infarction or, less technically, a heart attack. A severe attack often proves fatal unless emergency treatment is immediately given.

TRADITIONAL RISK FACTORS

Of course we must all die eventually of some disorder or other, but the distressing aspect of CHD is that many victims are only just entering middle age and are in the full swing of career and family life. What makes these people vulnerable to such illness? In terms of premature CHD there are several well-recognized risk factors: being male, being a smoker, having high blood pressure, having a family history of heart disease, having high levels of cholesterol in the blood, being diabetic. However, any one of these risk factors by itself explains only a minuscule portion of the variability in who does or does not suffer CHD, and epidemiological evidence often points to complexity in the way that risk is translated into effect. One particular high-smoking country, for example, may 'buck the trend' and produce low CHD statistics; similarly, a community known for its high consumption of saturated fats might nevertheless prove to have a low incidence of heart disease. Some of the anomalies disappear when we look at multiple risk. The risk factors do not simply add to each other but interact such that over all, risk is considerably increased for an individual who scores unfavourably on more than one single factor.

However, even the best predictive equation using traditional risk factors leaves most of the aetiology of CHD unexplained and this has led some researchers to ask whether additional *psychological* factors may exist.

CHD AND 'STRESS'

An obvious candidate, but one difficult to define with any exactitude, is social stress. Certainly researchers have looked at the role that certain life events may play in predicting CHD, particularly events which involve substantial change in a person's routine and which require a good measure of adjustment. Theorell (1984) showed that a measure of such life change effectively doubled in the three months prior to occurrence of ischaemic heart disease. Similar findings have been reported by Rahe and Lind (1971). Stressors such as overload at work and chronic conflict have also been implicated as risk factors for heart disease (Jenkins 1971, 1976).

Fisher (1986) cites indirect evidence of the role of stress by showing that heart-disease rates in the United States show a distributional pattern which parallels suicide rates rather than infant-mortality rates. In so far as suicide rates can be taken to reflect stress levels, whereas infant-mortality rates provide a control level of general deprivation, then one can plausibly infer that stress levels in different communities rather than differences in levels of physical deprivation partly underpin observed differences in the distribution of heart disease.

However, stress, assessed in various ways, has generally been implicated in illness of many kinds. The most promising developments in linking psychological factors to CHD in particular have undoubtedly arisen from the notion that certain people, by dint of certain characteristic behaviours, are more at risk of CHD than others. From such a notion has sprung the concept of a 'Type A' person. Although it is possible that Type A itself may have wider implications for risk of illness in general (see, for example, Rime *et al.* 1989; Woods and Burns 1984), this is an avenue which has remained for the most part unexplored and most research has been concerned with the relationship between Type A and CHD in adults.

THE TYPE A CONSTRUCT

The Type A construct was first invented by two cardiologists, Friedman and Rosenman, to describe a certain kind of individual who, they believed, tended to be overrepresented as clients in their clinical practice. Type A persons were depicted as people with a highly competitive craving for achievement and recognition, together with a tendency towards hostility and aggression, and a sense of tremendous time urgency and impatience. The Type A individual sees goals and challenges everywhere, wants to win every 'game' in life, speaks fast, acts fast, interrupts and manifests impatient gestures when faced with slower mortals, cannot abide queues, is only superficially interested in the aesthetic aspects of life and tends to measure success in terms of material gains, and number rather than quality of goals achieved.

One of the difficulties with the Type A construct is that it is a broad pen portrait which includes or suggests the presence of a number of different but perhaps interacting personality traits. Psychologists who have spent many years refining and measuring traits are quite understandably prone to regret that the research in this area has not developed around more tried and tested measures, which avoid the artificiality inherent in dividing people into broad types – a practice which is bound to ignore the dimensional nature of real traits (see Eysenck 1985). However, in so far as Type A has been measured as a general *behaviour pattern* rather than a personality measure in the true sense, we shall see that it has had some real success in predicting incidence of CHD. How, then, has Type A been measured and are such measures reliable and valid?

THE MEASUREMENT OF TYPE A

Friedman and Rosenman originally assessed Type A using a structured interview (SI) method. The interviewer in this procedure not only asks subjects about their behaviour but also observes and elicits behaviour in the actual interview. Thus, the subject's style of speaking – how fast or explosive it is, the subject's reactions to pauses by the interviewer, and other behavioural characteristics are all noted and recorded as part of the assessment. The structured nature of the procedure means that with adequate experience, two independent raters can achieve respectable reliability in terms of classification agreement. Raters have traditionally favoured the use of four categories. Type A1 and A2 simply differentiate degree of Type A and are often collapsed into a single category. Type B indicates a notable absence of Type A characteristics. Finally Type X is an 'unsure' middling category where Type A characteristics are not sufficiently in evidence to justify a Type A judgement but not so totally absent as to indicate a Type B judgement.

Although the SI method of Type A assessment remains a sort of 'gold standard' against which other measures are judged, many self-report measures have been used by researchers, not least because self-report instruments are less time consuming, more convenient to use, and their reliability is often, superficially at least, more easily established. Their validity has, as we shall see, proven in some cases to be more problematic. The most widely used self-report instruments have been the Jenkins Activity Survey (JAS), the Framingham Type A Scale (FTAS) and the Bortner Rating Scale (BRS).

THE PREDICTIVE VALIDITY OF TYPE A

The fact that so much research has been done on the Type A construct may lead one to suppose that its predictive validity as a genuine coronary risk factor has been established beyond doubt. Indeed, this was the authoritative view expressed by a review panel of distinguished American scientists gathered together in 1981 under the auspices of the National Heart, Lung and Blood Institute. Type A was duly added to the official list of traditional coronary risk factors which we mentioned earlier. Since then, however, there have been a number of negative findings in relation to Type A and CHD which has meant that any interpretation of the research as a whole is considerably complex and far from definitive in its conclusions. If we restrict ourselves solely to an examination of prospective research projects – ones which have taken measures of Type A and then followed up subjects over a period of years – what findings emerge?

The first major prospective study was the Western Collaborative Group Study (WCGS) in which a sample of over 3,000 Californian males, initially free of CHD and between the ages of 39 and 59, were followed up over a period of eight-and-a-half years. It was found that the subsequent incidence of CHD was twice as great among Type As (assessed by SI) than among Type Bs (Rosenman *et al.* 1975). To put this relative risk into some absolute perspective we can note that 7 per cent of the entire sample developed some signs of CHD and two-thirds of these were Type A. This degree of risk is comparable with the traditional physical risk factors to which we have referred earlier. Moreover, statistical analysis revealed that the risk associated with Type A was 'independent' risk. In other words researchers had not simply discovered something which predicted a traditional risk factor thereby suggesting a spurious link with CHD (for example, the Type As in the study might have been heavier smokers). It seemed that there was something about the Type A behaviour pattern itself which made people vulnerable to CHD.

Further support for the role of Type A as a coronary risk factor soon came from the opposite side of the United States, in Framingham, Massachusetts, where a large-scale investigation of CHD was under way. These researchers had got their subjects to fill in several psychosocial rating scales at the beginning of the study and certain key ratings were grouped to form a Framingham Type A measure. The FTAS succeeded to a similar extent in predicting CHD over a period virtually identical to that of the Californian study (S.G. Haynes *et al.* 1980). Two points can be added in regard to the Framingham study. First, it recruited both male and female subjects; thus it was the first major study to show Type A as a risk factor for women. Second, its predictive power in regard to CHD was better for angina than myocardial infarction.

Since these first major studies, the results of several further prospective investigations have been reported. Most of these have been considered in recent reviews (Booth-Kewley and Friedman 1987; Matthews 1988). Since several investigators have now reported negative or even contradictory results in relation to Type A, the major task of any reviewer is to try and determine what features distinguish supportive and non-supportive studies. Two such features seem to stand out.

First, studies which have used the SI method of assessing Type A have tended to indicate that it is a genuine risk factor, whereas studies that have assessed Type A using JAS have been particularly prone to negative conclusions. Since the classificatory agreement of the JAS with the SI is known to be little better than 60 per cent (one would expect agreement for 50 per cent of the time by chance), we might expect this measure to be problematic. Estimates of the variance shared by SI and the JAS seldom exceed 10 per cent and many researchers have explicitly cautioned that they should not be seen as substitute measures (Mayes *et al.* 1984). In at least one report JAS mean scores did not even linearly relate to SI categorization (Byrne *et al.* 1985). Both the FTAS and the BRS did appreciably better in their agreement with the SI. Little wonder, then, that Friedman and Booth-Kewley (1988) have now called for the virtual abandonment of the JAS as a research instrument.

The second distinguishing feature of the studies which have failed to show Type A as a risk factor for CHD is that they tend to be so-called 'high-risk' studies. Such studies typically select subjects who are already known to be at risk for CHD. The advantage of such studies is that they enable researchers to utilize smaller samples and still obtain enough CHD incidence to make statistical analysis possible. Many of these studies have taken subjects who have already suffered one episode of CHD and have followed them up over a further period in which subsequent mortality rates and recurrences of myocardial infarctions can be recorded. Other studies have selected subjects who are at greater risk of CHD by reason of another risk factor. One such British study reporting negative findings (Mann and Brennan 1987) used subjects exhibiting mild hypertension.

High-risk studies lead to several interpretative difficulties. For the most part the Type A measure is taken from subjects who are already aware of their greater risk and this may affect their response to assessment, particularly self-report measures. Some studies have indicated that there may be a higher prevalence of Type A persons in high-risk studies, thus perhaps limiting Type A differences to a degree where associations with CHD are difficult to demonstrate.

Survival itself may be a consideration. Type A subjects who have survived an initial episode of CHD may actually represent a subsample of Type A persons different in important respects from those who did not survive. They may be more likely to seek help for early warning symptoms. They may generally be better health monitors, or even complainers. This may be a particularly salient consideration when mortality rate is used as a key variable. Survivor Type As may also be precisely those who have suffered less atherosclerosis and therefore may not differ from Type Bs in regard to future CHD indices, or may even be at less risk.

On that note, one particular high-risk study (Ragland and Brand 1988) is worthy of special mention since it reports an apparently contradictory finding of greater risk for Type B subjects. It is particularly interesting because the group followed up consisted of the survivors of the original WCGS. Although this group included more Type A persons, by virtue of the original findings, it was nevertheless found that over a further follow-up period, mortality from CHD incidence was actually higher among the Type B persons who had survived their original incident. How can we account for this result? Any suggested answer must remain speculative, but at least two possibilities, not mutually exclusive, can be considered.

The first takes up the point that Type A survivors may be crucially different from Type As having fatal first incidents. Let us assume that Type A has two endangering effects in regard to CHD, first of all a chronic effect which aids the process of atherosclerosis, and second, an effect which makes the eventuality of an obstruction or blood clot more likely. The second effect may only be of major significance if atherosclerosis has advanced to a certain degree. If we suppose that the Type A persons who survived their first incident were those with less atherosclerosis, and, perhaps for a variety of reasons, were less prone to develop atherosclerosis, then we have invented a scenario in which the results of Ragland and Brand become more understandable.

The second line of reasoning suggests that the psychological impact of a heart attack may be different for Type As than it is for Type Bs. Type A persons may be more prone to reassess their life-style, modify their values and behaviour, and so on. At the very least one may argue that they have scope to do so, certainly more scope than their Type B opposites who seem to have suffered despite their laid-back manner! Although this may seem extremely speculative, it is worth noting that when we look at the figures provided by Ragland and Brand in more detail, it seems that their reported effect is apparent only for cases where an original myocardial infarction was 'overt', that is to say consciously registered at the time. The figures for so-called 'silent' myocardial infarctions, where damage only comes to light at some later time when for example an electrocardiographic record (ECG) is obtained, seem to show no difference between Type A and Type B subjects. Given that anecdotal reports from persons who have consciously suffered a heart attack often indicate a great sense of 'life-endangerment', it is not beyond the bounds of belief that Type A persons may resolve to re-assess their life-style and reduce their risk factors.

What, then, should we conclude in general, regarding the status of Type A as a risk factor for CHD? We could say that in population studies, as opposed to high-risk studies, and using Type A measures other than JAS, but preferably the SI, the evidence is strongly supportive. However, we have to recognize that the database for such a conclusion is considerably reduced in terms of sample size and also considerably narrowed. This means, I believe, that we are still, after several years of research, at the stage of requiring further prospective studies so that there is less need for the sport of speculative interpretations in which we have just indulged. However, there is bound to be a subjective element in deciding how convincing one finds a body of evidence. Reviewing essentially the same evidence, Friedman and Booth-Kewley (1988) conclude: 'By our reckoning, this adds up to convincing evidence that we should be asking how, why and for whom, not whether, Type A behaviour is an important element in heart disease.' Questions of 'how' and 'why' neatly take us on to a consideration of the more general construct validity of Type A. The measure not only seems to relate to CHD but to mechanisms which may explain the link with CHD. In other words the Type A literature has addressed the issue: how does behaviour influence physical pathology?

TYPE A, PSYCHOPHYSIOLOGICAL RESPONSE AND CHD

It has been thought for some time that psychophysiological response to stressors, particularly excessive neuroendocrine activity, may be implicated as a mechanism promoting premature CHD (Williams 1978). Reviews of such evidence (for example, Krantz and Manuck 1984) suggest, on the one hand, that psychophysiological response may indeed be an important factor and, on the other hand, caution us against accepting as meaningful any simple construct such as 'reactivity to stress'. Different patterns of physiological response exist and are manifested according to the exact nature of the task, challenge or situation. Such caution ought to be especially exercised when making the over-simplistic leap to the assertion that Type A persons are at risk because they are physiologically over-reactive to stress.

That said, suspicion has attached itself to neuroendocrine response for good reason, and enough is known at a more 'molecular' level (for example, effects of catecholamines on platelet aggregation) to draw plausible links with pathological processes such as atherosclerosis. A final synthesis in this area, if it is ever achieved, will probably involve fractionation of all of the three constructs which have variously been linked: Type A, reactivity, and coronary heart disease. But such dissection will be more profitable if it proceeds in an organized manner. Flawed positions with some apparent truth in them may indeed need refinement but at least they are temporary structures. In that spirit, we now consider the evidence from laboratory studies that Type A subjects on some physiological measures and in some situations do show heightened reactivity.

Numerous studies have now been done using SI or JAS assessment of Type A. They form the major focus of earlier reviews (Houston 1983; Matthews 1982). Most but by no means all have tended to differentiate Type A subjects from Type B subjects in the predicted direction. Measures have included heart-rate, blood pressure, skin conductance, and catecholamine response. The most consistent results have come from measures of systolic blood pressure. More recently, positive results have been found using the FTAS. Significant A/B differences have been found on systolic blood pressure (Smith *et al.* 1985) and heart rate (Evans and Fearn 1985; Evans and Moran 1987a).

An important question, given that positive findings have not been universal, is whether there are particular kinds of laboratory situation which favour the emergence of Type A/B differences. Broadly speaking, reviewers have emphasized the need for the task or situation to challenge the subjects sufficiently. However, unless we have a theory as to what constitutes effective challenge for Type A subjects there is a temptation simply to 'see' common denominators in just those studies which have produced positive results. It is therefore time to consider theories of what it is to be Type A.

TYPE A AND THE NEED TO BE IN CONTROL

That an overdeveloped need to control events lies at the core of the Type A behaviour pattern is a theory associated with Glass (1977). He suggests that in situations of challenge but where control is lacking or ambiguous, the Type A person exhibits relentless striving leading to frustration and exhaustion, when lack of control is eventually recognized. Type As will then decline into greater 'helplessness' than Type Bs. Thus he predicts that Type As will tend to be the victims of cycles of *hyper-responsiveness* and *hypo-responsiveness*, which are both associated with a pattern of physiological response linkable to processes which would favour the development of CHD.

Glass (1977) presents evidence using laboratory studies of induced 'helplessness' to support his theory. Brunson and Matthews (1981) similarly report that Type As exposed to repeated failure tend to exhibit significant helplessness effects. In our own laboratory we have also shown that Type A subjects will choose to monitor for a warning stimulus of a low probability electric shock even when they have little or no control over it and even though such monitoring is associated with higher cardiovascular arousal (Evans and Fearn 1985; Evans and Moran 1987a). Interestingly, in the same paradigm we have found (Evans and Moran 1987b) that the slow decline in heart rate at the end of the trial (slow 'unwinding') is particularly characteristic of those high on Type A and high on internal locus of control, i.e. a heightened tendency to see oneself as able to control events.

Although the control theory of Type A seems to capture an essential ingredient in the behaviour pattern, in practice it is not always easy to be precise as to what constitutes 'control' (see Thompson 1981). This was apparent for some male subjects in our own experiments who behaved counterintuitively: they proved more likely to *reject* control the more of it that was offered. This meant that our predictions about Type A and control seeking were effectively only confirmed for the female subjects in our sample. Similar seemingly irrational behaviour by male subjects has been reported before in a very similar experimental situation (Averill *et al.* 1977). What are we to make of it? One possibility which we suggested (Evans *et al.* 1984) was that these subjects may have been trying to show superordinate control over the situation and the experimenter by not doing what was expected of them. At the time we saw this in terms of Brehm's (1966) theory of 'reactance', that people react in certain predictable ways when they perceive a threat to their freedom. This in turn indicated to us, in regard to Type A hypotheses, that what subjects may at root be most concerned with controlling is the 'image' that they present and that control-seeking theories of Type A are perhaps secondary to theories which emphasize the importance of self-concepts. Such theories have in fact been developed.

TYPE A AND SELF-ESTEEM

Price (1982) puts forward a cognitive theory of Type A which seems to have parallels with Ellis's rational-emotive view of much neurotic disorder (Ellis 1984), in that the competitive relentless striving of Type A persons, their hostile emotions and so forth, stem from a belief that self-esteem is to be measured exclusively by accomplishments. Recognition by others is seen as a scarce and fluctuating resource for which a person must constantly battle. Beneath the superficial achievement-striving, there lies, on this view, a more profound sense of inadequacy and perhaps low self-esteem, although predictions in regard to such measures have to contend with the fact that Type A persons may be highly motivated not to reveal such weakness to others.

There is certainly evidence, direct and indirect, to support the sort of cognitive theory outlined by Price. In a study which actually used threat to self-esteem, Pittner and Houston (1980) showed that Type A subjects showed more denial responses than Type B subjects. Furnham and Linfoot (1987) report that Type As reveal a stronger need than Type Bs to 'prove themselves'. Henley and Furnham (1989) have demonstrated that Type A persons show higher actual–ideal self-discrepancy scores than Type B persons when asked to rate themselves, and their ideal selves on a list of forty trait-like adjectives. Interestingly, however, the study also suggests that low self-esteem is not necessarily synonymous with negative self-evaluation. It was found, for example, that Type A subjects were more likely than Type B subjects to rate their ideal selves as 'dominating', 'demanding' and 'conceited'.

BEYOND THE TYPE A CONSTRUCT

We have so far only considered Type A as a global construct. In doing so we have found that the crucial relationship with CHD is far from clear. The theories of what might underpin Type A which we have just considered might further suggest to us that certain more clearly defined personality measures, implicit in global Type A assessment, may be more important than others in predicting CHD. What findings emerge from the literature which give support to such a view?

The well-known theory of personality put forward by H.J. Eysenck proposes three principal and fundamental dimensions of personality, which are purported to have innate biological roots. Those dimensions are neuroticism ('anxiety-proneness'), extroversion and psychoticism (tough-mindedness). Eysenck and Fulker (1983) identify Type A individuals as high on neuroticism and extroversion, while Eysenck (1985) suggests that high psychoticism may also be linked to certain of the 'hostility' aspects of Type A behaviour pattern. From this perspective, however, we are still left with the question of trying to be more precise about CHD risk.

If Type A persons are more anxiety prone, this does not of itself seem related to risk of myocardial infarction, although anxiety measures do seem to predict angina (for a review of relevant studies see Eysenck 1985). Interestingly, the large Framingham study, described above, but not cited by Eysenck, could be interpreted as supporting his case. The overall significant predictive relationship between the FTAS and CHD relies heavily on incidence of angina. Moreover, the FTAS is more strongly and more consistently correlated with anxiety measures than any other Type A scale (Byrne et al. 1985; Evans and Moran 1987a). Unfortunately, the diagnosis of angina is far more 'subjective' than myocardial infarction and may be influenced by how much the person complains. Since anxiety-proneness measures such as Eysenck's neuroticism scale are also measures of 'complainer's syndrome', the interpretation of findings in this area is fraught with problems. Eysenck (1985) even cites one study (Elias et al. 1982) which reports a negative correlation between anxiety and the degree of arterial stenosis ('narrowing') objectively assessed by angiography, an invasive technique whereby the condition of artery walls can be directly inspected. Angiographic studies, in which the degree of coronary atherosclerosis is objectively determined, have however shed light on the role of other components of the Type A behaviour pattern. The background to such studies is similar to that in relation to CHD itself as an end-point measure. About half of the angiographic studies have found that global Type A measures do relate to degree of atherosclerosis and about half have found no significant relationship. In an important angiographic study using audio-tapes of SI assessments of Type A, Dembroski et al. (1985) rated their subjects on twelve distinct components of the global profile. Of these only two significantly predicted degree of atherosclerosis. They were:

'potential for hostility' and 'anger-in'. Moreover, the two interacted so that atherosclerosis was particularly pronounced in subjects high on both measures: someone with a lot of potential for hostility but uncomfortable about expressing angry emotions openly.

This study is important for two reasons. First, it does seem to offer some resolution of the ambiguities posed by angiographic findings as a whole. Second, it is in broad agreement with re-analyses of WCGS data concerning the relationship between Type A and CHD. Matthews *et al.* (1977) report that CHD cases in the original WCGS were primarily distinguished from controls on the basis of hostility, anger, irritation, competitiveness and vigorous voice stylistics. Prospective studies have also implicated a quite separate (MMPI) measure of hostility in CHD (Barefoot *et al.* 1983; Shekelle *et al.* 1983). It is therefore not surprising that most recent writers on the subject of Type A have tended to mention hostility as the most promising 'active' component of the Type A global pattern, perhaps especially what has been termed 'cynical' hostility (Williams 1989).

BEHAVIOURAL INTERVENTION? A CONCLUDING VIEWPOINT

If Type A is a behavioural risk factor for CHD then it might seem a reasonable course of action to devise 'treatments' to modify it. However, the evidence which we have reviewed in this chapter may lead us to a very different conclusion. It is at least possible that Type A is not a risk factor at all. If it is a risk factor we are still far from fully understanding which of its many components may be particularly 'malignant' and which may be quite 'benign'. Most seriously of all, the group at which any treatment would likely be targeted, i.e. survivors of an initial coronary incident, is the sort of high-risk group for whom evidence of Type A involvement is most lacking. Moreover, the wisdom of intervention to alter Type A must surely come under scrutiny when we consider that at least one study (Ragland and Brand 1988) has found worse survival rates for Type B individuals. Until the results of that study are more fully understood, I would think it quite premature to advocate Type A intervention studies on any great scale. Meanwhile, the efforts of health psychologists may perhaps be better directed towards devising broad treatment packages for the reduction of stress, and behavioural intervention to reduce the other known CHD risk factors such as cigarette smoking and high blood pressure.

Nevertheless, some studies already exist, dating from the more fair-weather days of Type A research, which suggest that intervention to reduce Type A behaviour can be beneficial. Behaviour modification trials are important tests of the validity of the Type A construct, even though we may at this stage have reservations about how enthusiastically we may recommend subjects to participate in them. The principal reason for their importance lies in the fact that such trials constitute the only research in which the key independent variable – Type A itself – is actually manipulated. Reduced CHD following reduced Type A behaviour thus directly argues in favour of a genuine causal link.

The results of a properly randomized trial of behaviour modification were reported by Friedman *et al.*(1984). The incidence of cardiac recurrence in patients allocated to an experimental treatment group was 7.2 per cent compared to 13 per cent in a routine cardiological counselling control group. However, as Eysenck (1985) points out, the effects are not large and there is a difficulty in knowing the specifics of the behaviour change which occurred. The latter is potentially an important matter. If cognitive theories of Type A of the kind we have discussed are correct in identifying core elements of the global construct, then it may be that some kind of 'cognitive therapy' will be more appropriate than simple behaviour modification in promoting the therapeutic goal of reducing risk for CHD.

Chapter 14

Social drugs: their effects upon health

Andrew Parrott

INTRODUCTION

The consumption of drugs which alter mood and behaviour form part of the habits and rituals of many societies. Aborigines smoked *Dubiosa* leaves for their narcotic effects; Aztec Indians smoked various psychoactive plants; chewing *Khat* leaves is part of Yemeni culture; while opium consumption is considered normal for the elderly in several far-eastern countries. Ingestion of three particular psychoactive drugs has however become ubiquitous – nicotine, alcohol and caffeine. Their modes of consumption, psychological effects, consequences for health and methods for reducing intake will be described.

NICOTINE

Tobacco (*Nicotinia tabacum*) was introduced into Europe from South America, although Europeans already smoked herbal mixtures for 'medicinal' reasons. Some of these remain available today, although why they are sold in 'health' shops, when their smoke is replete with cancer-inducing tars, remains a mystery. King James I in 1604 described smoking as: 'A custome lothsome to the Nose, hermful to the braine, dangerous to the Lungs, and in the blacke stinking fume therof, neerest resembling the horrible Stigian smoke of the pit that is bottomlesse' (Mangan and Golding 1984). He imposed a heavy import duty because: 'The health of our People is impayred and their bodies weakened.' Others claimed that smoking was medicinal: curing headaches, healing wounds, removing ulcers, getting rid of 'naughty breath' and an aphrodisiac (Ashton and Stepney 1982). Its addictiveness was recognized early; one Spanish conquistadore bishop reprimanded his soldiers in South America for 'drinking smoke', but they replied that it was not in their power to refrain.

The chewing of tobacco, snuff and nicotine bags is a rising concern for health in the USA, with around 12 million users, and increasing incidence of oral cancer (Glover *et al.* 1989; Surgeon General 1988), but tobacco is mostly consumed as cigarettes (93 per cent of UK tobacco consumption). The percentage of UK males who smoke fell from 65 per cent in 1950 to 40 per cent in 1980, but more females now smoke than previously (39 per cent in the UK in 1980), while consumption per female smoker has also increased (50 cigarettes per week in 1950, 114 cigarettes per week in 1980). This increase may reflect several factors: removal of social taboos, more socially assertive (drinking/smoking) role models, increased stress during adolescence and greater economic power. Rigotti (1989: 931) has summarized the current USA perspective:

> An estimated 56 million Americans still smoke, and the rate at which young people take up the habit has not declined since 1980. Rates of smoking are higher among less-educated, lower-income, and minority groups – groups already disproportionately burdened with illness. Equally disturbing, the gender gap among smokers is narrowing. If trends continue, women will outsmoke men by the mid-1990s.

In ethological terms smoking comprises a displacement activity: some purposeful activity during social uncertainty, and a form of social control or dominance. Psychoanalytic theories describe it as continuous oral self-gratification, penis or breast substitute, or death wish. However, a significant reason for smoking is the addictive properties of its active agent, nicotine (Surgeon General 1988). These are indicated by several types of evidence: Johnston (1942) self-administered nicotine, and after a while preferred the nicotine injections to his cigarettes; administration of a nicotine antagonist led to a 30 per cent increase in cigarette consumption (Stollerman et al. 1973); nicotine substitution can aid smoking cessation (Table 14.2); animals can be trained to self-administer nicotine, confirming its rewarding properties (Hanson et al. 1979); lastly, non-nicotine (herbal) cigarettes remain unpopular though they must fulfil equally the psychosocial and ethological functions.

Nicotine affects various psychological functions. Pomerleau et al. (1983) found that smoking led to an increase in beta-endorphin levels in CNS, the endogenous neuropeptides involved in pleasure and pain. Control of emotional states such as tenseness and aggression may be effected through the cholinergic synapses in the limbic system which is implicated in 'punishment' (Ashton 1987). Memory can be improved or impaired depending upon the conditions (Mangan and Golding 1984; Wesnes and Warburton 1983), while sustained attention and vigilance are often improved (Parrott and Winder 1989; Wesnes and Warburton 1983; Williams 1980). Nicotine's effects on arousal are biphasic, with low doses increasing EEG measures of alertness, and higher doses decreasing arousal. Smokers probably actively control their arousal level by manipulating nicotine intake (Ashton 1987; Mangan and Golding 1984). This is shown by their patterns of inhalation. Under conditions of high emotion or stress, inhalation is typically deep and frequent, thereby self-administering high (sedative) doses. In boring low-stress conditions, inhalation is shallow and less frequent, thus delivering low and alerting doses.

The burning cigarette produces hundreds of different gases and chemicals, including tar and carbon monoxide. Russell (1989) stated: 'People smoke mainly for nicotine but die mainly from tar, carbon monoxide and other components.' Tar comprises the organic chemicals suspended on the smoke droplets; on exhalation tar remains in the lungs as a sticky brown residue. Mangan and Golding (1984: 18) stated 'The position of tar as a cancer agent is clear. . .various tar components are cancer-initiating and cancer-accelerating . . .the carcinogenic role of cigarette smoke is causal and direct.' Doll and Peto (1976) demonstrated a direct relationship between cigarette consumption and cancer. Smokers taking 15–24 cigarettes per day had ten times the lung cancer rate of non-smokers, while those smoking more than twenty-five cigarettes per day had twenty-two times the incidence of cancer. Cancer takes time to develop, but other lung disorders are noticeable in new smokers. Lung capacity, as measured by the Forced Expiratory Volume (FEV) test, is reduced from the time smoking is started, and decreases the longer it continues (Royal College of Physicians 1983). Once smoking is stopped, the decline of FEV lung function becomes normalized, complaints of shortness of breath are reduced, and the capacity for strenuous physical activity gradually returns. Other smoking-induced lung disorders include mucus hypersecretion (persistent cough with voluminous phlegm), and chronic obstructive lung disease (airway passages constricted, with difficult breathing, and peripheral lung tissue death). Bronchitis or lung infection also becomes more common. Progressive disability leads slowly to death (Table 14.1). Pipe and cigar smokers, and tobacco chewers, tend to develop cancers of the lips, mouth and gum, rather than of the lung (Table 14.1), reflecting oral concentrations of nitrosamine and tar residues (Glover et al. 1989).

Carbon monoxide (CO) combines with haemoglobin in the blood to form carboxyhaemoglobin; it has 200 times greater affinity for haemoglobin than oxygen. Thus, the oxygen-carrying capacity of the blood is reduced, while diseases of the peripheral circulation increase. Arteriosclerosis in the lower limbs can cause leg pains; continued smoking can lead to tissue death and gangrene. Over 90 per cent of patients suffering from peripheral arterial disease are moderate or heavy smokers (Laing et al. 1981). When arterial bypass surgery is attempted, success is lower in those who continue to smoke, and leg amputation may be required. Arteriosclerosis may be followed by haemorrhage, thus cerebrovascular strokes are more frequent in smokers (Royal College of Physicians 1983). The most serious effect of this reduced blood supply, however, is upon the functioning of the heart. In a microscopic analysis of cardiac blood vessels, Auerbach et al. (1976) found that the smallest arteries supplying the heart were 'severely thickened' in 91 per cent of heavy smokers (more than forty cigarettes a day), in 48 per cent of moderate

Table 14.1 Medical and psychological effects of tobacco constituents: nicotine, tar and carbon monoxide

---

Nicotine
Arousal control: manipulate depth/frequency of inhalation.
Feeling states: reduced aggression/irritability, increased pleasure.
Information processing: attention increased, memory increased or decreased.
Heart function: increased heart rate and blood pressure, cardiac problems
 exacerbated.

Tar
Cancer of the lung associated with cigarettes.
Cancer of mouth and jaw associated with pipes, cigars and tobacco chewing.
Lung disease, e.g. bronchitis, chronic obstructive lung disease.
Lung capacity: progressive decline from initiation of smoking.
Colds and coughs: increased frequency/duration.

Carbon monoxide
Oxygen-carrying capacity of the blood: reduced.
Peripheral circulation impaired: tissue death, gangrene, amputation.
Blood supply to the heart reduced: heart attack.
Narrowed arteries: fatal haemorrhage, cerebrovascular stroke.
Foetal blood supply: reduced nourishment, below average birth weight.

---

smokers (more than twenty a day), and in 0 per cent of those who had never smoked regularly. Doll and Peto (1976) investigated the incidence of heart disease in British doctors. Among the under-45 year olds, for every 100,000 cases, 7 were non-smokers, 41 were smokers of between one and fourteen cigarettes a day, and 104 were smokers of more than twenty-five cigarettes a day. Within all age groups, the more cigarettes smoked, the higher the incidence of heart disease. Lee (1980) offered a reanalysis of these incidence rates, but the basic pattern remained unchanged. Overall, heart disease causes far more deaths than lung cancer.

Health concerns have recently been expressed about 'passive smoking', the uptake of smoke-impregnated air by non-smokers (Surgeon General 1986). An average room has three times the CO level when smoking has occurred, while in small confined spaces (cars, submarines, unventilated offices), concentrations can be raised thirty-fold. Carcinogenic tars enter the lungs of non-smokers and nicotine can be measured in their urine. Non-smoking wives of husbands who smoke have a doubled risk of lung cancer (Hirayama 1981). The health of the child is also impaired: bronchitis and pneumonia are increased in infants, older children suffer more respiratory complaints, time off school, are shorter in height, and score lower on standardized tests at age eleven (Royal College of Physicians 1983). During pregnancy, female smokers have an increased rate of antenatal problems, more spontaneous abortions, more abnormal placentas, and babies on average 200 gms lighter; this reflects retarded intra-uterine growth (Royal College of Physicians 1983).

Table 14.2 Smoking cessation methods

Pharmacological: nicotine substitution

Nicotine chewing gum: chewed slowly to generate serum nicotine 30–50 per cent of levels obtained with smoking. Cessation improved (Jarvis *et al.* 1982; Schneider *et al.* 1983).

Nasal nicotine: gel droplets in the nose. Higher plasma nicotine than with gum, but embarrassment at using it in company. Recent development (Jarvis *et al.* 1986).

Transdermal nicotine: sticky plaster with nicotine permeating slowly through the skin. Recent development (Abelin *et al.* 1989)

Nicotine antagonist: consumption of mecamylamine which blocks the actions of nicotine. Beneficial responses, but impractical due to adverse side-effects (Surgeon General 1988).

Change to lower nicotine brand: compensation by smoking more or inhaling more deeply or frequently, with nicotine, tar and carbon-monoxide levels only slightly reduced; therefore not very effective. Medium nicotine, low tar/carbon-monoxide cigarettes need to be developed (Benowitz *et al.* 1983; Russell 1989; Surgeon General 1988).

Behavioural treatments

Coping skills: cognitive coping strategies: remind self of negative consequences of smoking (e.g. cancer) and benefits of cessation (e.g. fitness).

Social skills: rejecting offered cigarettes, asking others not to smoke, or influencing work-place policy (Hall *et al.* 1984).

Relaxation training: learn alternative stategies for dealing with stress. Not adequately tested as a sole therapy, but important in many multicomponent programmes (Surgeon General, 1988).

Social support: an important factor. If partner/co-workers are non-supportive then cessation is difficult. However it is hard to generate social support empirically (McIntyre-Kingsolver *et al.* 1986).

Rapid smoking: inhalation deep and frequent (every 6 seconds instead of 90 seconds) leading to nicotine overdosing. The smoker begins to feel ill and then stops. Aversive conditioning generates negative feelings towards cigarettes. It comprises an aid to cessation, but other programme components are needed to forestall later relapse (Hall *et al.* 1984).

Financial contracting: pledge money to a 'disliked' organization should relapse occur. Short-term contracting improves initial cessation, but relapse follows. Need extended contracts over 1–2 years (Bowers *et al.* 1987).

Multicomponent programmes

Different behavioural principles, or pharmacological/psychological approaches combined. High success rates. Surgeon General (1988: 500): 'Multicomponent programs have been the principal target of recent research. This is both due to the relatively high clinical success of these programs, and the recognition that smoking is multidetermined and relatively invulnerable to any single intervention.' Examples in the text.

Many of the general population recognize that there are medical hazards from smoking (Rigotti 1989), while the majority of smokers report that they would like to give up (Klesges *et al.* 1987). But this is often difficult to achieve, since just as nicotine has some positive psychological effects, so equivalent negative effects can occur on cessation, including irritability, tenseness and craving (Surgeon General 1988).

A prime difficulty for research in this area is in defining cessation objectively. Follow-up measures must be for six or twelve months. Where studies simply telephone subjects and ask if they have remained non-smokers, far higher success rates are reported than when non-smoking compliance is objectively tested through blood assay of nicotine or expired-breath CO level. Two approaches that have been widely quoted as successful in popular magazines are hypnosis and acupuncture, but they are rarely tested adequately. The Surgeon General (1988) has concluded that 'There is little evidence that acupuncture (or hypnotic induction *per se*) relieves withdrawal symptoms or promotes smoking cessation.' Many of the individual techniques summarized in Table 14.2 improve initial cessation but long-term improvements are frequently only marginal. Multicomponent programmes are generally more successful. Hall *et al.* (1984) found rapid smoking to be beneficial, as long as treatment was given on an individual basis, the therapist–client relationship was warm, there was positive success expectation, and regular encouragement was given. Some studies have successfully combined lecture courses on smoking with skills training, desensitization with intensive follow-up, or financial contracting with support groups (Surgeon General 1988). The possible combinations of approaches are endless, but Lando (1981) warns against overwhelming clients with too many strategies.

Pharmacological and psychological combinations also demonstrate increased success for smoking cessation. With nicotine gum alone, the British Thoracic Study (1983) found comparatively low success (10 per cent), but many subjects were not actively seeking treatment, and gum use was only briefly explained to participants. Studies where general practitioners recommend the gum, only briefly describe its use, and hope that it will be effective, indicate similarly low success rates (Jamrozic *et al.* 1984) with many patients not using the gum properly. Smoking clinics have higher success. Schneider *et al.* (1983) achieved 30 per cent cessation, while Jarvis *et al.* (1982) found 47 per cent success at one-year follow-up. Both trials employed trained advisors, with gum-use techniques fully explained and practised, so that success under placebo gum was also high (20 per cent and 21 per cent respectively). Counselling and rapid smoking also complement nicotine gum use (Surgeon General 1988), while Killen *et al.* (1984) found coping-skills training improved cessation 23 per cent for gum alone to 50 per cent in the combined condition. Minimal intervention has, however, been advocated as a cost-effective approach to smoking cessation. Success in percentage terms may be low, but if every doctor simply asked all patients visiting the surgery to give up smoking, gave them a leaflet to help this, and warned that they will be followed up, then 5 per cent success at one year could be expected, compared with only 0.3 per cent for control patients. If every UK doctor followed this procedure, then 500,000 ex-smokers might be achieved in one year (Heather 1989; Russell 1989).

ALCOHOL

Most civilizations have discovered alcohol, since any sugary juice left in an open container will be fermented by airborne yeasts in a few days. The earliest known laws concerned the regulation of Babylonian drinking taverns, while most societies have developed rules concerning its consumption. These follow the recognition of its pleasant effects in low doses, but deleterious consequences when taken too liberally. The effects of alcohol are summarized in Table 14.3. Modifying factors can cause this profile to vary: body weight, proportion of body fat, speed of drinking and time of day. Two further factors of importance are acute and chronic tolerance. Acute pharmacodynamic tolerance can be demonstrated by comparing subjective effects and blood alcohol (BAC) level during the initial stages of drinking (when they correlate closely) with those during further drinking when subjective effects are lower than would be expected for the BAC level (Lowe 1984). This occurs because there are rapid neuronal changes following alcohol ingestion, so that subsequent drinks are acting upon an altered neurochemical substrate. Due to this acute alcohol tolerance, drinkers routinely underestimate their degree of intoxication after a few drinks. Chronic pharmacodynamic tolerance is described by Ashton (1987); infrequent drinkers are affected by small amounts of alcohol, while habitual drinkers need large amounts to experience equivalent subjective effects. This chronic tolerance partially explains the neurochemical basis of 'alcohol dependency'. Following regular drinking, dose and frequency have to increase to produce subjective feelings of intoxication. Abrupt withdrawal causes abstinence symptoms: sleep disturbance, nausea, panic, tremor and, more severely, convulsions, craving and hallucinations.

Alcohol is a central nervous system depressant 'producing a dose-dependent decrease in arousal in a manner similar to that of the general anaesthetics' (Ashton 1987: 178). All psychological functions are impaired by moderate to high doses of alcohol. Low doses affect sensory alertness, vigilance and psychomotor accuracy, while leaving response speed unchanged. Hansteen et al. (1976) assessed car driving on a 1.1 mile closed course, and found accuracy significantly impaired while course completion times were marginally faster. The frequency of car accidents is related to the BAC level of the driver. At 80mg/100ml BAC, the incidence of accidents is doubled, at 150mg/100ml it is ten times higher, while at 200mg/100ml car accidents are twenty times more frequent (Royal College of Psychiatrists 1986).

Table14.3 Psychological and physiological effects of alcohol in an 'average' drinker

Blood alcohol concentration	Typical psychological/physiological effect
(BAC; mg/100ml blood)	
30	relaxation
	increased talkativeness
50	impaired vigilance/concentration
	mild euphoria
70	reduced sensory alertness
	reduced mental/cognitive ability
	reduced motor co-ordination
100	feelings of intoxication
	pronounced decrements in skilled tasks
	clumsiness, walking affected
150	staggering with eyes open
	slurred speech
	severe mental/psychomotor impairments
200	nausea/vomiting
	unresponsive to most stimuli
300	anaesthesia/slow heavy breathing
	hypothermia
400–500	coma/death

After: Ashton, 1987; Lowe, 1984; and others.

Performance impairments are not restricted to car driving. Billings *et al.* (1973) compared flying a light aircraft by experienced and novice pilots. Flying ability showed a linear dose-response decrement, and it was concluded that there was no safe alcohol level. An analysis of hospital out-patients being treated for accidental falls in Finland, showed that 53 per cent of patients had been drinking, compared with 15 per cent of matched controls, with the probability of an accident again being dose related (Honkanen *et al.* 1983).

Drinking is a cause of considerable social disruption: drunkenness, mugging, wife and child battering, rape, murder (British Medical Journal 1982). Social behaviours are strongly dependent upon behavioural inhibition, which is released under alcohol's disinhibiting influence. The Royal College of Psychiatrists (1986) stated:

> The more one considers the woman who steals, the accountant who embezzles, the man who knives his wife in a quarrel, the more one sees common elements . . . lack of impulse control . . . which brings the individual nothing in the way of real gain or satisfaction.

Residential and business fires, deaths by drowning, transport disasters – each is more common under alcohol. Regulatory authorities concerned with health and welfare list alcohol as a major contributor to accident rates. McDonnell and Maynard (1985) estimated the 1983 costs to industry in England and Wales as £1,398 millions. These compared with £96 millions for the costs of the health service, £89 millions for traffic accidents, and £1 million for expenditure on national alcohol agencies and research. The indirect social costs of alcohol to health and happiness considerably outweigh its direct health costs.

The subjective effects of a small dose of alcohol are pleasant, with reduced tension, and increased sociability. The Royal College of Psychiatrists (1986) described an unpublished study, where a cocktail hour was introduced into an American hospital for the aged. Medical and sleep complaints diminished, while many hospital staff joined in during their meal breaks. Social cohesiveness can therefore be improved, but similar findings might have occurred from the introduction of a low-alcohol cocktail hour! Alcohol can also induce negative feelings including increased aggression, and arguments. The development of acute and chronic tolerance (see above) means that continued drinking may fail to relieve the anxiety and depression it originally dulled, and may exacerbate feelings of depression or worthlessness. Alcohol also increases the suicide potential of sedative antidepressant and anxiolytic drugs (see Chapter 6).

Alcohol is metabolized by the liver into waste products (for example, acetaldehyde) which are then excreted. Regular drinking can lead to a progression of liver diseases, probably initiated by these breakdown products. Fatty liver is indicative of early disorder, and although it can be detected by metabolic tests, otherwise it is often symptomless. Inflammation of the liver or alcoholic hepatitis may next develop. It can cause severe problems: jaundice, abdominal pain and intestinal bleeding, but again may be symptomless. Further drinking may lead to cirrhosis, when the liver becomes shrunken, hard and knobbly with scar tissue. At this stage liver functioning is severely impaired, and eventual death may be hastened by liver cancer. This progressive decline in liver function takes years to develop, and may be stopped if drinking is halted (Sherlock 1982). The national incidence of liver cirrhosis correlates closely with per capita consumption of alcohol. It is most frequent in countries with high alcohol consumption (for example, France), and is increasing in other affluent nations where consumption is rising (UK). Stomach and intestines can also be adversely affected, both by occasional binge drinking, and moderate regular drinking. Inflammation of the endothelium ('lining') of the gut, lesions of the gut wall and ulcer exacerbation can all occur. The pancreas can also be damaged, causing potentially lethal pancreatitis. Excess drinking can also affect heart functioning, leading to hypertension and increased heart disease (Sherlock 1982). This occurs for all age groups, but is particularly noticeable in young, and otherwise apparently healthy, heavy drinkers.

Regular drinking is often associated with irregular eating and poor nutrition. This leads to general debilitation and proneness to disease. In extreme cases drinkers may not eat for long periods, leading to thiamine vitamin deficiency. This produces Wernicke's encephalopathy, which can progress to Korsakoff's Psychosis (Joyce 1987). Confusion and profound memory loss predominate, with lesions in many brain areas, and only the former disease responds to thiamine replacement. Impaired brain function also occurs in many heavy drinkers with no clinical signs of intellectual decline. Lee *et al.* (1979) found cortical atrophy in 49 per cent of young adult male heavy drinkers when assessed by computed tomography brain scan, with degeneration accompanied by deficits in psychometric test performance. Leonard (1989: 54) described alcohol as a neurotoxin which directly destroys neural tissue: 'Chronic alcohol consumption is associated with progressive degeneration and death of cortical neurones.' This may be caused by alcohol altering the lipid composition of nerve-cell membranes. Drinking leads to the 'Foetal Alcohol Syndrome', characterized by foetal maldevelopment (particularly in the CNS) in around 40 per cent of heavy-drinking pregnant mothers (Ashton 1987). Contributing factors include social deprivation, malnourishment and multiple drug use. The whole area of the health consequences of alcohol consumption is made difficult by the absence of reliable markers for early disease states. In the absence of clear criteria for foetal damage, it is therefore best to advise caution about drinking alcohol during pregnancy.

Two models are currently used to conceptualize problem drinking and alcoholism, the medical and social-learning models. Although often seen as contrasting, each describes elements of the overall problem. The social-learning model concentrates on environmental cues for alcohol (Heather and Robertson 1981; Peele 1985). Industrialized societies are replete with such cues, almost all of them positive. The deleterious effects of alcohol are rarely presented. In view of alcohol's pervasive position within society, the social-learning model sees it as unrealistic to expect any drinker to abstain totally, so 'controlled drinking' is advocated (Heather and Robertson 1981; Peele 1985). Problem drinkers are helped to learn more appropriate drinking responses, are presented with accurate information about its ill-effects, and encouraged to learn from their own and others' personal experiences.

The medical model sees the problem drinker or alcoholic as having a metabolism where normal control over alcohol is lost or reduced. Variants of the medical model suggest a genetic predisposition (an endogenous 'liking' for alcohol), or some other natural metabolic hypersensitivity (Blum and Trachtenberg 1988). Evidence for these predisposition models is weak. There is, however, more evidence for those medical models which state that alcoholism results from heavy drinking. Tolerance to the repeated ingestion of alcohol and other psychoactive drugs is well established. Numerous changes in the brain chemistry of alcoholics have been described, some of which remain after months or even years of abstinence (Ashton 1987; Blum and Trachtenberg 1988; Cicero 1978). Treatment along medical-model lines is often based upon the 'Minnesota' method, which requires total abstinence.

Following initial drying out (detoxification), support, encouragement, group discussion and experience sharing are provided by ex-alcoholics as co-therapists. Once stablilized as non-drinkers, follow-up support along the same lines is provided by Alcoholics Anonymous; everyone has a group of fellow ex-drinkers whom they can contact at any time for support in their abstention. These self-help groups have provided the model for many other successful organizations concerned with habitual behaviours i.e. overeating, narcotics abuse and gambling.

The basic principles of therapy proposed by the medical and social-learning models are not dissimilar: group support, open discussion of problems, the necessity for changed self-image and response repertoire. Their main differences are in their conceptualization (metabolic disease versus learned response), and advocated goal (abstinence or controlled drinking). This polarization into two opposing camps is comparatively recent. Davies (1962) described a group of alcoholics, some of whom had adopted a successful 'problem-free' style of drinking. This report led to heated exchanges in academic circles, and the emerging division between approaches (Peele 1985). Ojehagen and Berglund (1989) have stated, 'Whether engagement in non-problem drinking is possible for alcoholics is still one of the most controversial questions in the alcoholism treatment and research areas.' Theoretical *rapprochement* has been occurring, with both chronic drug tolerance and learned factors accepted as important, and therapeutic goal often chosen by the client. Heather and Robertson (1981) suggested that therapeutic goal could vary, depending upon the severity of the drinking problem, and whether the clients believed they had control over alcohol. Miller (1983) related the therapeutic goal to the initial drinking problem; with severe alcoholics, 'abstinence' often produced the best outcome, while with less severely affected drinkers 'controlled drinking' was generally superior.

CAFFEINE

'Caffeine is the most widely used behaviourally active drug in the world' (Griffiths and Woodson 1988: 437). It occurs in over 60 plant species, several of which are used to form beverages: tea (using leaves of *Thea sinensis*), coffee (seeds of *Coffea arabica*), chocolate and cocoa (berries of *Theobroma cacoa*), cola-flavoured drinks (berry of *Cola acuminata*), and others such as mate and yoco. It is also present in many over-the-counter medicines (Table 14.4). World consumption of caffeine averages 50 mg per person per day, with 90 per cent consumed in the form of tea or coffee (Gilbert 1981). Consumption in the west is higher, with an average daily intake of 200 mg in the USA (Gilbert 1981), 444 mg in the UK, and 425 mg in Sweden (Griffiths and Woodson 1988).

Caffeine is a weak CNS stimulant, leading to increased feelings of alertness (Clubley *et al.* 1979; Goldstein *et al.* 1969; Lieberman *et al.* 1987; Pacey and Parrott, unpublished; Seashore and Ivy 1953), and anxiety, jitteriness and

Table 14.4 Average caffeine content of various beverages, foods and proprietary medicines

Dietary source	Average caffeine concentration (5oz cup)
	mg
Tea	40
Real coffee	100
Instant coffee	70
Decaffeinated coffee	3
Cola drink	20
Hot chocolate	10
Milk chocolate (small bar)	20
Cojene	95
Phensic	50
Beecham's Hot Lemon	50
Lucozade	35
Anadin	15

From Barrone and Roberts 1984; Bruce and Lader 1986; Kenny and Darragh 1986 and others.

muscular tremor (Loke *et al.* 1985; Veleber and Templer 1984). Variation in response relates to whether the person is a high-caffeine user (HCU) or low-caffeine user (LCU). Goldstein *et al.* (1969) found that HCUs reported irritability and sleepiness when changed to placebo, whereas LCUs reported shakiness, jittery feelings and upset stomach when given caffeine. Self-rated alertness levels in HCUs and LCUs over twenty-four hours are shown in Figure 14.1. Caffeine maintained the alertness of HCUs, while with decaffeinated coffee alertness was decreased. Caffeine maintained the 'clear head' of HCUs, whereas after decaffeinated coffee 'headache' levels increased over the twenty-four hours (Pacey and Parrott, unpublished). In addition to headache and fatigue, sudden caffeine reduction can also lead to nausea and coffee craving, particularly with very high consumers, although this rarely lasts more than forty-eight hours (Griffiths and Woodson 1988).

In terms of behavioural effects, Dews (1984: 87) stated that 'Caffeine in the amounts that are given has effects so slight and subtle that the investigator is usually glad to be able to detect them.' During the Second World War, caffeine was assessed to see if it enhanced the performance of soldiers. It led to 'desirable subjective effects, but negligible improvements in sensori-motor coordinations' (Seashore and Ivy 1953: 13). Laboratory studies have tended to confirm the above (Bruce and Lader 1986; Kenny and Darragh 1986), although sensitive vigilance tasks are sometimes improved (Lieberman *et al.* 1987; Regina *et al.* 1974).

In terms of health effects, three main areas of concern have been raised concerning caffeine: impaired sleep, increased anxiety and irritability, and as a contributing factor to heart disease. The deleterious effects of caffeine upon sleep have been demonstrated in many studies (Bruce and Lader 1986; Kenny

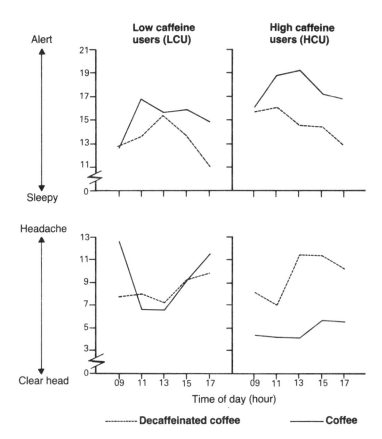

Figure 14.1 Self-rated feelings of alertness and headache incidence following decaffeinated and caffeinated coffee in low and high users of caffeine.

and Darragh 1986). Karacan *et al.* (1976) found sleep duration decreased, and time to fall asleep increased, in a dose-dependent manner. It increases subjective perceptions of time taken to get to sleep, while sleep feels less sound and with more restlessness (Goldstein *et al.* 1969). This occurs with many low- and high-caffeine users, although some HCUs report sleep improvements under caffeine. High rates of coffee consumption have been shown to produce a state characterized by anxiety, nervousness, restlessness, tremor and shakiness, and insomnia. These symptoms may be misdiagnosed as 'anxiety neurosis', since only when the high level of caffeine intake is revealed can it be identified correctly as 'caffeinism' (Greden 1974), or 'caffeine intoxication' (Bruce and Lader 1986).

Caffeinism is associated with regular high intake of caffeine in the region of 700–1,000 mg/day. It is remedied by the reduction of caffeine, but re-emerges if caffeine intake is restored (Bruce and Lader 1986; Greden 1974; Kenny and Darragh 1986). Since caffeinism is rarely recognized, those misdiagnosed as 'anxiety disorder' will often be treated with benzodiazepines or low-dose antidepressants (see Chapter 6). Both are inappropriate. The side-effects of benzodiazepines include drowsiness, and those of antidepressants dry-mouth in addition to drowsiness; and both may lead to increased caffeine intake. Hospital in-patients on antidepressant or neuroleptic medications often consume high levels of liquid in its most readily obtainable form, i.e. tea or coffee. When hospital supplies of normal coffee have been changed to decaffeinated, there have been indications of improved patient behaviour (De Freitas and Schwartz 1979; Podboy and Mallory 1977).

The third area of medical concern is cardiovascular effects, with reports of an increased risk from coronary heart disease (CHD). Several large-scale studies have been undertaken, and the current position is that these earlier reports of increased risk from heart attack have not been replicated (Bergman and Dews 1987; Robertson and Curatolo 1984). This area illustrates well some of the difficulties in undertaking health research. Much of the evidence is epidemiological, based on association between selected variables, for example coronary disease and caffeine intake. The problem is that an association may reflect common correlation with some third factor (for example, cholesterol, nicotine, blood pressure, social class or some other unknown factor).

In one of the earliest of the large-scale studies, Paul et al. (1968) noted a positive correlation between coffee consumption and heart disease, but a more detailed analysis found that this may have been caused by an association with tobacco, since the high coffee drinkers also smoked more cigarettes. The Boston Drug Surveillance Group also reported that coffee consumption was associated with CHD, but although smoking was controlled, other factors remained uncontrolled. A later study by the same group confirmed the association between caffeine and myocardial disease, having controlled for sugar use, past heart disease, obesity, smoking, age and sex. Coffee consumption of more than six cups a day was associated with a doubled risk of heart attack (Jick et al. 1973). Since then, however, several large-scale studies have failed to confirm any link between caffeine and heart disease. Heyden et al. (1978) found no association between caffeine and heart disease. In another prospective study, Tibblin and Wilhelmsen (1975) found no association between coffee intake and later heart disease in Sweden. Other negative findings are listed in Robertson and Curatolo (1984). They also suggested factors in the Boston research which may have caused a spurious association; the control group comprised discharged medical patients who may have previously reduced their caffeine for other reasons (for example, gastrointestinal problems), retrospective recall may have wrongly estimated the real level of caffeine consumption, and in addition, physical activity was not controlled in the study.

While current evidence therefore suggests that caffeine is not associated with coronary heart disease, it may exacerbate cardiac arrhythmias. The evidence is under debate. Bergman and Dews (1987: 207) concluded that 'No hazard from caffeine consumption in persons with cardiac arrhythmias has been established.' Robertson and Curatolo (1984) suggest that the problem needs more thorough investigation. Myers (1987) concluded that caffeine was not an exacerbating factor. Despite the absence of firm evidence, it remains medical practice to recommend caffeine reduction. Such advice is easy to give, appears sensible and logical, can be readily implemented, and perhaps comprises good 'placebo' treatment (see Chapter 6).

There have been suggestions that other medical conditions are caused by caffeine including cancer of the pancreas, fibrocystic disease of the breast, arteriosclerosis, and others (Bergman and Dews 1987; Robertson and Curatolo 1984; Somani and Gupta 1988). These reports sometimes originate from studies employing mega-doses of caffeine (40–250 mg/kg/day) given to animal species. These are equivalent to 2,800–17,500 mg per person per day, and have few implications for normal dietary intake. Caffeine has been shown to elevate free fatty acid metabolism, but the health implications of this remain unclear (Somani and Gupta 1988). The effects of caffeine during pregnancy have also been investigated; no studies have found any relationship between caffeine and birth weight, or birth abnormalities (ibid.). In their review of dietary caffeine and human health and disease, Bergman and Dews (1987: 199) concluded that 'There has continued to be a perhaps never-ending series of suggestions of adverse effects which further investigation shows to be ill-founded. . . . There is much more substantial evidence that dietary consumption is harmless in normal people.'

FUTURE PROSPECTS FOR HEALTH

Many smoking and alcohol programmes have been advocated by health agencies, but their implementation by governments is poor. A government may even scrap or limit a national health agency which starts to become effective, as reportedly happened recently in the UK (Farrell 1989a). Economic arguments which emphasize tax and excise revenue would, however, be short sighted, since reduced consumption would lead not only to improved health budgets, but to massive financial savings throughout industry. Many programmes for improved health have been proposed by international (WHO Expert Committees on Alcohol and Tobacco) and national agencies (Royal College of Psychiatrists 1986; Surgeon General 1988). These emphasize the roles for governments in defining policy concerning factors that determine consumption. These include: taxation, access, advertising images, education, legislation, and health-promotion campaigns. Many current programmes are based on models that emphasize individual responsibility, which may be inadequate in the absence of appropriate support systems.

Chapter 15

Diabetes

Brenda May

INTRODUCTION

There is no cure for diabetes, but modern medical procedures can 'manage', or control the symptom – high blood-sugar – so that near-normal physiological uptake of glucose can be achieved.

Reporting in 1988, Nabarro estimates that diabetes is a heavy burden on the resources of the National Health Service, with an annual cost of £350 million. This results from increased use of acute hospital beds which are needed when failure of management occurs. Nabarro suggests that if this cost is to be reduced, diabetic patients must be better educated on how to look after their condition. This would result in the economical use of health-care professionals' time. Most diabetics attend a hospital clinic two or three times a year, but the everyday management of the diabetes is in their own hands. The management involves diet and insulin injections (Type I diabetics), or diet and tablets (Type II diabetics). Blood testing (or urine testing) is undertaken by the diabetic as a way of monitoring the success of the management. Before considering the issue of education further it is necessary to understand the condition of diabetes itself.

THE NATURE OF DIABETES

Diabetes mellitus is a chronic disorder of carbohydrate, lipid and protein metabolism which results from the inadequate production, or utilization, of insulin. Insulin is a hormone produced by the Beta Cells of the pancreatic Islets of Langerhans and it acts at the cell membranes to promote the transportation of glucose, amino acids and potassium. Its action is crucial for the efficient synthesis and storage of energy from carbohydrate foods, for protein synthesis, for the synthesis and storage of fats and for the mobilization of energy reserves in the liver, muscles and adipose tissues.

Deficiency of insulin soon leads to a state similar to starvation. Since glucose cannot be converted into energy, the body turns to protein and fat metabolism. This in turn results in two dangerous outcomes: the build-up of high levels of sugar (glucose) in the blood, and high blood levels of toxic ketone bodies and free fatty acids. Due to this metabolic pathology, the untreated diabetic shows signs of weakness, weight loss, and constant thirst and urination as the kidneys attempt to deal with the pathological blood composition.

The concentration of blood sugar or glucose is also crucial because it is the only nutrient that can be used by the brain. In the non-diabetic, this concentration is maintained by what might be best construed as a 'negative-feedback control system' (Guyton 1976). According to this view, an 'error detector' compares the actual blood-sugar level with the normal range. When the blood sugar exceeds this range, for example after a meal, corrective action is taken – insulin is secreted, and the blood-sugar concentration is lowered. If the blood sugar falls below the normal range, then glucagon, which opposes insulin, is secreted by the Alpha cells of the pancreatic Islets of Langerhans and the blood-sugar level is brought back into normal limits. In diabetics, this negative-feedback control system has failed. Diabetics have to become their own 'self-regulator' so as to control the level of sugar in the blood, and provide insulin to facilitate the utilization of glucose. This task is a very complex one which necessitates the learning of new knowledge, new skills and changes in life-style.

The goal of the management of diabetes is to approximate as closely as possible to the physiological negative-feedback control system. How, then, does the diabetic detect an 'error' in the concentration of blood sugar? Many diabetics assert that they can 'tell' if their blood sugar is too high or too low. Certainly, at the extreme ends of the continuum it is likely they are aware of the error, but the accuracy of their subjective estimates is very poor. Clinical descriptions of the symptoms of high and low blood sugar are common: very high blood sugar is said to result in extreme thirst, frequent urination, headaches, tiredness and feelings of irritability. Very low blood sugar is described as resulting in sweating, hunger, visual disturbances, weakness, the disruption of motor co-ordination, mental confusion and feelings of anxiety (Eastman et al. 1983; Mutch and Dingwell-Fordyce 1985). Studies examining the relationship between physical symptoms and reported blood-sugar levels, and between mood and reported blood-sugar levels, have found low accuracy. Diabetics are not always aware that a deviation has occurred from normal ranges of blood-sugar levels; they cannot give an accurate estimate of their blood-sugar level. Nor is there any consistent relationship between the symptoms and levels of blood sugar. Accurate 'error detection' is important. High blood sugars are in the long term associated with complications such as retinopathy, neuropathy and kidney dysfunction; low blood sugar can lead very quickly to accidents due to cognitive confusion and, if unremedied, to unconsciousness.

THE MANAGEMENT OF DIABETES

So how can the diabetic accurately detect an 'error'? This is best achieved by home blood testing. Most clinics require their diabetic patients to test their blood at least once a day, and at a different time on different days so that a good profile of levels is obtained. Home blood testing is a complex skill involving finger pricking to obtain a drop of blood, accurate timing and then colour matching to obtain a measure, but most patients can be taught successfully. Schiffrin et al. (1983), for example, found a correlation of 0.96 between laboratory results and home blood testing carried out by adolescents.

Once the 'error' has been detected, corrective action must be taken; the diabetic must do something to bring the level back into the normal range. The action taken will depend on the direction of the error. There are a number of variables that can influence blood-sugar levels, all of which interact, and the corrective action will vary according to the perceived cause of the error, but all actions will be aimed at either raising or lowering the blood-sugar level. Some of these variables will now be examined.

First, the timing and amount of insulin injected will influence the blood-sugar level. Most diabetics are on a combination of slow- and fast-acting insulin so as to control the blood-sugar level throughout the twenty-four hours. Insulin is usually injected twice a day, once before breakfast and again before the evening meal. A more recent regimen is to inject four times a day: slow-acting insulin, usually injected before bed, acts as a background level, and injections of quick-acting insulin before each main meal cope with the intake of food. Insulin pumps are now available which are in place throughout the twenty-four hours and they administer small frequent amounts of insulin with larger amounts before meals. Whichever regimen the diabetic is on, the goal is the same: a balance must be maintained between the food eaten and the insulin injected. Too much insulin in relation to the food will result in too low a blood-sugar level (hypoglycaemia), and too little insulin in too high a level (hyperglycaemia).

Not all food is important in maintaining this balance; it is dependent upon the amount of carbohydrates eaten. The diabetic must acquire knowledge about the carbohydrate values of different foods, for example an egg-sized potato has 10 gm and bangers-and-mash about 90 gm! A constant amount of carbohydrate must be eaten at each meal each day, even if the diabetic is feeling ill. Meals must also be eaten on time. The quick-acting insulin starts its action about twenty minutes after injection. If the timing is wrong, the end-product of carbohydrate metabolism (glucose) and the action of the insulin will not coincide and either hypoglycaemia (if the meal is late) or hyperglycaemia (if the meal is early) will result.

Exercise reduces blood-sugar levels and extra carbohydrates must be taken to prevent the blood sugar dropping too low. A game of football or a day's shopping may demand preventive measures to avoid hypoglycaemia. Illness, on the other hand, increases insulin requirements even when food intake is reduced.

STRESS AND DIABETES

The role of stress in disrupting blood-sugar levels is a complex one. An association between psychological stress and blood-sugar levels, or diabetic control as it is termed, has been suggested for some time. An early though unreplicated study by Hinkle and Wolfe (1952) showed that blood-sugar levels fluctuated in both diabetics and non-diabetics in response to stressful conversation topics, the level either increasing or decreasing. Bradley (1978) gave diabetic subjects a demanding fifteen-minute tracking task under noise conditions and found that the direction of blood-sugar-level changes were dependent on initial levels – those with high initial levels showed an increase, and those with low levels a decrease. Chase and Jackson (1981) studied eighty-four insulin-dependent children and adolescents and found a significant positive correlation between common stress factors and blood-sugar levels in both the short and the long term. Bradley (1979) also studied the relationship between the experience of stressful life events and measures of diabetic control (defined as poorly controlled blood-glucose levels, and changes in insulin requirements as shown in clinic records). Factor analysis of the data from 114 diabetics provided support for the hypothesis that the occurrence of stressful life events is associated with problems in the good management of diabetic control.

More recent experimental studies (Delamater et al. 1988; Gilbert et al. 1987; Kemmer et al. 1984; Stabler et al. 1987) have failed to demonstrate the effects of stress on various indices of diabetic control. Future research on stress effects must be more sophisticated in its methodology. Given the demonstrated individual effects of stress on blood-sugar levels, and the suggestion that the effects are a function of initial blood levels at the onset of the stressor, and other methodological problems inherent in examining the effects of naturally occurring stressors (for example, retrospective data gathering), it is difficult to evaluate this area of research satisfactorily. Research must be multivariate, prospective and longitudinal in design, in order to accommodate the complexities of the several variables involved. This particularly applies to studies of young diabetics, as the hormonal changes occurring in adolescence may contribute to poor control (Amiel et al. 1986).

A further conceptual problem is that of specifying the mechanisms whereby stress affects blood-sugar control. It is possible, and likely, that stress acts both directly and indirectly. Directly, it results in the production of pituitary hormones and catecholamines which result in increased blood-sugar levels in both diabetics and non-diabetics. The termination of the stressor results in a return to normal blood-sugar levels in non-diabetics, but continued elevated levels in the diabetics. Indirectly, stress acts to change behaviour. These changes are likely to interfere with regimen adherence in various ways. Eating more, or less, when upset is a common experience. Forgetting to do blood tests, or even injections, can occur. Data from the self-reports of fifty-seven adult diabetics showed that negative emotions (19 per cent of violations) and conflict (7 per cent) were thought to be the cause of eating too much, or eating the wrong types of food (Kirley 1982).

So far, stress has been seen as the cause of poor control, but it is possible that the causality may be in the other direction. Poor control might interfere with general functioning, thus exacerbating the effects of various stressors or even precipitating stress reactions. For example, low blood sugars may result in poor coping skills, or poor co-ordination may result in accidents. Frequent absences from work may result in loss of job, and altered moods in marital problems. Effective functioning depends upon cognitive skills and an interesting study by Pramming et al. (1986) highlights the difficulties that might occur during episodes of low blood sugar. Sixteen insulin-dependent men were given neuropsychological tests at four levels of blood sugar. The levels were controlled under medical supervision, and were normal (6.3 mmol/l), low (2.9 mmol/l) and very low (1.8 mmol/l). The experimental group's test results were compared with those of a control group who were subjected to the same insulin-infusion techniques but whose blood sugar was kept at normal levels throughout. The tests were chosen so as to be sensitive to small changes and had low practice effects. The skills tested ranged from simple motor tasks to complex memory and control, and an elapsed time estimation task was included. Subjects scored the intensity of their hypoglycaemic symptoms on a check-list. As was hypothesized, lowering the blood sugar to below 3 mmol/l resulted in cognitive dysfunction in twelve out of the sixteen subjects, and when the levels dropped to less than 2 mmol/l, dysfunction in all. The tests showed gradual deterioration (except for the simple psychomotor tests), and the deterioration was characterized by diminished 'attention'. At low blood-sugar levels, considerable prompting and encouragement was needed to complete the test. Patients' estimation of elapsed time showed underestimation. Most importantly, 25 per cent of the subjects did not recognize that their blood sugar was low, even though their dysfunction was very marked.

The important question, of course, is how these cognitive dysfunctions affect the ability to take action to reduce the blood-sugar 'error' and so avert severe hypoglycaemic episodes and eventual unconsciousness. The results suggest that tasks requiring planning, problem solving, control, attention, motivation and appreciation of the passage of time will be difficult even at levels of blood sugar that do not produce noticeable symptoms recognized by the diabetic. Even if symptoms are recognized and the relevant remedial steps are known, the ability to execute the action is likely to be reduced. It is not unknown for the author to go into the kitchen to eat glucose, knowing low blood-sugar is present, only to be found later doing something quite different.

When asked if action has been taken, the reply is often that there hasn't been time yet, even though some ten minutes has elapsed!

Food intake, insulin dosage, exercise and stress can all affect blood-sugar levels. The goal of the 'controlling response' is to return these to optimum levels. In the short term this will involve reducing or increasing food intake, increasing or reducing insulin dosage, or adjusting carbohydrate intake to overcome the effects of exercise. Returning blood-sugar levels to optimum depends upon accurate estimations by home blood testing. The choice of which error-reduction strategy to use will depend on the attribution made as to the cause of the disruption. This in turn will depend upon accurate self-observation of behaviour and adequate knowledge of causal effects. For example, adjusting the insulin dosage will depend on observation of the amount of food eaten over the past few days ('Is my blood sugar too high because I had too much to eat at the party?'), on the timing of the injections ('Was I late with my morning injection because I am on holiday?'), on an understanding of the action of the various insulins ('As my bedtime blood sugar is too low, should I change the fast- or slow-acting insulin, and at the morning or evening injection?'). An attribution that the change in blood-sugar level is due to stress will depend upon monitoring of events, and corrective action might be to increase or decrease the insulin, or to develop a strategy for dealing with the stress itself. The decision to change the insulin dose will, of course, depend on the chronicity of the disruption and the stress, and on the individuals' knowledge of their previous responses to such events.

STRESS MANAGEMENT IN DIABETICS

The most frequently reported direct intervention strategy for dealing with stress has been the application of relaxation techniques. By reducing sympathetic-nervous-system activity and promoting parasympathetic dominance, relaxation should encourage the storage of glucose, so reducing the levels in the blood. Research into the effectiveness of relaxation techniques has provided mixed results. Fowler et al. (1976) reported a single case-study of a 20-year-old female whose diabetic control became disrupted by physical and emotional stress. Twice-daily practice of relaxation for six months resulted in indirect support for improved control: there were fewer hospitalizations and insulin requirements were halved. Seeburg and DeBoer (1980), using similar relaxation techniques with a 24-year-old woman, also found reduced insulin needs, but the relaxation training produced instability in blood-sugar levels and had to be abandoned. A multiple-baseline, across-subjects, design was used by Rose et al. (1983) to study the effects of anxiety-management training with six adolescent girls: one patient had to be dropped from training, but the other five showed some improvement in control.

There are a number of considerations when assessing the clinical usefulness of relaxation or anxiety-management training. These are not entirely specific to this area, but apply to research on diabetes in general. Scientific methodology would necessitate random allocation to experimental and control groups in assessing effects. In clinical research this is hardly ever possible, but at the very least the characteristics of the subjects should be defined so that replications can be used to clarify the important variables related to outcome. Information about length of diagnosis, age, knowledge and skills, adherence to the regimen and other environmental factors is essential.

COMPLIANCE AND DIABETES

So far, then, it would seem that for the diabetic there are a number of rules of management which should govern their attempts to be their own 'negative-feedback control system'. Some of the basic rules might be:

1 give myself the correct insulin at the right time;
2 eat the correct foods at the right time;
3 monitor how I am doing by testing my blood;
4 if I am not doing well, find out why, and adjust things.

It is not very surprising to discover that diabetics on the whole do not comply with these 'rules' very well. It is not easy to discover the exact levels of compliance; estimates vary according to the methods used. The most common method is to ask diabetics how well they are keeping to their diet, how many blood tests they have done and what the results of the tests are. Recently a test has been developed, the glycosylated haemoglobin test (HbA1C) which is laboratory based, and this is used as an indirect measure of compliance. The test gives a measure of the average blood-sugar level over the preceding three months. More direct assessments of compliance have been attempted using a variety of methods ranging from self-report to observation of behaviour. The most thorough surveys of diabetes self-care have been carried out by Watkins and his associates (Watkins, Roberts, Williams, Martin and Coyle 1967; Watkins, Williams, Martin, Hogan and Anderson 1967). Their results showed that 80 per cent of adult diabetics administered insulin in an unhygienic manner, 77 per cent tested their urine for sugar incorrectly and interpreted the results 'in a manner likely to be detrimental to their treatment', 75 per cent did not eat the prescribed foods, nor did they eat regularly. Wilson and Endres (1986) found that 40 per cent of a group of adolescents failed to record their blood-tests results. In a recent survey of 282 diabetic children (Wing et al. 1986), it was found that 74 per cent of the children had been taught how to do the blood tests, but only two-thirds of them were doing at least one blood test a day.

The nature of the illness, and its treatment, are two important correlates with compliance. Greater non-compliance is found when illnesses are long-lasting, the condition is asymptomatic, and the prescribed regimen is complex (Haynes *et al.* 1979). Diabetes fulfils all of these – it is chronic, the regimen is certainly complex and when control is good, it is often asymptomatic. One could predict, then, that low compliance would be shown, but such a prediction does not identify the mechanisms responsible. There are problems in measuring compliance. Epstein and Cluss (1982) discuss several methods: self-report has already been discussed and has been shown to be unreliable. Another indirect method, that of therapeutic outcome, is of equally doubtful utility. The use of therapeutic outcome, in this case satisfactory blood-sugar levels, is based on the assumption that if patients obey the medical instructions their condition will be improved. It has already been suggested that in diabetes there are many intervening variables related to good control, adherence to the regimen being only part of 'good control'. Many empirical attempts have been made to increase adherence to the prescribed regimen, mostly without great success. As recently as 1987, Glasgow *et al.* reached the conclusion that 'We know little about what particular psychosocial variables are significantly related to the management of, adjustment to, or course of diabetes' (p. 406). Studies up to the present have used modest numbers of subjects and again, their design is inappropriate for such a complex interaction. So far the relationship between compliance and control has been assumed to be linear, yet clinical experience suggests that it may not be so – there are some overzealous diabetics who adhere to perfection so having little time for life, and still do not show good control!

IMPROVING COMPLIANCE

Initial attempts to improve compliance were based on the assumption that failure was due to a lack of knowledge. This has face validity: the management of diabetes requires extensive information about the condition, the action of insulin and skill acquisition. However, many studies failed to find any significant relationship between knowledge and the diabetic control measures used as the dependent variable (Graber *et al.* 1977; Watkins, Williams *et al.* 1967; Watts 1980). A study by May (1988) examined the relationship between the HbA$_1$C measures of diabetic children and adolescents, and the knowledge levels of both the diabetics and their parents. No significant relationships were found with either. Many explanations have been suggested for these disappointing research findings. The measures used to test the knowledge of diabetes have been unstandardized and have been compiled on an *ad hoc* basis; the researcher and the clinic staff choosing the areas to be tested. This lack of consistency makes it difficult to compare across studies. Dunn *et al.* (1984) have devised three parallel forms of Diabetes Knowledge Scales which may meet the needs. The item format and selection have been pilot-tested on over 300 diabetic subjects and good reliability analysis has been found.

A second problem is the infamous 'knowledge–action' gap (Drury 1984), a term which describes the finding that knowledge is no guarantee of performance. The end-point of knowledge acquisition must be behaviour change. This is not to deny that knowledge is essential, but motivation to change behaviour is the essential element. The goal of diabetic education has been well expressed by Gay (1984), an educationalist who is also a diabetic:

> For me the ultimate goal of educating diabetics is to *provide the possibility* for each person's development into an active (thinking) diabetic who is *trying to understand his/her diabetes*, rather than passively following the last orders of the doctor with little or no understanding of what is happening.
>
> (p. 24)

This admirable aim needs to be operationalized so as to provide attainable goals for educational programmes. The format of education is also important. Dunn (1986) supports other studies by showing that group, self-directed education programmes provide the greatest knowledge acquisition, and more importantly, the greatest behaviour change.

Direct attempts have been made by psychologists to change levels of compliant behaviour (Wing *et al.* 1986). Behavioural interventions have been targeted at urine and blood-sugar monitoring, insulin adjustment and administration, anxiety about needles, diet, exercise and, as already discussed, the control of responses to stressful events. Behaviour change strategies that have been used include modelling, stimulus control, reinforcement and self-monitoring.

Schafer et al. (1982) used behavioural techniques to improve compliance to urine or blood-sugar monitoring. They sequentially introduced self-monitoring, goal-setting and contingency contracting (self-reinforcement for achieving goals) with three adolescents, using a multiple baseline across behaviours design. For two of the diabetics, goal-setting procedures increased adherence on five out of the six targeted behaviours. Carney et al. (1983) implemented a similar design with three children aged 10–14 years of age to increase the frequency of blood testing. Parents gave praise and points contingent on these behaviours. High levels of compliance were maintained at four-month follow-up and HbA_1C measures improved.

The studies described are representative of attempts directly to change the behaviour of diabetics. They are mostly single-case or small sample studies, and in general, follow-up data are unavailable or of only short duration. Behaviour *can* be changed, but the goal of this type of intervention must be long-term change. Up to the present, research has not been aimed at examining the persistence of any changes achieved.

The aim of blood testing is to use the results so as to bring the levels of blood sugar as near as possible to that of non-diabetics. In other words, what is the use of testing the blood if high readings, or low ones, do not lead to changes? It would seem obvious that a target for behaviour change would be optimum levels of control via adapting behaviour, *not* compliance to, for example, requested blood-testing frequency.

The decision-making process regarding insulin adjustment is a difficult one and is likely to be confounded by the health beliefs about, and the attitudes towards diabetes held by the individual, as well as knowledge and skills. Given the complexity of factors affecting diabetic control, it would seem that a more appropriate model for intervention would be that of a functional analysis of behaviour (Owens and Ashcroft 1982), rather than an *ad hoc* attempt to 'change behaviour'.

MODELS OF DIABETIC CONTROL

The control of diabetes is moving away from being seen as a 'medical problem' towards a view that encompasses the complete individual. Psychological constructs such as 'motivation', 'attitudes', 'beliefs' and 'locus of control' are assuming greater importance in attempts to understand the difficulties faced by the diabetic, and it is to this area that the focus must turn.

In the general medical literature on adherence (Haynes and Sackett 1976), health beliefs have appeared to provide an interesting and fruitful line of approach. According to Becker and Maiman's (1975) health belief model of compliance, the likelihood of an individual taking action to adhere to the prescribed regimen is determined by five psychological 'readiness' variables. Applied to diabetes, these can be interpreted as:

1 the person's perceived susceptibility to the disease process ('I won't get diabetic complications');
2 the perceived severity of the condition ('Diabetes is serious'). These two together are termed the 'perceived threat posed by the illness';
3 the perceived benefits of taking action ('If I stick to my diet, everything will be OK');
4 the perceived physical, psychological and financial costs of taking action ('evening injections mean I can't go to the cinema with my friends');
5 the degree to which cues to action are present to activate the above psychological readiness variables ('I feel OK, even if the doctor says my sugar is too high'). These cues may be internal such as symptoms, or external such as advice from doctors and family.

This approach attempts to explain an individual's behaviour in terms of the cognitions about the disease. Studies which have examined the role of health beliefs in predicting diabetic compliance have provided ambiguous support for the model (Brownlee-Duffeck *et al.* 1987). Different measures of the five categories of health beliefs and compliance have been used. This reflects differing conceptual content. For example, 'cues to action' have been defined in the following ways: 'the subjects' ability to detect reactions in themselves' (Brownlee-Duffeck *et al.* 1987); 'the intensity of symptoms that would lead the patient to seek medical intervention' (Harris and Linn 1985); and 'the subject's intention to comply' (Cerkoney and Hart 1980). This conceptual confusion makes it impossible to conclude that certain health beliefs have any explanatory power. Studies also vary in the methodology used, some using a combination of direct observation and self-report, and others questionnaires.

The statistically significant relationships found between the five psychological variables of the health-belief model and diabetic compliance or metabolic control have on occasion been in the opposite direction from that predicted by the model. Brownlee-Duffeck *et al.* (1987), Harris and Linn (1985) and Marteau and Johnston (1986) all found that greater perceived susceptibility predicted poor adherence, though the model predicts exactly the opposite. Brownlee-Duffeck *et al.* (1987) discuss why this might be so: it could be that the model is wrong, i.e. patients who perceive themselves as susceptible do not alter their behaviour but instead react with denial. Alternatively, this could be a realistic appreciation by patients who are in poor control that they *are* more susceptible to complications! The implications of this are that it is not the health beliefs that result in particular patterns of adherence, but that health beliefs are actually determined by levels of adherence.

The usefulness of the health-belief model in predicting compliance and, more importantly, control in diabetes seems limited. As Marteau and Johnston (1986) point out, the non-independence of the main independent and dependent variables may render the model redundant as it stands. Beliefs may affect behaviour, but they may be affected by behaviour. The non-independence may also mean that any relationship between the variables may change over time. If diabetics start off with a belief that the condition is serious, they will be likely to comply (positive correlation), and this adherence might result in good control and a move towards seeing the condition as less serious (negative correlation). The relationship would vary according to the time point at which it was measured. It is also important to recognize that diabetes is not a static disease. Not only are there environmental variables that influence control, but there are times of known deterioration in both diabetic control and adaptation to the condition (Dunn 1986). The first two years after diagnosis is termed the 'honeymoon period'. During this time there is a reduction in symptoms and improved, more stable control. This initial improvement then reverses and many diabetics find this hard to deal with as it follows a time of easy control. Control also deteriorates at adolescence, possibly due to hormonal changes which coincide with the developmental tasks of increased independence at this time. Finally, fifteen to twenty years after onset, the serious complications begin to occur. Research has yet to document the psychological impact of these changes, or their effect on compliance, control and adherence.

Diabetics who perceive the disease as serious might also feel dependent upon the medical profession and see themselves as having little personal control over the outcomes of their behaviour or 'locus of control'. The relevance of locus of control to diabetic control is also ambiguous. No differences were found in locus of control between poorly controlled and well-controlled groups of adolescent diabetics (Kellerman *et al.* 1980). Hamburg and Inoff (1982) related internal locus of control to good metabolic control in girls, but to poor control in boys. Johnson (1984) points out that although an internal locus of control is held to be desirable in determining diabetic control ('It's what I do that counts'), it is possible that it may not be so desirable in practice. Such individuals might become resentful and unable to cope with what they see as 'undeserved' spontaneous poor control and this might lead to 'learned helplessness' (Seligman 1975). Internality might also be associated with delay in seeking medical advice. Wallston and Wallston (1981) reviewed and summarized numerous studies showing that adults with a chronic illness consistently state lower internal beliefs, and higher beliefs in control by chance and powerful others than do healthy adults. It would appear that the same criticisms are applicable to the locus-of-control research as to that of the health belief model. Research comparing those with chronic illness to those without, or those looking at the relationship between locus of control and adherence or diabetic control, have little to say yet to improve the life of the diabetic. We need to know the direction of causality, if the psychological construct predicts the behaviour, or vice versa. Even more important, we need to know how to change whatever it is that is measured by this psychological construct if it proves causal. More sophisticated experimental designs are the only way to clarify these issues.

EMOTION AND CONTROL

One area where promising research is developing concerns the emotional components of attitudes associated with diabetes (Dunn 1986). Earlier attempts at measuring emotions had used the judgements of 'experts' (usually doctors) as criteria for good and bad adjustments. Such experts frequently disagreed. Dunn's solution to this problem was to make no *a priori* assumptions, but to score patients' responses relative to the norms of a large representative sample. The measurement instrument was a questionnaire consisting of thirty-nine items, each being a short statement such as 'Hypos are not really as frightening as people think.' The diabetic is asked to indicate agreement with the statement on a five-point scale. Factor analysis developed six factors which Dunn suggests are best understood by analogy to a common thermometer – very high body temperatures are as pathological as very low ones, and extreme emotions and attitudes are seen as equally pathological. Standardization of the factors infers that scores above or below a cut-off point (above or below one standard deviation from the mean) represent abnormality. The factors are as follows:

1 High stress/low stress: (the degree to which the diabetic feels diabetes creates stress);
2 Poor coping/good coping: (the degree to which the diabetic feels able to cope with this stress);
3 High guilt/low guilt: (guilt and embarrassment associated with diabetes);
4 Alienated/co-operative: (measures both the degree of disenchantment with the medical profession and a conviction that one can cope independently);
5 Rejects disease/accepts disease: (measures denial and acceptance of diabetes);
6 Low tolerance/high tolerance: (measures flexibility and openness to new input, and tolerance of the ambiguities of diabetes).

A position at either end of a factor is considered maladaptive. For example, extreme scores on factor 4 would indicate that individuals who are over-dependent on the medical profession, turning to them for decisions and advice at every minor difficulty, are as maladaptive as those who do not attend the clinic at all, and feel that no one knows as much about their diabetes as they do. The scales were administered before and after an educational programme and again three months later. Two sets of results are of particular interest. First, changes in the relationship between profiles on the factors and HbA_1C measures were found as a result of the education programme. Cluster analysis produced ten distinct profile patterns, and diabetics showing a profile of co-operative adjustment – i.e. scores within the positive range on all except coping, which was just negative – showed only slight knowledge gains after the programme, and their control, which was excellent at the outset, improved even further. In contrast, initial unbalanced profiles showing low guilt and good tolerance, but negative scores on all the other factors, showed the smallest knowledge gain and their poor control deteriorated over the months following the programme. These results are initial support for the causal direction of the relationship between control, attitudinal emotions and education.

Changing attitudes, according to the model, should affect changes in control: multivariate analysis of interaction effects showed that the programme *did* produce changes in attitudes which were associated with control measures. Regression analysis showed a tendency for scores to converge towards normal during the programme.

The second set of interesting results was the differential effects due to the educational format. Group programmes produced greater knowledge and attitude change than individual education, the greatest convergence of attitudes occurring in those diabetics attending groups which allowed more time for group interaction. As ever, this study needs replication, and more information is required as to the exact educational methods and content that are effective.

It has been hypothesized that patients' perceptions and understandings of their situations can account for differences in adaptation – that is, the implicit and explicit causal explanations for their circumstances and behaviour may affect how they deal with events. These phenomena have been termed 'attribution'. As attributions are often made following negative and un-expected events, and in situations of high uncertainty, it is not surprising that the attributions made by diabetics about why their blood sugars are high or low have been of interest. Attributions which are perceived by the individual as valid and helpful in avoiding future upsets provide a working hypothesis for the future control ('Last time I sat an exam, my blood sugar went very low, so tomorrow I will give myself less insulin, or perhaps I should just eat more breakfast?'). The problem arises when the attributions are invalid. In the example given, the low sugar may have been due to getting up early to do last-minute revision and thus altering the timing of the pre-breakfast injection – something not planned for the coming exams. Valid attributions, like other hypotheses, then, need the opportunity for refutation before they can be accepted. This will depend upon information gathering such as that from measures of blood tests, and from observations of the effects of differing injection times.

One other factor that might affect compliance and control is the discrepancy between the goals and attributions of the doctors and the diabetics. Although diabetologists are now aware of the effects of psycho-logical factors on diabetic control, it is likely that their discrepant attitudes, values and attributions are transmitted to the patient during clinic attend-ances. The doctors, aware of the importance of good control in the development of complications, focus on normative blood-sugar levels as goals. The lower the blood-sugar is kept, however, the more likely it is that hypoglycaemia will occur, and this is a problem for diabetics and not likely to be an acceptable goal. Marteau and Baum (1984) obtained information from physicians as to their preferences between different blood-sugar profiles, and 90 per cent preferred a consistent, low level. Comparison of similar data from the parents of diabetic children demonstrated different goals and preferences. Significantly more parents than doctors preferred a higher than normal blood-sugar profile, and the children's level of control was closely related to their parents' rather than the doctors' goals. In line with other studies of communication effectiveness during consultations, those conducted with diabetics show that there are significant discrepancies between what the doctors tell the patients during clinic visits and what the patient recalls (Hulka et al. 1975; Page et al. 1981).

Gillespie and Bradley (1988) provide data showing that, in routine consultations, there was considerable disagreement between adult diabetics and their doctors in other areas. The diabetics and the doctors disagreed about the focus of the problem being discussed, and the causes of that problem. An example of this discrepancy was when the doctor saw fluctuating blood sugars as due to 'poor control' whereas the patient saw it as owing to not being able to go to the pub with his friends if he had to stick to his diet and go home first to do his evening injection.

These studies suggest that a number of factors during the clinic visits might be hindering the attainment of good control. First, the patient finds it difficult to recall accurately the information and instructions given by the doctor. With such a complex regimen, it is easy to see how this will lead to non-compliance. Second, the understanding of the nature of the problem may be discrepant; and third, acceptable goals may not be agreed. The study by Gillespie and Bradley (1988) showed that coaching the doctors to elicit and agree the main problem and its cause reduced the discrepancy. Disappointingly, neither satisfaction with the consultation nor diabetic control was affected by the increased congruence!

ATTRIBUTIONS AND CONTROL

The mechanisms whereby attributions contribute towards adaptation and, more particularly, good control, are not clear (Turnquist et al. 1988). Preservation of self-esteem has been suggested as a mediator. Individuals are seen as accepting greater causal responsibility for positive outcomes than for negative ones. However, the research on diabetics suggests that patients, and also medical staff attribute negative outcomes to the diabetic.

The most popular mechanism for attributional effects has been perceived locus of control over oneself and one's environment. By making 'self-attributions' one can hope to control current and future events. The concept of 'locus of control' has been applied to diabetic compliance and metabolic control, with ambiguous results. The psychological construct of 'locus of control' is concerned with the extent to which people believe that their actions influence events. People with an external locus of control tend to believe that the outcome is in the hands of chance or powerful others; in the case of diabetes, this is likely to be the doctor. Those with internal locus of control perceive that events are more contingent on their own behaviour (Rotter 1966). Bradley et al. (1984), noting that the more general locus-of-control scales had been unable to predict diabetics' behaviour (Alogna 1980; Lowery and DuCette 1976), developed a diabetes-specific locus-of-control and attributes-of-responsibility measure for adults requiring insulin. The scale divides the perception of control for positive and negative outcomes concerning diabetes management. Six descriptions of hypothetical events, three positive and three negative, were given to 186 patients who were asked to write down the likely cause of the particular outcome. They then rated this cause on seven seven-point Lickert scales, labelled Internality, Treatment, Externality, Chance, Personal Control, Medical Control or Foreseeability. An example of a negative outcome description is, 'Imagine that for several days you have found high levels of sugar when you tested your blood or urine.'

Principal-component analysis confirmed two independent factors: one characterized by Internality/Externality and the other by Medical Treatment. Results showed that, in this sample, the diabetics were predominantly Internal in their attributions. There was considerable reluctance to give responsibility to the medical treatment for negative outcomes. So far, relationships to diabetic control for this scale have not been reported.

These studies would suggest that doctors and patients see the control as within the diabetic. This may be realistic: diabetics certainly have to manage the day-to-day control – be their own 'negative-feedback control system'. However, it is also possible that this belief in Internality, if not accompanied by clear definition of the problem, the goals and, even more importantly, discussion and clarification of the changes that will end in achieving the goals, will create 'learned helplessness' in the diabetic, which would lead to reduced motivation to act (Seligman 1975). It is not unreasonable to suggest that 'out-of-control' diabetics will avoid consultations with the health carers at the clinics and remain without more adaptive strategies for dealing with their problems.

HEALTH PROFESSIONALS AND THE MANAGEMENT OF DIABETES

Health professionals have been found to vary in their beliefs about diabetes (Marteau and Baum 1984; Redmond and Gordon 1982). In a study of 61 physicians and 428 adult diabetics, Hiss et al. (1983) found significant differences between the management of patients looked after by doctors under 40 years of age and those over 40. The patients of the younger group of doctors had lower HbA_1Cs and they more frequently monitored their blood sugar. Patients may have chosen a physician whose treatment and beliefs were compatible with their own, but this is unlikely, given clinic practices and the unlikelihood of seeing the same doctor over visits to the clinics.

Evidence for the contribution of attitudes, beliefs and knowledge to diabetic control suggests that education of medical staff should focus on all these areas. Newton (1985: 26) writes, 'Clinic staff have become pre-occupied with the technical aspects of diabetes and we have neglected efforts to improve social aspects of diabetes, which may be at least as important as a comprehensive diabetic education.' Particularly with adolescent diabetics, difficulties in relating to clinic staff who are usually of a different generation, and not often themselves diabetic, do not help them to adapt to diabetes. These sentiments have increasingly led to self-support groups being formed, particularly for adolescents (Dunn 1986; Steel 1985).

CONCLUSIONS

A number of areas of research on diabetes have been considered. At this point some conclusions are necessary about the contributions that have been made

by psychological research. It is sad to read in a recent editorial article
(Williams *et al.* 1988: 211) the following:

> Psychological and emotional factors undoubtedly affect diabetes, directly
> or indirectly, and a holistic approach to diabetes management demands an
> understanding of the mind as well as the body. Unfortunately, the
> psychological aspects of diabetic management have been largely neglected
> by diabetologists. We suggest that this is because physicians find much of
> the psychological literature difficult to understand and to apply to clinical
> practice. . .the large literature on the topic has so far done little to improve
> our understanding of the nature, diagnosis or consequences of
> psychological problems in diabetic patients.

What answers do psychologists have to these criticisms? It would be easy
to reply with the well-worn phrase, 'more research is needed', and of course
that is true, there are still very few psychologists working alongside diabetologists. But what of the existing research? Bradley and Marteau (1986) put
forward the view that the integration of psychology into diabetic management
is difficult because a medical perspective guides the formulation of questions,
the design of the investigation and the analysis and interpretation of the data.
There has often been too much emphasis on metabolic control. Most studies
use HbA_1C as the dependent variable, yet blood-sugar levels are not the whole
picture. As a diabetic, my basic premiss is that a satisfactory life-style is one
where my diabetes does not prevent me from doing things, I can only do things
if I can manage my diabetes well, and this depends on three components:
understanding and information, adaptive attitudes and beliefs, and an ability
to problem solve. These are all psychological components.

Another reason why psychology has not yet had a greater impact may be
down to poor communication. The models and methods of psychology are not
easily understood by non-psychologists, but if the aim is to help the effective
management of diabetes, then this problem must be overcome. The
management of diabetes should not be the application of scientific facts to
'patients', but an interaction between two individuals who share the same
goal. If this approach is to be supported, then the behaviour of the health-care
professionals will have to be changed. If emotional attitudes are important in
adaptation to diabetes, then we need to be clear where these arise, and how to
change them. Finally, it is not accurate to say that psychology has 'done little
to improve our understanding'. The fact that a holistic approach is now
accepted constitutes a conceptual change. This holistic approach necessitates
adoption of more sophisticated research designs where psychological aspects
are integral rather than after-thoughts.

Chapter 16

Health, illness, and the family

Jacky McGuire

INTRODUCTION

In this chapter we consider ways in which the behaviour or circumstances of families interact with the health status of children. Characteristics of parents relevant to child health will be examined by looking at influences prenatally and within the context of subsequent prevention of illness or accident. Next, coping with a sick child and the impact of parental mental-health problems on child health are reviewed. Finally, an environmental model for studying the influence of the family on child health is presented.

Health psychology admirably illustrates the interdependency between biological and environmental influences on development, and issues of child health provide a particularly focused view of this process. While children may be encouraged to make independent choices early in life within some spheres (for example, toys, playmates, preferred games or school activities), the child is not usually able to make health-related decisions independently for a number of years. Many factors within the environment may have far-reaching effects upon a child's health but parental behaviour is likely to be crucial, and is one part of a child's experience that health professionals may be able to influence directly.

Styles of parenting have been the focus of a considerable amount of psychological research and it has become clear that some styles are more conducive to optimal child development than others. Authoritative inter-actions seem to be the most beneficial while neglecting, authoritarian or indulgent styles may lead to problems for children (Baumrind 1967; Maccoby and Martin 1983). The authoritative parent is child centred, accepting of child behaviour and responsive when needed while at the same time demanding high standards and wanting some control over the child's life. In contrast the indulgent style is very child centred but without many demands being imposed. The authoritarian pattern is demanding and controlling but within a parent-centred context, while the neglecting style also tends to be adult centred but low in control and making few demands upon the child. Cognitive development, academic achievement or personality characteristics are the outcome measures usually considered in relation to parenting styles, but do these dimensions also have implications for child health? And what other aspects of the family are relevant?

It has been shown that in families which support autonomous decision making, provide reasons for requests and reward good behaviour, children have high levels of health-care practice (Pratt 1973). This parenting style corresponds well with the authoritative style of management. Children of parents who punished 'bad' behaviour and provided less choice or justification for demands (authoritarian) were less likely to care for their own health. Thus, parental behaviour can influence child health-related behaviour once children begin to make their own decisions about health-care practices. The foundations for these decisions are likely to be laid down during early childhood. Even 4–6 year olds can understand and explain simple health-care practices such as eating green vegetables, exercising or brushing teeth (Lasky and Eichelberger 1985). Thus, the behaviour of parents in early childhood is likely to be crucial in establishing children's ideas about health.

Not only do parents influence the attitudes which their children take, they also have an active role in maintaining the health of their families. Children are in a unique position in their early years in that many of the causes of mortality or morbidity can be attributed in part to the behaviour of other people. For example, a growing number of infants are being born addicted to drugs or suffering from AIDS (see Chapter 10 in this volume). Cases of child abuse are said to be increasing and abuse is a leading cause of infant death in societies such as the United Kingdom or United States, which have adequate food supplies and medical services. In addition to maintaining the health status of their children, parents also have an impact prenatally upon the child's future health prospects.

BEFORE BIRTH

While prenatal behaviour or attitudes do not teach the child directly, it has become clear that studying parental behaviour at this time can be a very useful way of understanding which aspects are likely to be most relevant to subsequent child health. Prolonged maternal stress and anxiety during pregnancy have traditionally been linked with a number of infant health problems such as hyperactivity, restlessness, feeding problems, sleep problems and colic (Hurlock 1980), not to mention birthmarks and other physical blemishes (Reading 1983). The association between maternal anxiety and the child's health and development is thought to be mediated by physiological mechanisms. The mother's experience of stress may lead to hormonal imbalance and the release of steroids into the bloodstream. Reading suggests that the release of catecholamines into maternal circulation leads to higher blood pressure and by implication reduced placental blood flow. Thus, it is not that the hormones pass through the placenta to influence the growing child but that they influence growth and development indirectly via the oxygen supply to the foetus.

Hurlock further suggests indirect influences after birth. A child who is of low birth weight or born early owing to poor uterine environment is often irritable, restless and a poor feeder. This in turn may arouse some unfavourable attitudes from family members, feelings of hostility and rejection, which may then be associated with continued below average physical development. While these relationships are not easily validated, research has shown that attitudes formed before having a child are associated with the mother's subsequent feelings about her infant and behaviour with the child.

A recent longitudinal study has shown that in particular a mother's ability to visualize herself as a mother and express confidence in herself and her ego strength were predictive of infant development at twelve months (Heinicke *et al.* 1983). Families in the Los Angeles area having their first child were given extensive interviews prenatally and the mother–child dyads were observed throughout the first year. Infant characteristics such as persistence or goal directedness during play, alertness and skill in manipulation at 12 months could be predicted by the prenatal maternal Ego Strength Index of the Minnesota Multiphasic Personality Inventory (Dahlstrom *et al.* 1972, 1975) and by a confident attitude shown in responses to interview questions such as 'Can you picture yourself as a mother?'. Parental stimulation of the child during play sessions could also be related to these prenatal maternal characteristics. Thus, mothers who were prepared for parenthood and expressed confidence had responsive children with appropriate developmental skills. It is likely that their children were also healthier, since alertness and persistence would not be so typical of an underweight or sickly child.

Work with adolescent mothers, an 'at-risk' group for potential parenting difficulties (McAnarney *et al.* 1986; Taylor *et al.* 1983; Wadsworth *et al.* 1984), has shown that they are likely to form stable ideas about their child's behaviour before its birth. A group of expectant young women was asked at 32 and 36 weeks' gestation to complete infant temperament questionnaires, with instructions to imagine what their infant would be like (Zeanah *et al.* 1987). The questionnaire covered behaviours such as regularity, activity, excitability and mood. Those mothers who imagined that their infants would be difficult to predict had children who were less responsive during videotaped feeding sessions when the infants were 4 months old. The babies also looked, smiled and vocalised less to their mothers. While problems with feeding are the most directly relevant to future health and physical development, the quality of interactions could be important for predicting the development of a mutually satisfying mother–child relationship, relevant to subsequent mental health. These findings are particularly interesting to health-care professionals concerned with improving infant health care since they indicate ways in which intervention can be developed to prevent later problems. For instance, it has been shown that social support provided during pregnancy has an identifiable effect upon improved parenting and infant development at 4 months of age (Crnic *et al.* 1983). In the same way one could provide counselling for at-risk groups such as pregnant teenagers to boost their confidence and provide a positive image of their infant.

Women who lack confidence and expect their baby to be difficult to manage are likely to become anxious. While this may be harmful in itself, coping strategies used to alleviate the anxiety such as smoking or drinking or overeating might be even more detrimental to child health. The implications of high maternal anxiety should be considered very carefully by any health-care practitioner but especially by those involved in prenatal screening for child disorders such as Down's syndrome. While procedures such as amniocentesis will eventually reduce anxiety about possible chromosomal problems for the majority of mothers, it will also highlight and potentially increase state anxiety related to their pregnancy for a large part of the pregnancy (up to twenty-two weeks in most cases) which might be detrimental.

Maternal anxiety can in fact be reduced significantly, in both medically high-risk and normal pregnancies, by scanning procedures providing immediate feedback, for example foetal echocardiography. Changes were noted in attitudes to the pregnancy, to the baby and to the baby's health, though not in *trait* anxiety for twenty-four mothers at increased risk of having a baby with cardiac problems and twenty-six matched controls (Barton *et al.* 1987). Trait anxiety is the general level of anxiety shown by the individual in most circumstances. It is considered to be a relatively stable characteristic whereas state anxiety refers to worry and nervousness which is very specific, directed at one particular situation or experience – in this case, the pregnancy.

The relevance of state rather than trait anxiety is stressed by Reading (1983). He suggests that the level of state anxiety will influence the type of coping used. High levels may lead to behaviours such as maternal smoking, drinking or decreased health care, which in turn influence the uterine physiology and the infant's well-being (Toubas *et al.* 1986). The traditional approach to changing maternal smoking habits has been educational, stressing risks to the child. In order to improve the efficacy of such interventions Baumrind's model of parenting can usefully be applied to the question of why some mothers are able to give up potentially harmful behaviours such as smoking, drinking or drug taking during pregnancy while others are not. Those with a child-centred frame of reference are likely to be more committed to change in their own habits for the sake of the child's welfare than those who are adult (i.e. self-) centred. They may also reflect a certain style of health prevention behaviour, which has been found to be a very useful explanatory variable for a number of preventive child health behaviours (Butler and Golding 1986).

Overall, many parental characteristics may be relevant to prenatal child health, but a key area to focus on is a mother's attitudes both to herself as a potential parent and to the developing child. Changes at that attitudinal level may lead to subsequent changes in other relevant characteristics such as smoking, drug taking or poor eating habits.

PREVENTION OF INJURY AND ILLNESS

Information on the rates of childhood accidents and deaths suggests that psychological factors are implicated, though it is difficult to distinguish between the contributions of child and parents. Wright (1979), for example. points out that in the USA one child in 500 is involved in the preschool years in a poisoning accident. The chances that a child would be involved a second time should also be one in 500 if such accidents were random. However, incredibly the chance rises by 125 times, to one in four for a second poisoning. He suggests that since neither parental storage practices nor knowledge of toxicity seem to be related to the chance of an accident, something may be identifiable in the psychological characteristics of the families of repeat poisonings.

Similarly, data on the use of preventive health services for children (for example, immunizations, developmental checks, dentists) strongly suggest that aspects of the family functioning and maternal attitudes are again relevant. Beattie (1985) proposes that the mother's self-esteem 'may be the most important factor in determining the health and welfare of the preschool child'. There are many factors that could influence self-esteem. It would seem to be important to look beyond the current maternal state to areas of experience that might be relevant, such as educational level, living conditions, social support, family dynamics or social-class status of her own or her partner's work. In addition, specific behaviours related to personal health care are relevant to prevention of child health problems.

For example, in the longitudinal Child Health and Education Survey (Butler and Golding 1986), maternal smoking was a significant factor in explaining the take-up of preventive child health services; even more powerful as an explanatory variable than social class. Information was obtained from more than 12,000 mothers of 5 year olds, the majority of a cohort of children born in England, Scotland and Wales during one week in 1975. They were asked a variety of questions concerned with the use of preventive health services such as health-visitor visits, attending child health clinics and the take-up of immunizations.

While absence of the health visitor following birth could be explained most effectively by practical variables such as many moves of the household, the best predictor of mothers making no visits to the child health clinic (true for more than 10 per cent of the sample) was maternal smoking. The risk of non-attendance rose in direct relation to the number of cigarettes smoked daily, with those children whose mothers smoked more than twenty-five per day at most risk. This was an independent effect, taking into account other variables which might relate to maternal smoking, such as poor housing, lack of support or social status. Use of dental health services also conformed to this pattern. By the age of 5 only 22 per cent of non-smokers' children had never visited a dentist, while this was true for almost twice as many children (39 per cent) of heavy smokers. However, in relation to dental visits social class was also a significant factor, with 45 per cent of children from social class V homes never having seen a dentist compared with only 8 per cent in social class I.

Finally, the proportion of children who had received immunizations, particularly the most contentious one – pertussis (or whooping cough) – but also the measles vaccine, could be associated with maternal smoking habits. Almost 10 per cent of heavy smokers had not obtained any immunizations for their 5 year old (compared with 2 per cent for light or non-smokers) and the figures relating just to the pertussis immunization were similar, 16 per cent compared with 5 per cent. These results lead to the hypothesis that the parental behaviour most relevant to child health may be specifically their own health-related behaviour, rather than indirect characteristics such as social class. It would seem that poor health practices may endure within families and be transmitted between generations.

Mayall (1986) interviewed 135 London mothers, each with a first child between 18–36 months, about many aspects of health care. She did not find any social-class differences in mothers' ideas about what a healthy child was or how to promote child health. However, knowledge of how to prevent illness did indicate differences. More working-class mothers followed the 'thermal theory', that illness was related to temperature change and that they therefore should keep their child warmly dressed to remain free from colds and coughs. In contrast more middle-class mothers mentioned diet in relation to preventing such illnesses (60 per cent versus 21 per cent). Educational level may be another aspect of parents which is very important for their child's health. Mayall found that mothers make decisions about immunizations on the basis of their own experiences and ideas rather than on information in the literature given out by child health clinics. Mayall's study was conducted after the national Child Health and Education Survey (Butler and Golding 1986), and at a time when many concerns were being aired in the British media about immunizations, particularly pertussis and measles. Only 58 per cent had received the recommended series of three pertussis vaccinations but there was still a clear social-class trend (as in the Butler and Golding study). However, within classes III, IV and V those mothers with the lowest educational qualifications were unlikely to have had the immunizations done. Additionally, mothers with less education were more likely to give medical (but usually unfounded) reasons for not having immunizations done (for example, that a cousin had one convulsion). She suggests that the lack of education makes mothers more vulnerable to scare stories concerning health.

There is disagreement about how to change parent perceptions on the necessity for preventing illness or accident to their children. Kellmer Pringle (1980) emphasized parent education, reporting that more than 50 per cent of mothers thought their 5 year old could cross a main road safely without adult help. However, as mentioned earlier, poisonings and other preschool accidents seem to be unrelated to parents' knowledge of toxicity or their storage practices (Wright 1979). It may be more effective to intervene at an environmental level with practical changes rather than trying to change beliefs, since attitudes are notoriously difficult to alter. Intervention at an environmental level avoids the problem of which parents will respond if it is provided for all.

An example of this is the introduction of child-proof tops for many household items such as aspirins or other medications, bleach and cleaning fluids. The rate of childhood ingestion of poisons has been reduced most dramatically in recent years following this marketing change (Cataldo *et al.* 1986). Alternatively the environmental change might be provided for a specific high-risk population such as residents of high-rise flats. The installation of free window guard rails in a New York high-rise complex led to a 50 per cent reduction in children falling from windows within a two-year period (ibid.).

Data on attempts to reduce child deaths in car accidents clearly illustrate the problems of changing parental behaviour. In the USA in 1984 there were 532 deaths of children aged 0–4 years. Within this group of fatalities the principal cause of death was injury resulting from a car accident, far outnumbering deaths from cancer, heart disease or from poisoning (Faber 1986). The main problem is identified by Faber as parent motivation since most parents report knowledge of the protective capability of restraints but do not use them, giving many spurious reasons (for example, they will be able to grab the child in time if they are held on someone's lap; they only drive in town so there is no danger) or reasons relating to inconvenience and expense. Social class was relevant, with more middle-class parents using child seats, but parents' behaviour in relation to their own safety was also a factor. Most parents who used child seats also used seat belts themselves and were concerned about other preventive health measures such as visiting the dentist. Faber recommends that the time before birth is the most 'teachable moment' and she suggests that health-care professionals should demonstrate the use of infant seats in the hospital, along with the baby bath.

There is thus a pattern in many of the studies of prevention of childhood illness that the most relevant parental behaviours are those that concern their own health care, such as smoking, visiting the dentist or using safety measures. In addition, social class seems important, though with such a nebulous concept it is difficult to link this directly with parental behaviour. It could mean having the time and resources to be child centred, it could be having a higher level of education or it could be an interaction between social class, knowledge and health care. While parental beliefs are a significant factor in explaining preventive child health practices, intervention may be more successful at a level beyond individuals, in their environment.

THE SICK CHILD

Take-up of preventive health provision is rather an indirect way of examining the influence of the family on child health. Coping with a sick child is more clear cut in that most parents would agree that some medical intervention is important. Ways in which parents cope with childhood illnesses can provide useful information, relevant to education for the prevention of child illness. As with other stressful life events, the onset of serious illness in a child can bring into focus the dynamics within the family, as they try to cope. Studies are generally of two kinds; those which investigate children with an acute condition that requires a hospital visit (for example, tonsillectomy) or those of children with chronic conditions (for example, asthma, diabetes, eczema).

Coping with hospitalization

The majority of paediatric hospital settings are now considering or already offering some form of preparation involving the parents before a child is hospitalized. This has been linked theoretically with Escalona's emotional contagion hypothesis (Melamed 1988). The basis of this is that parental anxiety (usually maternal) is communicated to children by non-verbal and verbal channels, leading to anxiety and nervousness in them, which is likely to make them more distressed and less co-operative during their stay in hospital.

Visitainer and Wolfer (1975) designed a preparation programme to help parents cope with stress and anxiety. They provided information to the child and mother together, explaining to the child the role which the mother could take (for example, holding the child's hand and talking while a blood test was going on). Overall the preparation focused on the mother's importance to the child and her control over it during the hospital visit. This proved to be successful not only in gaining the child's co-operation during procedures but also in lowering parental anxiety.

While this style of intervention is designed to help the child to cope by emphasizing the mother's role to the child, Melamed (1988) suggests that it may be more effective to teach the mother how to cope rather than the child. She and colleagues observed mothers and children in a paediatric out-patient clinic in a tertiary referral hospital (Bush et al. 1988). Their observations were based on attachment theory and included measuring behaviours such as maternal responsiveness, use of distraction, providing information, and child exploration and approach to their mothers. It was found that the behaviour shown by the mothers did influence the child's tolerance of the medical experience. Those who made use of distraction, were informative on non-medical matters (for example, read books or chatted about the toys) and attentive (i.e. unlikely to ignore child approaches) had children who coped better. Their children explored the waiting area more and did not show high levels of distress or clinging. In contrast, mothers who provided a lot of reassurance, talking about medical topics, were likely to have children who displayed more 'attachment' behaviour such as approaching or touching the parent and also more distress, which could be crying and running about or quiet withdrawal and unease. In line with the 'emotional contagion' theory, those mothers who were themselves overtly agitated had children who showed more distress.

This work corresponds closely with work on parenting in a broader perspective. The mothers whose children coped best could be described as child centred in their responsiveness, but also demanding in that they read books and expected their children to play productively. The parents who were 'neglecting' by ignoring or those who were very adult centred, concentrating upon their own distress, had children who coped less adequately, as did those who were too child centred (indulgent) providing lots of reassurance and comfort. While this particular study cannot show clearly whether the parent influences the child or vice versa, it does suggest that intervention directed at parent behaviour is a most useful way for practitioners to proceed, particularly with young children who might be less able to benefit from an educational form of preparation such as describing what will happen to them.

Chronic illness

A number of studies have shown how psychological characteristics of the parents, and of the family, will influence the course of children's illnesses, both acute and chronic. Possibly the most pervasive problem encountered by practitioners in the delivery of health care to children is the non-compliance of parents with professional recommendations (Parrish 1986). Not only might therapeutic effects be minimized by such parent action but it could lead to further complications and the necessity for additional diagnostic or treatment procedures. Parrish reports surprisingly low levels of compliance with prescribed medication ranging from 18 to 58 per cent for children with ear or throat infections and from 11 to 89 per cent for those with chronic conditions such as asthma, epilepsy or cancer. While he outlines a number of features of the therapeutic regimen which might hinder or promote parental compliance, he also notes that parents' perceptions of their child's vulnerability, their own health beliefs, their perceptions of the severity of the illness, their child's vulnerability and the potential effectiveness of medical treatment are very important when trying to understand parental behaviour in relation to the sick child. In attempting to reconcile inconsistencies in the research, he suggests that parental compliance with medical recommendations is related to the perceived severity of the child's illness in a U-shaped curve. Compliance is low both when the severity is seen to be low and high, and compliance is high when severity is moderate. He also highlights the parental relationship, and the extended social environment of the family. Shared responsibility and the presence of social support have been found to improve compliance with treatment programmes for children.

There is a great deal to cope with, both for the child and for other family members, when one child has a chronic illness. Parents may experience a range of emotions such as guilt, helplessness, anxiety, shame, anger or misery, all of which could influence child-care practices. Over-protection, rejection, leniency or excessive strictness may be the result. Mattson (1972), in an overview of studies of coping with chronic illness, proposes that children who cope most successfully have parents who have mastered feelings of guilt or fear and treat them as much like a healthy child as possible. While over-indulgence and lack of discipline may lead to management problems, Mattson suggests that the opposite – parental rejection, criticism or neglect – may potentially be more harmful to the child's physical and mental well-being.

The nature and quality of interactions within the family appear to be relevant to a number of chronic childhood illnesses. The illness itself may lead to styles of interaction that are then associated with further psychological and physical difficulties. For example, families of children with epilepsy were compared with children who had another chronic illness, diabetes, and a second comparison group with no health problems (Ferrari et al. 1983). The children ranged in age from 6 to 13 years and were seen at home. Based on structured interviews with parents and children it was reported that children with epilepsy saw themselves as less close to parents than those with diabetes or no health problems. The parent–child communications were more often about problems than general issues and the epileptic children tended to lack autonomy and show immature emotional reactions. Other work, reviewed by Hoare (1987), has shown that families of children who had both epilepsy and behavioural problems resembled families of children with behavioural disturbance but no epilepsy in that there was poor communication between parents and children. He describes the paradigm of the psychosomatic family often associated with children who have epileptic seizures, developed on the basis of family therapy (for example, Minuchin et al. 1978). It generally takes the form of over-protective parents who are rigid in their behaviour to the child, unable to accept developing needs. The parents and children are likely to be 'enmeshed', lacking the usual generational boundaries, with a tendency to avoid disagreement, overprotective with the child but rigid and lacking adequate means of resolving conflict. These maladaptive styles of family interactions are associated with the risk of emotional problems in children, whether or not they are sick. Thus, chronic ill-health can become further complicated by socio-emotional difficulties as a consequence of environmental, family influences.

The Ferrari et al. (1983) study found that interactions in families of a diabetic child were similar to those of children with no health problems.

Other work has shown that in some ways they may function more effectively, though some conflict between parents may occur. Hauser and colleagues (1986) studied families with a diabetic child, and those with a child who had an acute illness which had required some change in daily activities such as missing school or frequent visits to the doctor (for example, fractures, appendicitis, infections). The children ranged from 10 to 14 years and were observed in a family task. They were given questionnaires concerned with typical parent–child dilemmas not related to illness but concerned with autonomy, privacy, honesty and support. Instances were found in which the mother and child agreed, but the father did not and vice versa. They were then asked to defend positions and finally reach a consensus. Overall, the mothers of the diabetic children were more 'enabling', explaining, attempting to clarify the other person's point of view and trying to come to agreement than the control mothers, while the fathers of diabetic children were slightly more judgemental than the control fathers, whose children had an acute illness.

The authors suggest that the 'we'll fight it together' spirit of the mothers may be beneficial to parent–child relationships in diabetic adolescents, although they caution that it may also be an indication of the 'enmeshed' over-protection that Minuchin described. Additionally, some potential conflict within the family is indicated by the behaviour of the fathers. They may be less able to cope with the daily work of coping with a sick child and show more guilt and sadness, possibly withdrawing in the way that some fathers of mentally handicapped infants tend to react (McConachie 1982). This study shows that when one is attempting to understand the influences of the family on the child's illness, one must consider both parents separately, since their roles in relation to home and the outside world may lead to quite different interactions within the family.

It has been suggested that the onset of asthmatic symptoms in genetically vulnerable children is related to emotional stressors such as parental disagreements or problems in parent–child relationships (Graham et al. 1967). However, the issue is still a matter of keen debate (Mrazek 1986). One recent longitudinal study in fact found no relationship between onset of illness and major life events in the family (Horwood et al. 1985). Nevertheless, clinical reports of three cases of fatal asthma attacks in teenagers pin-point the role of the family (Fritz et al. 1987). In all three cases a supportive family environment was lacking. Instead, they were either over-demanding, unaccepting or overtly abusive. The clinicians involved suggest that the children might have used their asthma to defuse tense family situations, to manipulate family members or to mask troubled relationships. However, these data are merely suggestive in view of the small sample size.

While more work is needed to resolve the role played by emotional stress on asthmatic symptoms, it is more clearly established that children with severe asthma are at risk of mental-health problems in addition to their physical illness. Mrazek et al. (1985) found that 35 per cent of a sample of twenty-six middle-class preschool-age children with moderate to severe asthma had significant emotional and behavioural difficulties compared with none of a comparison sample of twenty-two healthy children. An interaction between parental behaviour and child problems was strongly suggested. Observations showed that the asthmatic sample were much more confrontative and non-compliant than the healthy children and that many of the confrontation episodes were preceded by crying and whining. Mothers of the asthmatic children revealed in their interviews that they were often unable to gain compliance, relating incidents in which emotional conflict led to an asthma attack. In contrast most mothers of the healthy children were able to persuade their young children to comply when there was a confrontation. In addition to style of discipline and control, Mrazek (1986) stresses the importance of family discord and parental psychopathy which need to be taken into account as risk factors for emotional problems in a child with asthma.

Family factors are implicated not only in the development of emotional or behavioural problems but also in the severity of symptoms for some chronic conditions. A study of children with atopic dermatitis clearly illustrates this effect (Gil et al. 1987). The aim of the study was to see how stress and the family environment influenced indices of symptom severity such as the extent of inflammation or the amount of antihistamine cream which had to be used to alleviate distress. The family environment was assessed using a ninety-item scale with ten subscales. These were further reduced by factor analysis to four dimensions of family behaviour. The largest factor was called 'active support', families were cohesive, intellectually orientated, expressed feelings and took part in recreational activities together. The second factor, called 'aggression', was typified by high control, high conflict and an emphasis on achievement (similar to Authoritarian). The third was an orientation to autonomy and organization and the fourth characterized a moral or religious orientation within the family. Contradicting predictions, major stressors or 'life events' were not found to influence symptom severity but the family environment revealed many relationships.

Six of the seven measures of symptom severity were significantly lower in children whose parents were said to be active and supportive, with a similar but less marked pattern for families with a focus upon independence and organization. The aggressive (authoritarian) factor was not related to symptoms but those children with families that were reported to have a moral/religious emphasis had significantly more symptoms. These results correspond quite well with the more broadly based research of the effects of parenting styles upon child development. The active, supportive parents in the study of children with eczema and those concentrating upon independence could be described as placing demands upon the children, but within a child-centred focus (i.e. authoritative). The authors suggest that the moral/religious families had strong views on what was right and wrong, believed in punishment and were rigid in their style of coping, relying heavily on medication. This could also be described as a demanding but adult-centred strategy, similar to Baumrind's authoritarian style.

Thus, many aspects of parent behaviour have relevance to a sick child, both in terms of how well parents cope and how well the child develops emotionally and physically. Parents' perceptions of their child's vulnerability are implicated in the take-up of medical advice and in their tendency towards an indulgent over-protective style of child rearing. While this is implicated in the development of children's emotional problems, a child-centred but demanding approach appears to facilitate acute situations such as a brief hospital visit and long-term conditions such as epilepsy or eczema.

THE SICK PARENT

In the same way that studies of pathological behaviour elucidate processes of normal development, so the influence which the family might have upon child health can be understood more clearly by examining families in which a parent is emotionally ill. A great deal of research has been carried out examining the influences of parental mental illness upon their children (Earls 1987; Rutter and Quinton 1984). Generally there is agreement that children are most at risk when they are the victims of aggressive or hostile acts, the target for parental delusions or when neglected for pathological reasons. Adult psychiatrists are increasingly being encouraged to consider the whole family for potential adverse effects when a parent has a major psychiatric illness (Mander *et al.* 1987).

Certain influences which parents may have upon children's health are of particular interest either because they are widespread – for example, depression, alcoholism – or because the abusive parental behaviour may seem initially to be directed at good health care (Munchausen by proxy – see below). These selected topics will be discussed in detail to illustrate the way that family behaviour can influence the well-being of young children.

By far the most widespread mental-health problem experienced by mothers of young children is depression (Brown and Harris 1978; Richman 1978), and several studies have shown that children with depressed mothers have an increased likelihood of experiencing emotional and behavioural disturbance (Ghodsian *et al.* 1984; Hammen *et al.* 1987; Pound *et al.* 1985; Richman *et al.* 1982). The situation is clearly very complex and a number of explanations are possible. The same stresses that contribute to the mother's feelings of depression might be influencing the child, the child might be influencing the mother or vice versa. While all of these possibilities may be operating together, recent work has highlighted the importance of the quality of the relationship between mother and child to the child's well-being.

By using detailed observations in homes, distinctive features have been identified in the interactions between depressed women and preschool-aged children, characterized in particular by a lack of synchrony (Mills *et al.* 1985).

In other words the depressed mother was not so likely to respond appropriately to her child's comments or actions and might herself initiate exchanges when the child was not attending, making it unlikely that the child will respond. Observations of a group of depressed mothers with older children, aged between 8 and 16, in a family discussion about a topic of disagreement revealed that the depressed women were more critical and negative to their children than non-depressed mothers (Gordon *et al.* 1988). They were also less likely to stay on task and made fewer positive confirming statements. The tendency to step back from involvement in their children's development was evident in the comments of a sample of middle-class depressed women. While non-depressed and affectively ill mothers were equally satisfied with their children, the depressed women expressed helplessness, feeling that the outcomes of child development were determined by uncontrollable factors (Kochanska *et al.* 1987).

Inattentiveness, unresponsiveness or criticisms about ideas can be fairly easily observed in play or a family session, but the implications of this style of parenting for health-related issues may not be so easy to identify. For example, this style of interacting may also be associated with ignoring symptoms of child illness such as fussiness, lethargy or loss of appetite, or by accusing them of malingering, possibly putting the child at risk of complications developing. Thus, children of depressed mothers (there is little information about fathers) are at risk for both emotional and physical well-being.

Another fairly common family problem is parental alcoholism, which has been associated with a number of child health problems. Again, the research literature is vast and space limitations prevent a full review being presented here (for some comprehensive reviews see Jacob 1975; Jacob *et al.* 1978; West and Prinz 1987). Parental alcoholism has been found to relate to hyperactivity and conduct disorders in younger children, substance abuse, truancy and delinquency in older children. What is more relevant to note is that the effects of parental problems need to be viewed within the context of an ecological model, considering multiple stresses upon the child, parents and other family members rather than an effect of parent upon child (West and Prinz 1987). While possible genetic effects cannot be ignored, by looking at parental alcoholism within the context of a model focusing upon stress, risk and protective factors (Garmezy and Rutter 1983) it can be seen that neither all nor even a majority of children from alcoholic homes are inevitably doomed to psychological disorder or similar addiction (West and Prinz 1987). They are, however, particularly at risk when they are experiencing multiple stresses. For instance the risk of truancy or delinquency is much greater when the child is from economically disadvantaged circumstances, when parental divorce has occurred, when living with only one parent or when the father has been imprisoned. It is suggested that the disruptions in the home related to parental alcoholism may drive the child out of the home to seek other sources of support. Being vulnerable to the influences of peers may increase the likelihood of delinquency and associated substance abuse.

Although much rarer than depression or alcoholism, the parental mental-health problem most clearly related to child health is Munchausen syndrome by proxy (Meadow 1977) named after Munchausen syndome. In this extreme form of hypochondria individuals seeks out for themselves repeated medical treatment and invasive diagnostic procedures or operations, faking evidence and moving from one hospital to another in order to gain more medical attention, usually without having any definite illness. In Munchausen by proxy the parent, invariably the mother, takes her child from doctor to doctor complaining of symptoms in the child. Thus, the over-concerned protective mother–child relationship sometimes seen in families with a sick child is distorted to one which becomes abusive.

In some cases the maternal behaviour may be the extreme exaggeration of an existing child illness such as asthma (Masterson *et al.* 1988). High levels of medication are used, often contrary to the physician's advice, and the parent does not recognize improvements in symptoms. In a more pathological pattern, mothers go to such extreme measures as injecting their children with contaminating material, poisoning and suffocating (Orenstein and Wasserman 1986). Libow and Schreier (1986) suggest that the parental behaviour takes three general forms. The 'help seeker' may actually want to give up the child, feeling unable to cope, so fictitious symptoms are described but nothing more. 'Doctor addicts' are similarly passive in that their behaviour is limited to falsifying medical histories in order to get medical attention. They may be using their child to project personal hypochondria. The most hazardous pattern of behaviour they label 'active inducers', mothers who have been found to put blood on their infants, inject them with excreta, induce unconsciousness through suffocation or poison with laxatives and barbiturates. Libow and Schreier pin-point the relationships within the families of active inducers, noting that the marital relationships are often disturbed, with peripheral uninvolved fathers. The resulting feelings of anxiety are coped with by the use of paranoid projection and denial, the child's supposed illness becoming the focus of the mother's life in order to divert her anxiety from other problems. The level of denial is such that the parent is able to sustain her statements about the child's illness even when confronted with falsehoods. Orenstein and Wasserman (1986) describe such a case. The mother had gone so far as to place advertisements requesting that she could meet families with a child suffering from cystic fibrosis in order that she could gain additional information about what symptoms to describe, and she obtained specimens of sputum from patients in order to present them for laboratory analysis, instead of her child's own specimens. When confronted by doctors and people she had contacted, she denied most of her actions. In this particular case it was decided that the mother's behaviour posed such a risk to her child that legal guardianship should be taken from her, but many less marked cases may go unnoticed. Munchausen by proxy illustrates very vividly how overconcern with child health could become detrimental to the child's well-being.

CONCLUSIONS – AN ECOLOGICAL MODEL OF CHILD HEALTH

The effects of family characteristics upon the child are best understood within a system such as Bronfenbrenner's ecological model (1979) or Belsky's (1984) model of parenting. In both these theoretical formulations parental behaviour and child development are seen within a wider context, encompassing not just the immediate family characteristics but also the neighbourhood and the social structure. Bronfenbrenner proposed that a child's world could be seen as a 'set of nested structures, each inside the next like a set of Russian dolls'. Several layers are proposed starting with the immediate influences such as parents, siblings and peers and moving through services available in the neighbourhood and extended family systems to situations in which the child is not directly involved (such as a parent's work-place) to an outer 'layer' representing the attitudes and beliefs of the culture in which they live. Stresses in any part of that system at any level are likely to have an impact upon other levels. Belsky's model was developed to analyse not child development but the development of maladaptive parenting, seen in child abuse. He takes a similar view to Bronfenbrenner in that he suggests that parenting is multiply determined, by past history, by personality, work situation, marital relationships, the child characteristics and the social network available. Applying this type of model to the influence of the family on child health, a child's illness might lead to a change of financial circumstances and living conditions for a whole family. But it is just as possible that poor living conditions (for example, overcrowding, damp) might lead to child ill-health. Illness of one parent might be associated with depression in the other partner and either of these could place their children at risk of emotional or physical illness.

Green (1983, 1986) recommends to paediatricians just such an environmental approach, that they use the concept of vulnerability to stress when planning preventive or therapeutic interventions with children. He outlines a 'Homeogram', a chart which can be used to list strengths and weaknesses of the child, the family and the environment. Thus, the child with severe asthma but a responsive family with good resources living in a town which has extra teachers available for home or hospital teaching may need to be treated quite differently from a milder case whose parents are divorced and whose mother has recently been depressed, living in a poor neighbourhood.

The example of divorce illustrates very clearly the complex interactions between child health, family and wider social factors. A large-scale study in the USA found that children in families whose parents were divorced were said by parents to have significantly more health problems than those from intact families (Guidubaldi and Cleminshaw 1985). This study gathered no information about parent behaviour, but based on the research described in this chapter one can think of any number of explanations for their findings. Financial factors might be implicated, leading to a poorer diet with less fresh produce, poorer living conditions, or not enough money for the kinds of medicines needed for minor coughs, colds or other infections. The parent caring for the child may not be able to afford to miss work in order to see the doctor, or to obtain preventive measures such as immunizations. If the child is living in a single-parent household, a stressful move away from the family home might have taken place. The parents might have been preoccupied with their personal difficulties and missed children's symptoms, leading to more serious conditions. Alternatively the children may be highlighting their health problems as a way of diverting parents or gaining attention, leading their parents to believe they may be more ill than was in fact the case. Many more explanations are possible, but could not be resolved without a more detailed study in which the children were examined by medical personnel, rather than relying on parental information. However, it does seem that doctors are taking a more ecological perspective in the care of children.

From the studies reviewed here one can say that several aspects of the family, and specifically parents, are particularly relevant to child health. Social class is a concept that has been applied to many health issues, showing the inequalities which exist in the rate of infant deaths, childhood accidents, take-up of services, extent of child illnesses and emotional problems (Black Report 1980). However, it may be more useful to look more specifically at parental characteristics such as their own self-esteem, confidence to be parents, health-related behaviours such as smoking or overeating, views on how to protect their children and emotional well-being. It is also notable that a style of resolving parent–child disputes or setting limits which is conscious of child needs, but within a framework setting definite guidelines, is beneficial not only when coping with children once they are ill but to prevent physical or emotional problems from arising. Nevertheless, these need to be interpreted within a model which takes into account the environment in which the family lives.

From the preceding review many ways in which parents can influence child health can be identified. Apart from the immediate relevance to the children's well-being the influence of the family is likely to persist into adulthood. The health practices, beliefs and experiences of childhood will be the basis of adult styles of health and health beliefs. Styles of parenting have strong inter-generational influences, and ways in which parents promote good health or cope with illness may have even farther-reaching implications for optimal development than methods of toilet training, discipline techniques, rules about tidying the house or encouragement to succeed academically. Child health can only be properly understood within the ecology of the family and its environment.

References

Abelin, T., Buehler, A., Muller, P., Vesanen, K. and Imhof, P.R. (1989) 'Controlled trial of transdermal nicotine patch in tobacco withdrawal', *Lancet* i: 7–10.

Abrams, M. (1985) 'Birth control use by teenagers: one and two years post abortion', *Journal of Adolescent Health Care* 6: 196–200.

Acton, T. (1989) 'In your hands: a psychological view of the human immunodeficiency virus (HIV)', *Royal Society of Medicine. The AIDS Letter* 12 (April–May): 1–3.

Ader, R. (ed.) (1981) *Psychoneuroimmunology*, New York: Academic Press.

Adler, N. (1982) 'The abortion experience: social and psychological influences and after effects', in H.S. Friedman and M.S. DiMatteo (eds) *Interpersonal Issues in Health Care*, New York: Academic Press.

Aggleton, P.J., Hart, G. and Davies, P. (eds) (1989) *AIDS: Social Representations and Social Practice*, Lewes: Falmer Press.

Aggleton, P., Homans, H., Mojsa, J., Watson, S. and Watney, S. (1989) *AIDS: Scientific and Social Issues. A Resource for Health Educators*, Edinburgh: Churchill Livingstone.

Agras, W.S., Horne, M. and Taylor, C.B. (1982) 'Expectation and the blood-pressure-lowering effects of relaxation', *Psychosomatic Medicine* 44: 389–95.

Agras, W.S., Southam, M.A. and Taylor, C.B. (1983) 'Long-term persistence of relaxation-induced blood pressure lowering during the working day', *Journal of Consulting and Clinical Psychology* 51: 792–4.

Agras, W.S., Taylor, C.B., Kraemer, H.C., Southam, M.A. and Schneider, J.A. (1987) 'Relaxation training for essential hypertension at the worksite: II. The poorly controlled hypertensive', *Psychosomatic Medicine* 49: 264–73.

Ajzen, I. (1985) 'From intentions to actions: a theory of planned behaviour', in J. Kuhl and J. Beckmann (eds) *Action-Control: From Cognition to Behavior*, Heidelberg: Springer-Verlag.

Ajzen, I. and Fishbein, M. (1980) *Understanding Attitudes and Predicting Social Behavior*, Englewood Cliffs, NJ: Prentice-Hall.

Alexander, A.B. (1975) 'An experimental test of the assumptions relating to the use of electromyographic biofeedback as a general relaxation training technique', *Psychophysiology* 12: 656–62.

Alexander, A.B., White, P.D. and Wallis, H.M. (1977) 'Training and transfer of training effects in EMG biofeedback-assisted muscular relaxation', *Psychophysiology* 14: 551–60.

Alexander, F. (1939) 'Emotional factors in essential hypertension', *Psychosomatic Medicine* 1: 175–9.

Alexander, F. (1950) *Psychosomatic Medicine: Its Principles and Applications*, New York: Norton.

Alfredsson, L., Bergamn, U., Eriksson, R., Gronskog, K., Norell, S.E., Schwartz, E. and Wiholm, B.E. (1982) 'Theophyllines three times daily – when are the doses actually taken? Pharmokinetic ideals versus clinical practice', *European Journal of Respiratory Diseases* 63: 234–8.

Allan, D. and Armstrong, D. (1984) 'Patient attitudes towards radiographic examinations involving contrast media', *Clinical Radiology* 35: 457–9.

Allen, I. (1981) *Family Planning, Sterilisation and Abortion Services*, London: The Policy Studies Institute, No. 595.

Alogna, M. (1980) 'Perception of severity of disease and health locus of control in compliant and non-compliant diabetic patients', *Diabetes Care* 3: 533–40.

Amiel, S.A., Sherwin, R.S., Simonson, D.C., Lauritano, A.A. and Tamborlane, W.V. (1986) 'Impaired insulin action in puberty: a contributing factor to poor glycaemic control in adolescents with diabetes', *New England Journal of Medicine* 315: 215–19.

Andersen, J., Aabro, E., Gulmann, N., Hjelmstead, A. and Pederson, H.E. (1980) 'Anti-depressant treatment in Parkinson's disease: a controlled trial of the effect of nortriptyline in patients with Parkinson's disease treated with L-Dopa', *Acta Neurologica Scandinavica* 62: 210–19.

Andrasik, F. and Holroyd, K.A. (1983) 'Specific and non-specific effects in the biofeedback treatment of tension headache: three year follow-up', *Journal of Consulting and Clinical Psychology* 51: 634–6.

Andreassi, J.L. (1980) *Psychophysiology. Human Behavior and Physiological Response*, Oxford: Oxford University Press.

Antonovsky, A. (1979) *Health, Stress and Coping. New Perspectives on Mental and Physical Well-Being*, San Francisco: Jossey-Bass.

Appel, M.A. (1986) 'Hypertension', in K.A. Holroyd and T.L. Creer (eds) *Self-Management of Chronic Disease*, New York: Academic.

Apter, M. (1982) *The Experience of Motivation. The Theory of Psychological Reversals*, London: Academic Press.

Aranko, K., Mattilla, M.J. and Seppala, T. (1985) 'Development of tolerance and cross-tolerance to the psychomotor actions of lorazepam and diazepam in man', *British Journal of Clinical Pharmacology* 15: 545–52.

Arber, S. and Sawyer, L. (1985) 'The role of the receptionist in general practice: "a dragon behind the desk"?', *Social Science and Medicine* 20: 911–21.

Ashton, H. (ed.) (1987) *Brain Systems, Disorders, and Psychotropic Drugs*, Oxford: Oxford University Press.

Ashton, H. and Golding, J.F. (1989) 'Tranquillisers. Prevalence, predictors and possible consequences: data from a large United Kingdom survey', *British Journal of Addiction* 84: 541–6.

Ashton, H. and, Stepney, R. (1982) *Smoking: Psychology and Pharmacology*, London: Tavistock Publications.

Atwell, J.R., Flanagan, R.C., Bennett, R.L., Allan, D.C., Lucas, B.A. and McRoberts, J.W. (1984) 'The efficacy of patient-controlled analgesia in patients recovering from flank incisions', *Journal of Urology* 132: 701–3.

Auerbach, D., Carter, H.W., Garfinkel, L. and Hammond, E.C. (1976) 'Cigarette smoking and coronary heart disease: a macroscopic and microscopic study', *Chest* 70: 697–705.

Averill, J.R., O'Brien, L. and De Witt, G.W. (1977) 'The influence of response effectiveness on the preference for warning and on psychophysiological stress reactions', *Journal of Personality* 45: 395–418.

Avorn, J., Dreyer, P., Connelly, K. and Soumerai, S.B. (1989) 'Use of psychoactive medication and the quality of care in rest homes', *New England Journal of Medicine* 320: 227–32.

Badia, P., Harsh, J. and Abbott, B.A. (1979) 'Choosing between predictable and unpredictable shock conditions: data and theory', *Psychological Bulletin* 86: 1107–31.

Baker, G.H.B. (1987) 'Invited Review: Psychological factors and immunity', *Journal of Psychosomatic Research* 31: 1–10.

Baldwin, J.D. and Baldwin, J.I. (1988) 'Factors affecting AIDS-related sexual risk-taking behavior among college students', *Journal of Sex Research* 25: 181–96.

Bandura, A. (1977) *Social Learning Theory*, Englewood Cliffs, NJ: Prentice-Hall.

Bandura, A. (1986) *Social Foundations of Thought and Action: A Social Cognitive Theory*, Englewood Cliffs, NJ: Prentice-Hall.

Barefoot, J.C., Dahlstrom, W.G. and Williams, R.B. (1983) 'Hostility, CHD incidence, and total mortality: a 25 year follow-up study of 255 physicians', *Psychosomatic Medicine* 45: 59–63.

Barone, J.J. and Roberts, H. (1984) 'Human consumption of caffeine', in P.B. Dews (ed.) *Caffeine. Perspectives from Recent Research*, Berlin: Springer-Verlag.

Barr, M., Pennebaker, J.W. and Watson, D. (1988) 'Improving blood pressure estimation through internal and environmental feedback', *Psychosomatic Medicine* 50: 37–45.

Barton, T., Harris, R., Weinman, J., Allan, L. and Crawford, D. (1987) 'Psychological effects of prenatal diagnosis: the example of foetal echocardiography', *Current Psychological Research and Reviews* 6: 57–68.

Bartrop, R.W., Luckhurst, E., Lazarus, L., Kihlo, L.G. and Penny, R. (1977) 'Depressed lymphocyte function after bereavement', *Lancet* i: 834–6.

Baumrind, D. (1967) 'Child care practices anteceding 3 patterns of preschool behavior', *Genetic Psychology Monographs* 75: 43–88.

Beach, L.R., Campbell, F.L. and Townes, B.D. (1979) 'Subjective expected utility and the prediction of birth planning decisions', *Organizational Behavior and Human Performance* 24: 18–28.

Beard, R.W., Belsey, E.M., Lal, S., Lewis, S. and Greer, H.S. (1974) 'Contraceptive practice before and after out-patient termination of pregnancy. Kings Termination Study II', *British Medical Journal* i: 418–21.

Beattie, A. (1985) 'Self esteem, self help, and community education', in P. Belson (ed.) *Health Inequalities and the Under Fives*, London: Voluntary Organisations Liaison Council for the Under Fives (VOLCUF).

Beck, A.T. (1976) *Cognitive Therapy and the Emotional Disorders*, New York: International Universities Press.

Beck, J.G. and Davies, D.K. (1987) 'Teen contraception: a review of perspectives on compliance,' *Archives of Sexual Behaviour* 16: 337–68.

Becker, M.H. (ed.) (1974) 'The health belief model and personal health behaviour', *Health Education Monographs* 2: 324–508.

Becker, M.H. and Joseph, J.G. (1988) 'AIDS and behavior change to reduce risk: a review', *American Journal of Public Health* 78: 462–7.

Becker, M.H. and Maiman, L.A. (1975) 'Sociobehavioral determinants of compliance with health and medical care recommendations', *Medical Care* 13: 10–24.

Beecher, H.K. (1959) *Measurement of Subjective Responses: Quantitative Effects of Drugs*, New York: Oxford University Press.

Belloc, N.B. (1973) 'Relationship of health practices and mortality', *Preventive Medicine* 2: 67–81.

Belloc, N.B. and Breslow, L. (1972) 'Relationship of physical health status and health practices', *Preventive Medicine* 1: 409–21.

Belsky, J. (1984) 'The determinants of parenting: a process model', *Child Development* 55: 83–96.

Benowitz, N.L., Hall, S.M., Herning, R.I., Jacob, P., Jones, R.T. and Osman, A.L. (1983)

'Smokers of low-yield cigarettes do not consume less nicotine', *New England Journal of Medicine* 309: 129–42.

Ben-Sira, Z. (1984), 'Chronic illness, stress and coping', *Social Science and Medicine* 18: 725–36.

Benson, A.J. (1984) 'Motion sickness', in M.R. Dix and J.D.Hood (eds) *Vertigo*, Chichester: Wiley.

Bentler, P.M. and Speckart, G. (1979) 'Models of attitude–behaviour relation', *Psychological Review* 86: 452–64.

Bentler, P.M. and Speckart, G. (1981) 'Attitudes "cause" behaviors: a structural equation analysis', *Journal of Personality and Social Psychology* 40: 226–38.

Berg, R.L. (1976) 'The high cost of self deception', *Preventive Medicine* 5: 483–95.

Bergman, J. and Dews, P.B. (1987) 'Dietary caffeine and its toxicity', *Nutritional Toxicology* 2: 199–221.

Biddle, S. (1989) 'Self-efficacy and health-related exercise: a review', paper presented at the Annual Conference of the British Psychological Society, St Andrews.

Billings, C.E., Wick, R.L., Gerke, R.J. and Chase, R.C. (1973) 'The effects of alcohol upon pilot performance', *Aerospace Medicine* 44: 379–83.

Birk, L. (1973) *Biofeedback: Behavioral Medicine*, New York: Grune & Stratton.

Black Report (1980) *Inequalities in Health: Report of a Research Working Group*, London: Her Majesty's Stationery Office.

Blanchard, E.B. (1979) 'Biofeedback and the modification of cardiovascular dysfunctions', in R.J. Gatchel and K.P. Price (eds) *Clinical Applications of Biofeedback: Appraisal and Status*, New York: Pergamon Press.

Blanchard, E.B. and Abel, G.G. (1976) 'An experimental case study of the biofeedback treatment of a rape-induced psychophysiological cardiovascular disorder', *Behavior Therapy* 7: 113–19.

Blanchard, E.B. and Young, L.D. (1973) 'Self-control of cardiac functioning: a promise as yet unfulfilled', *Psychological Bulletin* 79: 145–63.

Blanchard, E.B. and Young, L.D. (1974) 'Clinical applications of biofeedback training: a review of evidence', *Archives of General Psychiatry* 30: 573–89.

Blanchard, E.B., McCoy, G.C., Musso, A., Gerardi, M.A., Pallmeyer, T.P., Gerardi, R.J., Cotch, P.A., Siracusa, K. and Andrasik, F. (1986) 'A controlled comparison of thermal biofeedback and relaxation training in the treatment of essential hypertension: I. Short-term and long-term outcome', *Behavior Therapy* 17: 563–79.

Blaney, P.H. (1986) 'Affect and memory: a review', *Psychological Bulletin* 99: 229–46.

Blaxter, M. (1983) 'The causes of disease: women talking', *Social Science and Medicine* 17: 59–69.

Block, A.R., Kremer, E.F. and Gaylor, M. (1980) 'Behavioral treatment of chronic pain: the spouse as a discriminative cue for pain behavior', *Pain* 9: 243–52.

Blum, K. and Trachtenberg, M.C. (1988) 'Alcoholism: scientific basis of a neuropsychogenetic disease', *International Journal of the Addictions* 23: 781–96.

Blumenthal, J.A. (1985) 'Relaxation therapy, biofeedback and behavioral medicine', *Psychotherapy* 22: 516–30.

Boddy, J. (1983) 'Information processing and functional systems in the brain', in A. Gale and J.A. Edwards (eds) *Physiological Correlates of Human Behavior. Volume 1. Basic Issues*, London: Academic Press.

Bongaarts, J. (1976) 'Intermediate fertility variables and marital fertility rates', *Population Studies* 30: 227–41.

Bonica, J.J. and Albe-Fessard, D. (eds) (1976) *Recent Advances in Pain Research and Therapy. Volume 1*, New York: Raven Press.

Booth-Kewley, S. and Friedman, H.S. (1987) 'Psychological predictors of heart disease: a quantitative review', *Psychological Bulletin* 101: 343–62.

Boureston, N.C. and Howard, M.T. (1965) 'Personality characteristics of three disability groups', *Archives of Physical Medicine and Rehabilitation* 46: 626–32.

Bower, G.H. (1981) 'Mood and memory', *American Psychologist* 36: 129–48.

Bowers, T.G., Winett, R.A. and Frederiksen, L.W. (1987) 'Nicotine fading, behavioural contracting and extended treatment: effects on smoking cessation', *Addictive Behaviours* 12: 181–4.

Boyle, C.M. (1970) 'Differences between patients' and doctors' interpretations of some common medical terms', *British Medical Journal* 2: 286–9.

Boyle, M.E., Pitts, M.K., Phillips, K.C., White, D.G., Clifford, B. and Woollett, E.A. (1989) 'Exploring young people's attitudes to and knowledge of AIDS: the value of focussed group discussions', *Health Education Journal* 48: 21–3.

Bradley, C. (1978) 'Psychophysiological aspects of stress in diabetic patients, ischemic heart disease patients and healthy subjects', unpublished doctoral dissertation, University of Nottingham.

Bradley, C. (1979) 'Life events and the control of diabetes mellitus', *Journal of Psychosomatic Research* 23: 159–62.

Bradley, C. and Marteau, T.M. (1986) 'Towards an integration of psychological and medical perspectives of diabetes management', in K.G.M.M. Alberti and L.P. Krall (eds) *The Diabetes Annual. Volme 2*, Amsterdam: Elsevier.

Bradley, C., Brewin, C.R., Gamsu, D.S. and Moses, J.L. (1984) 'Development of scales to measure perceived control of diabetes mellitus and diabetes-related health beliefs', *Diabetic Medicine* 1: 213–18.

Bradley, P.B. and Hirsch, S.R. (1986) *Psychopharmacology and Drug Treatment of Schizophrenia*, Oxford: Oxford University Press.

Brady, J.V. (1958) 'Ulcers in "executive monkeys"', *Scientific American* 199: 95–100.

Braken, M.B., Klerman, L.V. and Braken, M. (1978) 'Abortion, adoption or motherhood: an empirical study of decision making during pregnancy', *American Journal of Obstetrics and Gynecology* 130: 251–62.

Brehm, J. (1966) *A Theory of Psychological Reactance*, New York: Academic Press.

Brener, J.M. (1981) 'Control of internal activities', *British Medical Bulletin* 37: 169–74.

Brener, J.M., Phillips, K.C. and Connally, S. (1977) 'Oxygen consumption and ambulation during operant conditioning of heart rate increases and decreases in rats', *Psychophysiology* 14: 483–91.

Brennan, A.F., Barrett, C.L., and Garretson, H.D. (1987) 'The utility of McGill Pain Questionnaire subscales for discriminating psychological disorder in chronic pain patient', *Psychology and Health* 1: 257–72.

Brenner, M.H. (1987) 'Economic change, alcohol consumption and heart disease mortality in nine industrialised countries', *Social Science and Medicine* 25: 119–32.

Brewer, C. (1977) 'Incidence of post-abortion psychosis: a prospective study', *British Medical Journal* i: 476–7.

British Medical Journal (1982) *Alcohol problems*, London: BMJ Publications.

British Thoracic Study (1983) 'Comparison of four methods of smoking withdrawal in patients with smoking related diseases', *British Medical Journal* 286: 595–7.

Britton, B.J. (1987) 'A surgeon's view of day case surgery', in I. Hindmarch, J.G. Jones and E. Moss (eds) *Aspects of Recovery from Anaesthesia*, Chichester: Wiley.

Bronfenbrenner, U. (1979) *The Ecology of Human Development*, Cambridge, Mass.: Harvard University Press.

Brooks, N.A. and Matson, R.R. (1982) 'Social-psychological adjustment to multiple sclerosis: a longitudinal study', *Social Science and Medicine* 16: 2129–35.

Brorsson, B. and Herlitz, C. (1988) 'The AIDS epidemic in Sweden: changes in awareness, attitudes and behavior', *Scandinavian Journal of Social Medicine* 16: 67–71.

Brown, B.B. (1977) *Stress and the Art of Biofeedback*, New York: Harper & Row.

Brown, G.W. and Harris, T.O. (1978) *Social Origins of Depression. A Study of Psychiatric Disorder in Women*, London: Tavistock.

Brown, G.W and Harris, T.O. (1986) 'Establishing causal links: the Bedford College studies of depression', in H. Katschnig (ed.) *Life Events and Psychiatric Disorders*, Cambridge: Cambridge University Press.

Brownlee-Duffeck, M., Peterson, L., Simonds, J.F., Goldstein, D., Kilo, C. and Hoette, S. (1987) 'The role of health beliefs in the regimen adherence and metabolic control of adolescents and adults with diabetes mellitus', *Journal of Consulting and Clinical Psychology* 55: 139–44.

Bruce, M.S. and Lader, M.H. (1986) 'Caffeine: clinical and experimental effects in humans', *Human Psychopharmacology* 1: 63–82.

Bruch, M.A. and Haynes, M.J. (1987) 'Heterosocial anxiety and contraceptive behaviour', *Journal of Research in Personality* 21: 343–60.

Brunson, B.I. and Matthews, K.A. (1981) 'The Type A coronary prone behaviour pattern and reactions to uncontrollable stress. An analysis of performance strategies, affect and attributions during failure', *Journal of Personality and Social Psychology* 40: 906–18.

Budzynski, T.H., Stoyva, J.M., Adler, C.S. and Mullaney, D.J. (1973) 'EMG biofeedback and tension headache: a controlled outcome study', *Psychosomatic Medicine* 35: 484–96.

Buller, M.K. and Buller, D.B. (1987) 'Physicians' communication style and patient satisfaction', *Journal of Health and Social Behaviour* 28: 375–88.

Burnham, L. and Werner, G. (1979) 'The high-level tetraplegic: psychological survival and adjustment', *Paraplegia* 16: 184–92.

Bush, C., Ditto, B. and Feuerstein, M. (1985) 'A controlled evaluation of paraspinal EMG biofeedback in the treatment of chronic low back pain', *Health Psychology* 4: 307–21.

Bush, J.P., Melamed, B.G., Greenbaum, P.E. and Sheras, P.L. (1988) 'Mother–child patterns of coping with anticipatory medical stress', in B.G. Melamed, K.A. Matthews, D.K. Routh, B. Stabler and N. Schneiderman (eds) *Child Health Psychology*, Hillsdale, NJ: Lawrence Erlbaum Associates.

Butler, N.R. and Golding, J. (eds) (1986) *From Birth to Five. A Study of the Health and Behaviour of Britain's Five Year Olds*, Oxford: Pergamon Press.

Byers, E.S. and Lewis, K. (1988) 'Dating couples' disagreements over the desired level of sexual intimacy', *Journal of Sex Research* 24: 15–29.

Byrne, D. (1961) 'The repression–sensitization scale: rationale, reliability and validity', *Journal of Personality* 29: 334–49.

Byrne, D.G., Rosenman, R.H., Schiller, E. and Chesney, M.A. (1985) 'Consistency and variation among instruments purporting to measure the Type A behavior pattern', *Psychosomatic Medicine* 47: 242–61.

Cairns, D. and Pasino, J.A. (1977) 'Comparison of verbal reinforcement and feedback in the operant treatment of disability due to chronic low back pain', *Behavior Therapy* 8: 621–30.

Calnan, M. (1984) 'The health belief model and participation in programmes for the early detection of breast cancer', *Social Science and Medicine* 19: 823–30.

Capstick, N. (1980) 'Long-term fluphenazine decanoate maintenance dosage requirements of chronic schizophrenic patients', *Acta Psychiatrica Scandinavia* 61: 256–62.

Carlson, J.G., Basilio, C.A. and Heaukulani, J.D. (1983) 'Transfer of EMG training: another look at the general relaxation issue', *Psychophysiology* 20: 530–6.

Carney, R.M., Schechter, K. and Davis, T. (1983) 'Improving adherence to blood glucose testing in insulin-dependent diabetic children', *Behavior Therapy* 14: 247–54.

Caron, H.S. and Roth, H.P. (1968) 'Patients' cooperation with a medical regimen', *Journal of the American Medical Association* 203: 922–6.

Carroll, D., Hewitt, J.K., Last, K.A., Turner, J.R. and Sims, J. (1985) 'A twin study of cardiac reactivity and its relationship to parental blood pressure', *Physiology and Behavior* 34: 103–6.

Cartwright, A. (1967) *Patients and Their Doctors. A Study of General Practice*, London: Routledge & Kegan Paul.

Cassel, J. (1975) 'Studies of hypertension in migrants', in O. Paul (ed.) *Epidemiology and Control of Hypertension*, New York: Stratton.

Cassileth, B.R., Lusk, E.J., Strouse, T.B., Miller, D.S., Brown, L.L., Cross, P.A. and Tenaglia, A.N. (1984) 'Psychosocial status in chronic illness – a comparative analysis of six diagnostic groups', *New England Journal of Medicine* 311: 506–11.

Catalan, J., Gath, D., Edmonds, G., Ennis, J., Bond, A., Martin, P. (1984) 'The effects of non-prescribing anxiolytics in general practice: I. Controlled evaluation of psychiatric and social outcome', *British Journal of Psychiatry* 144: 593–610.

Cataldo, M.F., Dershewitz, R.A., Wilson, M., Cristophersen, E.R., Finney, J.W., Fawcett, S.B. and Seekins, T. (1986) 'Childhood injury control', in N.A. Krasegor, J.D. Arasteh and M.F. Cataldo (eds) *Child Health Behavior. A Behavioral Pediatrics Perspective*, New York: John Wiley.

Cavanagh, S. (1983) 'The prevalence of emotional and cognitive dysfunction in a general medical population: using the MMSE, GHQ and BDI', *General Hospital Psychiatry* 5: 15–24.

Cay, E., Philip, A. and Aitken, C. (1976) 'Psychological aspects of cardiac rehabilitation', in O.W. Hill (ed.) *Modern Trends in Psychosomatic Medicine. Volume 3*, London: Butterworths.

CDC (Center for Disease Control) (1981) 'Kaposi's sarcoma and pneumocystis pneumonia among homosexual men – New York City and California', *Morbidity and Mortality Weekly Reports* 30: 305–8.

CDC (Center for Disease Control) (1982) 'Unexplained immunodeficiency and opportunistic infections in children – New York, New Jersey, California', *Morbidity and Mortality Weekly Reports* 31: 665–7.

CDC (Center for Disease Control) (1985) *Education and Foster Care of Children Infected with Human T-lymphotropic Virus Type 3/lymphadenopathy Associated Virus*, Atlanta, Georgia.

CDC (Center for Disease Control) (1987) 'Classification system for human immunodeficiency virus (HIV) infection in children under 13 years of age', *Morbidity and Mortality Weekly Reports* 36: 225–30, 235–6.

Cella, D.F. and Holland, J.C. (1988) 'Methodological considerations in studying the stress–illness connection in women with breast cancer', in C.L. Cooper (ed.) *Stress and Breast Cancer*, Chichester: John Wiley.

Cerkoney, K.A. and Hart, L. (1980) 'The relationship between the health belief model and compliance of persons with diabetes mellitus', *Diabetes Care* 3: 594–8.

Chalmers, B.E. (1982) 'Stressful life events: their past and present status', *Current Psychological Reviews* 2: 123–38.

Chapman, S. and Hodgson, J. (1988) 'Showers in raincoats: attitudinal barriers to condom use in high risk heterosexuals', *Community Health Studies* 12: 97–105.

Chase, H.P. and Jackson, G.C. (1981) 'Stress and sugar control in children with insulin-dependent diabetes mellitus', *Journal of Pediatrics* 98: 1011–13.

Chesney, M.A., Black, G.W., Swan, G.E., and Ward, M.M. (1987) 'Relaxation training for essential hypertension at the Worksite: I. The untreated mild hypertensive', *Psychosomatic Medicine* 49: 250–63.

Chilman, C.S. (1985) 'Feminist issues in teenage parenting', *Child Welfare* 64: 225–34.

Christie, M.J. and Woodman, D.D. (1980) 'Biochemical methods', in I. Martin and P.H. Venables (eds) *Techniques in Psychophysiology*, Chichester: John Wiley and Sons.

Cicero, T.J. (1978) 'Tolerance to and physical dependence on alcohol', in W. Wuttke and R.R. Dries (eds) *Brain and Pituitary Peptides*, Ferring Symposium, Munich. Basle: Karger.

Cinciripini, P.M. and Floreen, A. (1983) 'An assessment of chronic pain behavior in a structured interview', *Journal of Psychosomatic Research* 27: 117–23.

Claus-Walker, J., Campos, R.J. and Carter, R.E. (1972) 'Longitudinal analysis of daily excretory rhythms in men with tetraplegia due to cervical cord transection', *Paraplegia* 10: 142–52.

Cleary, P.D. (1987) 'Why people take precautions against health risks', in N.D. Weinstein (ed.) *Taking Care: Understanding and Encouraging Self-Protective Behaviours*, Cambridge: Cambridge University Press.

Clubley, M., Bye, C.E., Henson, T.A., Peck, A.W. and Riddington, C.J. (1979) 'Effects of caffeine and cyclizine alone and in combination on human performance: subjective effects and EEG activity', *British Journal of Clinical Pharmacology* 7: 157–62.

Coates, T.J. (1982) 'Hypertension in adolescents', in A. Baum and J.E. Singer (eds) *Handbook of Psychology and Health. Volume II. Issues in Child Health and Adolescent Health*, Hillsdale, NJ: LEA.

Cobliner, W.G., Schulman, H. and Smith, V. (1975) 'Patterns of contraceptive failures: the role of motivation reexamined', *Journal of Biosocial Science* 7: 307–18.

Cohen, J.B., Hauser, L.B. and Wofsy, C.B. (1989) 'Women and IV drugs: parenteral and heterosexual transmission of human immunodeficiency virus', *Journal of Drug Issues* 19: 39–56.

Coles, M.G.H., Donchin, E. and Porges, S.W. (1986) *Psychophysiology: Systems, Processes, and Applications*, New York: Guilford.

Committee on the Review of Medicines (1980) 'Systematic review of the benzodiazepines', *British Medical Journal* 1: 910–12.

Connor, W.H. (1974) 'Effects of brief relaxation training on autonomic response to anxiety-provoking stimuli', *Psychophysiology* 11: 591–9.

Conviser, R. and Rutledge, J.H. (1989) 'Can public policies limit the spread of HIV among IV drug users?', *Journal of Drug Issues* 19: 113–28.

Coomber, J.A. and Parrott, A.C. (unpublished) 'Smoking reduction during premenstrual and midcycle periods: differential effects upon mood state', submitted for publication.

Cox, T. (1978) *Stress*, London: Macmillan.

Cox, T. (1983) 'The psychological and physiological response to stress', in A. Gale and J.A. Edwards (eds) *Physiological Correlates of Human Behaviour. Vol. 1: Basic Issues*, London: Academic Press.

Cox, T. (1988) 'Psychobiological factors in stress and health', in S. Fisher and J. Reason (eds) *Handbook of Life Stress, Cognition and Health*, Chichester: John Wiley and Sons.

Cox, T. and Mackay, C. (1982) 'Psychosocial factors and psychophysiological mechanisms in the aetiology and development of cancers', *Social Science and Medicine* 16: 381–96.

Crnic, K.A., Greenberg, M.T., Ragozin, A.S., Robinson, N.M. and Basham, R.B. (1983) 'Effects of stress and social support on mothers and premature and full-term infants', *Child Development* 54: 209–17.

Crue, B.L. Jr. and Carregal, E.J.A. (1975) 'Pain begins in the dorsal horn – with a proposed classification of the primary senses', in B.L. Crue, Jr. (ed.) *Pain: Research and Treatment*, New York: Academic Press.

Cunningham-Burley, S. and Irvine, S. (1987) '"And have you done anything so far?", An examination of lay treatment of children's symptoms', *British Medical Journal* 295: 700–2.

Cvetkovich, G. and Grote, B. (1981) 'Psychosocial maturity and teenage contraceptive use: an investigation of decision-making and communication skills', *Population and Environment* 4: 211–26.

Cvetkovich, G. and Grote, B. (1983) 'Adolescent development and teenage fertility', in D. Byrne and W.A. Fisher (eds) *Adolescents, Sex and Contraception*, Hillsdale, NJ: Lawrence Erlbaum.

Dahl, L.K. (1961) 'Possible role of excess salt consumption in the pathogenesis of essential hypertension', *American Journal of Cardiology* 8: 571–5.

Dahl, L.K. and Love, R.A. (1957) 'Etiological role of sodium chloride intake in essential hypertension in humans', *Journal of the American Medical Association* 164: 397–400.

Dahlstrom, W.G., Welsh, G.S. and Dahlstrom, L.E. (1972) *An MMPI Handbook. Volume I. Clinical Interpretations*, Minneapolis: University of Minnesota Press.

Dahlstrom, W.G., Welsh, G.S. and Dahlstrom, L.E. (1975) *An MMPI Handbook. Volume II. Research Developments and Applications*, Minneapolis: University of Minnesota Press.

Dakof, G.A. and Mendelsohn, G.A. (1986) 'Parkinson's disease: the psychological aspects of a chronic illness', *Psychological Bulletin* 99: 375–87.

Dalos, N.P., Rabins, P.V., Brooks, B.R. and O'Donnell, P. (1983) 'Disease activity and emotional state in multiple sclerosis', *Annals of Neurology* 13: 573–7.

Daly, L.E., Mulchaly, R., Graham, I.M. and Hickey, N. (1983) 'Long-term effect on mortality of stopping smoking after unstable angina and myocardial infarction', *British Medical Journal* 287: 324–6.

Dantzer, R. (1989) 'Neuroendocrine correlates of control and coping', in A. Steptoe and A. Appels (eds) *Stress, Personal Control and Health*, Chichester: Wiley.

D'Atri, D.A. and Ostfield, A.M. (1975) 'Crowding: its effects on the elevation of blood pressure in a prison setting', *Preventive Medicine* 4: 550–66.

Davies, D.L. (1962) 'Normal drinking in recovered alcoholics', *Quarterly Journal of Studies on Alcohol* 23: 94–104.

Davies, J.M. and Casper, R.C. (1978) 'General principles of clinical use of neuroleptics', in W.G. Clark and J. DelGuidice (eds) *Principles of Psychopharmacology*, 2nd edition, New York: Academic Press.

Davis, D.R. (1947) 'Psychomotor effects of analeptics and their relation to "fatigue" phenomena in aircrew', *British Medical Bulletin* 5: 43–5.

Davis, M.S. (1966) 'Variations in patients' compliance with doctors' orders: analysis of congruence between survey responses and results of empirical investigations', *Journal of Medical Education* 41: 1037–48.

Davis, R., Buchanan, B. and Shortliffe, E. (1977) 'Production rules as a representation for knowledge based consultation program', *Artificial Intelligence* 8: 15–42.

DeFrank, R.S., Jenkins, C.D. and Rose, R.M. (1987) 'A longitudinal investigation of the relationships among alcohol consumption, psychosocial factors, and blood pressure', *Psychosomatic Medicine* 49: 236–49.

De Freitas, B. and Schwartz, G. (1979) 'Effects of caffeine on chronic psychiatric patients', *Americal Journal of Psychiatry* 136: 1337–8.

Delamater, A., Bubb, J., Kurtz, S., Kuntze, J., Smith, J., White, N. and Santiago, J. (1988) 'Physiologic responses to acute psychological stress in adolescents with type 1 diabetes mellitus', *Journal of Pediatric Psychology* 13: 69–86.

Dembroski, T.M., MacDougall, J.M., Williams, R.B., Haney, T.L. and Blumenthal, J.A. (1985) 'Components of Type A, hostility, and anger-in: relationship to angiographic findings', *Psychosomatic Medicine* 47: 219–33.

De Rios, M.D. (1989) 'A modern day shamanistic healer in the Peruvian amazon: pharmacopoeia and trance', *Journal of Psychoactive Drugs* 21: 91–9.

Devine, E.C. and Cook, T.D. (1983) 'A meta-analysis of psychoeducational interventions on length of postsurgical hospital stay', *Nursing Research* 32: 267–74.

Devine, E.C. and Cook, T.D. (1986) 'Clinical and cost-saving effects of psychoeducational interventions with surgical patients: a meta-analysis', *Research in Nursing and Health* 9: 89–105.

Devins, G.M. and Seland, T.P. (1987) 'Emotional impact of multiple sclerosis: recent findings and suggestions for future research', *Psychological Bulletin* 101: 363–75.

Dews, P.B. (1984) 'Behavioural effects of caffeine', in P.B. Dews (ed.) *Caffeine. Perspectives from Recent Research*, Berlin: Springer-Verlag.

DHSS and Welsh Office (1987) *AIDS: Monitoring Response to the Public Education Campaign February 1986–February 1987*, London: HMSO.

DiMatteo, M.R. and DiNicola, D.D. (1982) *Achieving Patient Compliance*, New York: Pergamon Press.

Dinardo, Q.E. (1971) 'Psychological adjustment to spinal cord injury', doctoral dissertation, University of Houston.

Dockter, B., Black, D.R., Hovell, M.F., Engleberg, D., Amick, T., Neimier, D. and Sheets, N. (1988) 'Families and intensive care nurses: comparison of perceptions', *Patient Education and Counseling* 12: 29–36.

Dohrenwend, B.S. and Dohrenwend, B.P. (1974) *Stressful Life Events: Their Nature and Effects*, New York: Wiley.

Dolce, J.J. (1987) 'Self-efficacy and disability beliefs in behavioral treatment of pain', *Behaviour Research and Therapy* 25: 289–99.

Dolce, J.J., Doleys, D.M., Raczynski, J.M., Lossie, J., Pool, L. and Smith, M. (1986) 'The role of self-efficacy expectancies in the prediction of pain tolerance', *Pain* 27: 261–72.

Doll, R. and Peto, R. (1976) 'Mortality in relation to smoking: 20 years' observations on male British doctors', *British Medical Journal* ii: 1525–36.

Drury, M.I. (1984) 'Diabetic education: a physician's view – who, what, where, when and how?', *Diabetic Medicine* 1: 233–6.

Dubuisson, D. and Melzack, R. (1976) 'Classification of clinical pain description by multiple group discriminant analysis', *Experimental Neurology* 51: 480–7.

Dunbar, F. (1943) *Psychosomatic Diagnosis*, New York: Harper & Row.

Dunbar, M. (1989) 'The effects of psychological and educational interventions on the recovery of surgical patients: a meta-analysis', unpublished dissertation submitted in completion of B.Sc. Psychology, Polytechnic of East London.

Dunn, D. (1969) 'Adjustment to spinal cord injury in the rehabilitation hospital setting', doctoral dissertation, University of Maryland.

Dunn, S.M. (1986) 'Reactions to educational techniques: coping strategies for diabetes and learning', *Diabetic Medicine* 3: 419–29.

Dunn, S.M., Bryson, J.M., Hoskins, P.L., Alford, J.B., Handelsman, D.J. and Turtle, J.R. (1984) 'Development of the Diabetic Knowledge (DKN) Scales: forms DKNA, DKNB, and DKNC', *Diabetes Care* 7: 36–41.

Dworkin, B. (1988) 'Hypertension as a learned response: the baroreceptor reinforcement', in T. Elbert, W. Langosch, A. Steptoe and D. Vaitl (eds) *Behavioral Medicine in Cardiovascular Disorders*, Chichester: John Wiley and Sons.

Dyck, P.J., Lambert, E.H. and O'Brien, P. (1976) 'Pain in peripheral neuropathy related to size and rate of fibre degeneration', in M. Weisenberg and B. Tursky (eds) *Pain: New Perspectives in Therapy and Research*, New York: Plenum Press.

Earls, F. (1987) 'On the familial transmission of child psychiatric disorder', *Journal of Child Psychology and Psychiatry* 28: 791–802.

Eastman, B.G., Johnson, S.B., Silverstein, J., Spillar, R.P. and McCallum, M. (1983) 'Understanding of hypo- and hyperglycaemia by youngsters with diabetes and their parents', *Journal of Pediatric Psychology* 8: 229–43.

Eddy, D.M. and Clanton, C.H. (1982) 'The art of diagnosis: solving the clinicopathological exercise', *New England Journal of Medicine* 306: 1263–8.

Edwards, V. (1980) 'Changing breast self-examination behaviour', *Nursing Research* 29: 301–6.

Elias, M.F., Robbins, M.A., Rice, A. and Edgecombe, J.L. (1982) 'A behavioral study of middle-aged chest pain patients: physical symptom reporting, anxiety and depression', *Experimental Aging Research* 8: 45–51.

Ellis, A. (1962) *Reason and Emotion in Psychotherapy*, New York: Lyle Stuart.

Ellis, A. (1984) 'Rational emotive therapy', in R.J. Corsini (ed.) *Current Psychotherapies* 3rd edition, Itasca, Ill.: Peacock Press.

Elson, B.D., Hauri, P. and Cunis, D. (1977) 'Physiological changes in yoga meditation', *Psychophysiology* 14: 52–7.

Engel, B.T. and Bleecker, E.R. (1974) 'Applications of operant conditioning techniques to the control of cardiac arrhythmias', in P.A. Obrist, A.H. Black, J. Brener and L.V. DiCara (eds) *Cardiovascular Psychophysiology*, Chicago: Aldine.

Epstein, L.H. and Cluss, P.A. (1982) 'A behavioral medicine perspective on adherence to long-term medical regimens', *Journal of Consulting and Clinical Psychology* 50: 950–71.

Epstein, M. and Oster, J.R. (1984) *Hypertension: A Practical Approach*, Philadelphia; Saunders.

Ergonomics (1985) *Special Issue: Industrial Back Pain in Europe*, Volume 28 (Jan.): whole issue.

Evans, P.D. and Edgerton, N. (1989) 'Uplifts, hassles, and the common cold', paper delivered to the International Conference on Health Psychology, Cardiff, UK.

Evans, P.D. and Fearn, J.M. (1985) 'Type A behaviour pattern, choice of active coping strategy and cardiovascular activity in relation to threat of shock', *British Journal of Medical Psychology* 58: 95–9.

Evans, P.D. and Moran, P. (1987a) 'The Framingham Type A scale, vigilant coping and heart rate reactivity', *Journal of Behavioural Medicine* 10: 311–21.

Evans, P.D. and Moran, P. (1987b) 'Cardiovascular unwinding, Type A behaviour pattern and locus of control', *British Journal of Medical Psychology* 60: 261–5.

Evans, P.D., Phillips, K.C. and Fearn, J.M. (1984) 'On choosing to make aversive events predictable or unpredictable: some behavioural and psychophysiological findings', *British Journal of Psychology* 75: 377–91.

Evans, P.D., Pitts, M.K. and Smith, K. (1988) 'Minor infection, minor life events and the four day desirability dip', *Journal of Psychosomatic Research* 32: 533–9.

Eysenck, H.J. (1985) 'Personality, cancer and cardiovascular disease: a causal analysis', *Personality and Individual Differences* 6: 535–56.

Eysenck, H.J. and Fulker, D.W. (1983) 'The components of Type A behaviour and its genetic determinants', *Personality and Individual Differences* 4: 499–505.

Faber, M.M. (1986) 'A review of efforts to protect children from injury in car crashes', *Family and Community Health* 9: 25–41.

Farrell, M. (1989a) 'News and notes: On the misuse of drugs regulations', *British Journal of Addiction* 84: 703–6.

Farrell, M. (1989b) 'News and notes: The Health Education Authority', *British Journal of Addiction* 84: 949–51.

Fava, G., Pilowsky, I., Pierfederici, A., Bernardi, M. and Pathak, D. (1982) 'Depression and illness behavior in a general hospital: a prevalence study', *Psychotherapy and Psychosomatics* 38: 141–53.

Feldman, D.J. (1974) 'Chronic disabling illness: a holistic view', *Journal of Chronic Disorders* 27: 287–91.

Ferrari, M., Matthews, W.S. and Barabas, G. (1983) 'The family and the child with epilepsy', *Family Process* 22: 53–9.

Feuerstein, M., Labbe, E.E. and Kuczmierczyk, A. R. (1986) *Health Psychology. A Psychobiological Perspective*, New York: Plenum Press.

Finkel, M.L. and Finkel, D.J. (1975) 'Sexual and contraceptive knowledge, attitudes and behaviour of male adolescents', *Family Planning Perspectives* 7: 256–60.

Fischl, M.A., Dickinson, G.M., Scott, G.B., Klimas, N., Fletcher, M.A. and Parks, W. (1987) 'Evaluation of heterosexual partners, children and household contacts of adults with AIDS', *Journal of the American Medical Association* 257: 640–4.

Fishbein, M. (1972) 'Towards an understanding of family planning behaviours', *Journal of Applied Social Psychology* 2: 214–27.

Fishbein, M. and Ajzen, I. (1975), *Belief, Attitude, Intention and Behaviour: An Introduction to Theory and Research*, Reading, Mass.: Addison-Wesley.

Fisher, A.A. (1977) 'The health belief model and contraceptive behaviour: limits to the application of a conceptual framework', *Health Education Monograph* 5: 244–50.

Fisher, S. (1986) *Stress and Strategy*, London: Lawrence Erlbaum Associates.

Fitzpatrick, R., Hinton, J., Newman, S., Scambler, G. and Thompson, J. (eds) (1984) *The Experience of Illness*, London: Tavistock Publications.

Fletcher, B.C. (1988) 'The epidemiology of occupational stress', in C.L. Cooper and R. Payne (eds) *Causes, Coping and Consequences of Stress at Work*, Chichester: John Wiley & Sons.

Flodmark, A. (1986) 'Augmented auditory feedback as an aid in gait training of the cerebral-palsied child', *Developmental Medicine and Child Neurology* 28: 147–55.

Flor, H., Haag, G.. Turk, D.C. and Koehler, H. (1983) 'Efficacy of EMG biofeedback, psychotherapy, and conventional medical treatment for chronic back pain', *Pain* 17: 21–31.

Fontaine, R., Chouinard, G. and Annable, L. (1984). 'Rebound anxiety in anxious patients after abrupt withdrawal of benzodiazepine treatment', *American Journal of Psychiatry* 141: 848–52.

Fordyce, W.E. (1976) *Behavioral Methods for Chronic Pain and Illness*, St Louis: W.C. Mosby.

Fordyce, W., Caldwell, L. and Hongadarrow, G. (1979) 'Effects of performance feedback on exercise tolerance in chronic pain', unpublished manuscript, University of Washington.

Fordyce, W.E., Lansky, D., Calsyn, D. A., Shelton, J.L., Stolov, W.C. and Rock, D.L. (1984) 'Pain measurement and pain behavior', *Pain* 18: 53–69.

Foster, R.S., Lang, S.P., Constanza, M.C., Worden, J.K., Haines, C.R. and Yates, J.W. (1978) 'Breast self examination practice and breast cancer stage', *New England Journal of Medicine* 229: 265–70.

Fowler, J.E., Budzynski, T.H. and Vandenbergh, R.L. (1976) 'Effects of an EMG biofeedback relaxation programme on the control of diabetes: a case study', *Biofeedback and Self-regulation* 1: 105–13.

Fox, B.H. (1981) 'Psychosocial factors and the immune system in human cancer', in R. Ader (ed.) *Psychoneuroimmunology*, New York: Academic Press.

Fox, E.J. and Melzack, R. (1976) 'Transcutaneous electrical stimulation and acupuncture: comparisons of treatment for low back pain', *Pain* 2: 141–8.

Frank, J.W. and Mai, V. (1985) 'Breast self examination in young women: more harm than good?', *Lancet* ii (8456): 654–7.

Frank, R.G., Elliott, T.R., Corcoran, J.R. and Wonderlich, S.A. (1987) 'Depression after spinal cord injury: is it necessary?', *Clinical Psychology Review* 7: 611–30.

Frank, R.G., Kashani, J.H., Wonderlich, S.A., Lising, A. and Visot. L.R. (1985) 'Depression and adrenal function in spinal cord injury', *American Journal of Psychiatry* 142: 252–3.

Frank, R.G., Elliott, T.R., Wonderlich, S.A., Corcoran, J.R., Umlauf, R.L., Ashkanazi,

G.S. and Wilson, R. (1987) 'Gender differences in the interpersonal response to depression and spinal cord injury', *Cognitive Therapy and Research* 11: 437–48.

Frank, R.G., Wonderlich, S.A., Corcoran, J.R., Umlauf, R.L., Ashkanazi, G.H., Brownlee-Duffeck, M. and Wilson, R. (1986) 'Interpersonal response to spinal cord injury', *Journal of Social and Clinical Psychology* 4: 447–60.

Frankenhaeuser, M., Jearpe, G., Svan, H., Wrangsjea, B. (1963) 'Psychophysiological reactions to two different placebo treatments', *Scandinavian Journal of Psychology* 4: 245–50.

Freedman, R. and Ianni, P. (1985) 'Effects of general and thematically relevant stressors in Raynaud's disease', *Journal of Psychosomatic Research* 29: 275–80.

Freedman, R., Ianni, P. and Wenig, P. (1985) 'Behavioural treatment of Raynaud's disease: long-term followup' *Journal of Clinical and Consulting Psychology* 53: 136.

Freedman, R., Lynn, S., Ianni, P. and Hale, P. (1981) 'Biofeedback treatment of Raynaud's disease', *Biofeedback and Self-Regulation* 6: 355–65.

Freeman, E.W., Rickels, K., Huggins, G.R., Mudd, E.H., Garcia, C.R. and Dickens, H.O. (1980) 'Adolescent contraceptive use: comparisons of male and female attitudes and information', *American Journal of Public Health* 70: 790–7.

Friedman, H.S. and Booth-Kewley, S. (1988) 'Validity of the Type A construct: a reprise', *Psychological Bulletin* 104: 381–4.

Friedman, M., Thoreson, C.E., Gill, J.J., Powell, L.H., Ulmer D., Thompson, L., Price, V.A., Rabin, D.D., Breall, W.S., Dixon, T., Levy, R. and Bourg, E. (1984) 'Alteration of type A behavior and reduction in cardiac recurrences in post-myocardial infarction patients', *American Heart Journal* 108: 237–48.

Friedman, S., Southern, J.L., Abdul-Quader, A., Primm, D.C., Des Jarlais, D.C., Kleinman, P., Mauge, C., Goldsmith, D.S., El-Sadr, E., and Maslansky, R. (1987) 'The AIDS epidemic among blacks and hispanics', *Milbank Quarterly* 65: Supplement 2.

Fritz, G.K., Rubinstein, S. and Lewiston, N.J. (1987) 'Psychological factors in fatal childhood asthma', *American Journal of Orthopsychiatry* 57: 253–7.

Fullerton, D.T., Harvey, R.F., Klein, M.H. and Howell, T. (1981) 'Psychiatric disorders in patients with spinal cord injury', *Archives of General Psychiatry* 38: 1369–71.

Furnham, A. and Linfoot, J. (1987) 'The Type A behavior pattern and the need to prove oneself: a correlated study', *Current Psychological Reviews and Research* 6: 125–35.

Garber, J. and Seligman, M.E.P. (eds) (1980) *Human Helplessness: Theory and Applications*, New York: Academic Press.

Garmezy, N. and Rutter, M. (1983) *Stress, Coping and Development in Children*, New York: McGraw Hill.

Garrity, T.F. (1981) 'Behavioural adjustment after myocardial infarction: a selective review of recent descriptive, correlational and intervention research', in S.M. Weiss, J.A. Herd and B.M. Fox (eds) *Perspectives on Behavioural Medicine*, New York: Academic Press.

Gastaut, H. (1981) 'The effect of benzodiazepines on chronic epilepsy in man: with particular reference to clobazam', *Royal Society of Medicine International Symposium Series* 43: 141–50.

Gatchel, R., Korman, M., Weiss, C., Smith, D. and Clarke, L. (1978) 'A multiple response evaluation of EMG biofeedback performance during training and stress-induction conditions', *Psychophysiology* 15: 253–8.

Gay, N. (1984) In J-Ph. Assal, M. Berger, N. Gay, and J. Canivet, (eds) *Diabetes Education: How to Improve Patient Education*, Amsterdam: Excerpta Medica, Elsevier.

Geersten, H.R., Gray, R.M. and Ward, J.R. (1973) 'Patient non-compliance within the context of seeking medical care for arthritis', *Journal of Chronic Diseases* 26: 689–98.

Gentry, W., Foster, S. and Haney, T. (1972) 'Denial as a determinant of anxiety and perceived health status in the coronary care unit', *Psychosomatic Medicine* 34: 39–45.

Gentry, W.D., Chesney, A.P., Hall, R.P. and Harburg, E. (1981) 'Effect of habitual anger-coping pattern on blood pressure in black/white, high/low stress area respondents', *Psychosomatic Medicine* 43: 88–93.

Ghodsian, M., Zajicek, E. and Wolkind, S. (1984) 'A longitudinal study of maternal depression and child behaviour problems', *Journal of Child Psychology and Psychiatry* 25: 91–109.

Ghoneim, M.M., Mewaldt, S.P., Berie, J.L. and Himruchs, J.V. (1981) 'Memory and performance effects of single and 3-week administration of diazepam', *Psychopharmacology* 73: 147–51.

Gibbs, S., Waters, W.E. and George, C.F. (1989) 'The benefits of prescription leaflets', *British Journal of Clinical Pharmacology* 28: 345–51.

Gil, K.M., Keefe, F.J., Sampson, H.A., McCaskill, C.C., Rodin, J. and Crisson, J.E. (1987) 'The relation of stress and family environment to atopic dermatitis symptoms in children', *Journal of Psychosomatic Research* 31: 673–84.

Gilbert, B.D., Johnson, S.B., Silverstein, J.H. and Malone, J. (1987) 'Psychological and physiological responses to acute laboratory stressors in IDDM adolescents and non-diabetic controls', unpublished manuscript, Department of Psychiatry, University of Florida, Gainesville.

Gilbert, R.M. (1981) 'Caffeine: overview and anthology', in S.A. Miller (ed.) *Nutrition and Behaviour*, Philadelphia: Franklin Press.

Gillespie, C.R. and Bradley, C. (1988) 'Causal attributions of doctor and patients in a diabetic clinic', *British Journal of Clinical Psychology* 27: 67–76.

Giurgea, C. (1976) 'Piracetam: nootropic pharmacology of neurointegrative activity', in W.B. Essman and L. Valzelli (eds) *Current Developments in Psychopharmacology*, New York: Spectrum.

Glasgow, M.S., Engel, B.T. and D'Lugoff (1989) 'A controlled study of a standardized behavioral stepped treatment for hypertension', *Psychosomatic Medicine* 51: 10–26.

Glasgow, R.E., McCaul, K.D. and Schafer, L.C. (1987) 'Self-care behaviors and glycaemic control in type 1 diabetes', *Journal of Chronic Disorders* 40: 399–412.

Glass, D.C. (1977) *Behavior Patterns, Stress and Coronary Disease*, Hillsdale, NJ: Erlbaum.

Glover, E.D., Schroeder, K.L., Henningfield, J.E., Severson, H.H. and Christen, A.G. (1989) 'An interpretive review of smokeless tobacco research in the United States', *Journal of Drug Education* 19: 1–19.

Goffman, E. (1961) *Asylums*, Garden City, NY: Doubleday.

Goldsmith, S., Gabrielson, M., Gabrielson, I. Matthews, V. and Potts, L. (1972) 'Teenagers, sex and contraception', *Family Planning Perspectives* 4: 32–8.

Goldstein, I.B., Shapiro, D., Thananopavarn, C. and Sambhi, M.P. (1982) 'Comparison of drug and behavioral treatments of essential hypertension', *Health Psychology* 1: 7–26.

Goldstein, K., Kaiser, S. and Warren (1969) 'Psychotropic effects of caffeine in man, IV: Quantitative and qualitative differences associated with habituation', *Clinical Pharmacology and Therapeutics* 10: 489–97.

Golombok, S., Sketchley, J. and Rust, J. (1989) 'Condom use among homosexual men', *AIDS Care* 1: 27–33.

Goodman, L.S. and Gilman, A. (1985) *The Pharmacological Basis of Therapeutics*, New York: Macmillan.

Gordon, D., Burge, D., Hammen, C., Adrian, C., Jaenicke, C. and Hiroto, D. (1988) 'Observations of interactions of depressed women with their children', unpublished manuscript, Department of Psychology, University of California.

Gould-Martin, K., Paganini-Hill, A., Casagrande, C., Mack, T. and Ross, R.K. (1982)

'Behavioural and biological determinants of surgical stage of breast cancer', *Preventive Medicine* 11: 429–40.

Graber, A.O., Christman, B.D., Alogna, M.T. and Davidson, J.K. (1977) 'Evaluation of diabetic patient-education programmes', *Diabetes* 26: 61–4.

Graham, D.M. (1978) 'Caffeine – its identity, dietary sources, intake, and biological effects', *Nutritional Review* 36: 97–102.

Graham, P., Rutter, M., Yule, W. and Pless, I. (1967) 'Childhood asthma: a psychosomatic disorder? Clinical and epidemiological considerations', *British Journal of Preventive Social Medicine* 21: 78–85.

Greden, J.F. (1974) 'Anxiety or caffeinism: a diagnostic dilemma', *American Journal of Psychiatry* 131: 1089–92.

Green, E.E., Green, A.N. and Norris, P.A. (1979) 'Preliminary observations on the new non-drug method for control of hypertension', *Journal of the South Carolina Medical Association* 75: 575–86.

Green, L.W. (1970) 'Status identity and preventative health behaviour', *Pacific Health Education Reports* #1: 130.

Green, M. (1983) 'Coming of age in developmental pediatrics', *Pediatrics* 72: 275–82.

Green, M. (1986) 'Developmental psychobiologic implications for pediatrics', in N.A. Krasnegor, J.D. Arasteh and M.F. Cataldo (eds) *Child Health Behavior. A Behavioral Pediatrics Perspective*, New York: John Wiley and Sons.

Greenshaw, A.J., Sanger, D.J. and Blackman, D.E. (1984) 'Introduction to psychopharmacology and basic neuropharmacology', in D.J. Sanger and D.E. Blackman (eds) *Aspects of Psychopharmacology*, London: Methuen.

Greenstadt, L., Shapiro D.A. and Whitehead, R. (1986) 'Blood pressure discrimination', *Psychophysiology* 23: 500–9.

Greer, H.S. and Morris, T. (1975) 'Psychological attributes of women who develop breast cancer: a controlled study', *Journal of Psychosomatic Research* 19: 147–53.

Greer, H.S., Morris, T. and Pettingale, K.W. (1979) 'Psychological response to breast cancer: effect on outcome', *Lancet* ii: 785–7.

Greer, H.S., Lal, S., Lewis, S.C., Belsey, E.M. and Beard, R.W. (1976) 'Psychosocial consequences of therapeutic abortion. Kings Termination Study III', *British Journal of Psychiatry* 128: 74–9.

Griffiths, R.R. and Woodson, P.P. (1988) 'Caffeine physical dependence: a review of human and laboratory aniumal studies', *Psychopharmacology* 94: 437–51.

Guidubaldi, J. and Cleminshaw, H.K. (1985) 'Divorce, family health and child adjustment', *Family Relations* 34: 35–41.

Guyton, A.C. (1976) *Textbook of Medical Physiology*, 5th edition, Philadelphia, Penn.: Saunders.

Guyton, A.C. (1977) 'Personal views on mechanisms of hypertension', in J. Genest, E. Koiw and O. Kuchel (eds) *Hypertension: Physiopathology and Treatment*, New York; McGraw-Hill.

Guyton, A.C., Coleman, T.G., Bower, J.D. and Grainger, H.J. (1970) 'Circulatory control in hypertension', *Circulation Research* 27 (Suppl. II): 135–47.

Hackett, T.P. and Cassem, N.H. (1975) 'Psychological intervention in myocardial infarction', in W. Gentry and R. Williams (eds) *Psychological Aspects of Myocardial Infarction and Coronary Care*, St Louis: Mosby.

Hadlow, J. and Pitts, M.K. (1990) 'The understanding of common health terms by doctors, nurses and patients', *Social Science and Medicine* (in press).

Hall, R.G., Sachs, D.P.L., Hall, S.M. and Benowitz, N.L. (1984) 'Two year efficacy and safety of rapid smoking therapy in patients with cardiac and pulmonary disease', *Journal of Consulting and Clinical Psychology* 52: 574–81.

Hallal, J.C. (1982) 'The relationship between health beliefs, health locus of control and self concept on the practice of breast self examination in adult women', *Nursing Research* 31:137–42.

Hamburg, G.A. and Inoff, G.E. (1982) 'Relationships between behavioral factors and diabetic control in children and adolescents. A camp study', *Psychosomatic Medicine* 44: 321–39.

Hamill, E. and Ingram, I.M. (1974) 'Psychiatric factors in the abortion decision', *British Medical Journal* i: 229–32.

Hammen, C.L., Adrian, C., Gordon, D., Burge, D., Jaenicke, C. and Hiroto, D. (1987) 'Children of depressed mothers: maternal strain and symptom predictors of dysfunction', *Journal of Abnormal Psychology* 96: 190–8.

Hannay, D.R. (1980) 'The "iceberg" of illness and "trivial" consultations', *Journal of the Royal College of General Practitioners* 30: 551–4

Hanson, H.M., Ivester, C.A. and Morton, B.R. (1979) 'Nicotine self-administration in rats', *National Institute of Drug Research Monograph* 23: 70–89.

Hansteen, R.W., Miller, R.D., Lonero, L., Reid, L.D. and Jones, B. (1976) 'Effects of alcohol and cannabis on closed course car driving', *Annals of the New York Academy of Science* 282: 240–6.

Harburg, E., Blakelock, E.H. and Roper, P.J. (1979) 'Resentful and reflective coping with arbitrary authority and blood pressure: Detroit', *Psychosomatic Medicine* 41: 189–202.

Harris, D.M. and Guten, S. (1979) 'Health protective behaviour: an exploratory study', *Journal of Health and Social Behavior* 20: 17–29.

Harris, R. and Linn, M.W. (1985) 'Health beliefs, compliance, and control of diabetes mellitus', *Southern Medical Journal* 78: 162–6.

Hart, J.T. (1987) *Hypertension. Community Control of High Blood Pressure*, 2nd edition, Edinburgh: Churchill Livingstone.

Hassett, J. (1978) *A Primer of Psychophysiology*, New York: W.H. Freeman and Co.

Hathaway, D. (1986) 'Effect of pre-operative intervention on post-operative outcomes: a meta-analysis', *Nursing Research* 35: 269–75.

Hauser, S.T., Jacobsen, A.M., Wertlieb, D., Weiss-Perry, B., Follansbee, D., Wolfsdorf, J.I., Herskowitz, R.D., Houlihan, T. and Rajapart, D.C. (1986) 'Children with recently diagnosed diabetes: interactions within their families', *Health Psychology* 5: 273–96.

Hawkes, C. (1974) 'Communicating with the patient – an example drawn from neurology', *British Journal of Medical Education* 8: 57–63.

Haynes, R.B. (1979) 'Strategies to improve compliance with referrals, appointments, and prescribed medical regimens', in R.B. Haynes, D.W.Taylor and D.L.Sackett (eds) *Compliance in Health Care*, Baltimore, Md.: Johns Hopkins University Press.

Haynes, R.B. (1987) 'Patient compliance, then and now. Guest Editorial', *Patient Education and Counseling* 10: 103–5.

Haynes, R.B., Taylor, D.W. and Sackett, D.L. (1979) *Compliance in Health Care*, Baltimore, Md.: Johns Hopkins University Press.

Haynes, R.B., Taylor, D.W., Sackett, D.L., Gibson, E.S., Bernholz, C.D. and Mukherjee, J. (1980) 'Can simple clinical measurements direct non-compliance?', *Hypertension* 2: 757–64.

Haynes, S.G., Feinleib, M. and Kannel, W.B. (1980) 'The relationship of psychosocial factors to coronary heart disease in the Framingham study III. Eight year incidence of coronary heart disease', *American Journal of Epidemiology* 111: 37–58.

Health and Public Policy Committee, American College of Physicians (1985) 'Biofeedback for neuromuscular disorders', *Annals of Internal Medicine* 102: 854–8.

Heather, N. (1989) 'Psychology and brief interventions', *British Journal of Addiction* 84: 357–70.

Heather, N. and Robertson, I. (1981) *Controlled Drinking*, London: Methuen.

Heinicke, C.M., Diskin, S.D., Ramsey-Klee, D.M. and Given, K. (1983) 'Pre-birth characteristics and family development in the first year of life', *Child Development* 54: 194–208.

Henley, S. and Furnham, A. (1989) 'The Type A behaviour pattern and self-evaluation', *British Journal of Medical Psychology* 62: 51–9.

Henry, J.P. and Stephens, P.M. (1977) *Stress, Health and the Social Environment*, New York: Springer-Verlag.

Herbert, M. (1987) 'The duration of post-anaesthetic mental impairment', in I. Hindmarch, J.G. Jones and E. Moss (eds) *Aspects of Recovery from Anaesthesia*, Chichester: Wiley.

Hermann, F. (1973) 'The outpatient prescription label as a source of medication errors', *American Journal of Hospital Pharmacy* 30: 155–9.

Herold, E.S. (1981) 'Contraceptive embarrassment and contraceptive behaviour among young single women', *Journal of Youth and Adolescence* 10: 233–43.

Herold, E.S. (1983) 'The Health Belief Model: Can it help us to understand contraceptive use amongst adolescents?', *Journal of School Health* 53: 19–21.

Hersh, E.M. and Petersen, E.A. (1988) 'Editorial. The AIDS epidemic: AIDS research in the life sciences', *Life Sciences* 42: i-iv.

Hettinger, T. (1985) 'Statistics on diseases in the Federal Republic of Germany with particular reference to diseases of the skeletal system', *Ergonomics* 28: 17–20.

Heyden, S., Tyroler, H.A., Heiss, G., Hames, C.G. and Bartel, A. (1978) 'Coffee consumption and mortality', *Archives of Internal Medicine* 138: 1472–5.

Hill, J. (1937) 'Benzedrine in seasickness', *British Medical Journal* ii: 1109–12.

Hindmarch, I. (1985) 'The psychopharmacology of clobazam', *Royal Society of Medicine International Symposium Series* 74: 3–10.

Hindmarch, I. and Parrott, A.C. (1978) 'A repeated dose comparison of the side effects of five antihistamines', *Arzneimittel-Forschung (Drug Research)* 28: 483–6.

Hindmarch, I., Parrott, A.C. and Lanza, M. (1980) 'The effects of an ergot alkaloid derivative (Hydergine) on aspects of psychomotor performance, arousal and cognitive processing ability', *Journal of Clinical Pharmacology* 19: 726–32.

Hinkle, L.E. and Wolf, S. (1952) 'A summary of experimental evidence relating life-stress to diabetes mellitus', *Journal of Mount Sinai Hospital* 19: 537–46.

Hirayama, T. (1981) 'Non smoking wives of heavy smokers have a higher risk of lung cancer: a study from Japan', *British Medical Journal* 282: 183–5.

Hiss, R., Hess, G., and Lockwood, D. (1983) 'Differences in diabetic care practices of younger vs. older physicians', *Diabetes* 32: A119.

Hoare, P. (1987) 'Children with epilepsy and their families', *Journal of Child Psychology and Psychiatry* 28: 651–6.

Hobbs, P., Haran, D., Pendleton, L.L., Jones, B.E. and Posner, T. (1984) 'Public attitudes and cancer education', *International Review of Applied Psychology* 33: 565–86.

Hochstadt, N.J. and Trybula, J. (1980) 'Reducing missed appointments in a community health centre', *Journal of Community Psychology* 8: 261–5.

Hoelscher, T.J., Lichstein, K.L., Fischer, S. and Hegarty, T.B. (1987) 'Relaxation treatment of hypertension: do home relaxation tapes enhance treatment outcome?', *Behavior Therapy* 18: 33–7.

Hohmann, G.W. (1966) 'Some effects of spinal cord lesions on experienced emotional feelings', *Psychophysiology* 3: 143–56.

Holmes, T.H. and Rahe, R.H. (1967) 'The social readjustment rating scale', *Journal of Psychosomatic Research* 11: 213–18.

Honkanen, R., Ertama, L., Kuosmanen, P., Linnoila, M., Ahla, A. and Visuri, T. (1983) 'The role of alcohol in accidental falls', *Journal of Studies on Alcohol* 44: 231–45.

Horn, S. (1974) 'Some psychological factors in parkinsonism', *Journal of Neurology, Neurosurgery and Psychiatry* 37: 27–31.

Horwood, L.J., Fergusson, D.M. and Shannon, F.T. (1985) 'Social and familial factors in the development of early childhood asthma', *Pediatrics* 75: 859–68.

Houston, K.B. (1983) 'Psychophysiological responsivity and the Type A behavior pattern', *Journal of Research in Personality* 17: 22–39.

Hubley, J.H. (1988) 'AIDS in Africa: a challenge to health education', *Health Education Research* 3: 41–7.

Hulka, B.S., Kupper, L.L., Cassel, J.C. and Mayo, F. (1975) 'Doctor-patient communication and outcomes among diabetic patients', *Journal of Community Health* 1: 15–27.

Hunt, S.M. and Macleod, M. (1987) 'Health and behavioural change: some lay perspectives', *Community Medicine* 9: 68–76.

Hurlock, E.B. (1980) *Developmental Psychology. A Life-Span Approach*, New York: McGraw-Hill.

Ingham, J.G. and Miller, P. McC. (1986) 'Self referral to primary care: symptoms and social factors', *Journal of Psychosomatic Research* 30: 49–56.

Ingham, R. (1988) 'Behaviour change and safe sex: a social psychology approach', *Proceedings of the First Conference of the Health Psychology Section*, Leicester: British Psychological Society.

Irvine, M.J., Johnston, D.W., Jenner, D.A. and Marie, G.V. (1986) 'Relaxation and stress management in the treatment of essential hypertension', *Journal of Psychosomatic Research* 30: 437–50.

Isen, A.M., Shalker T.E., Clark M. and Karp L. (1978) 'Affect, accessibility of material in memory, and behaviour: a cognitive loop?', *Journal of Personality and Social Psychology* 36: 1–12.

Jaccard, J.J and Davidson, A.R. (1972) 'Towards an understanding of family planning behaviors: an initial investigation', *Journal of Applied Social Psychology* 2: 228–35.

Jacob, T. (1975) 'Family interaction in disturbed and normal families: a methodological and substantive review', *Psychological Bulletin* 82: 33–65.

Jacob, T., Favorini, A., Meisel, S. and Anderson, C. (1978) 'The alcoholic's spouse, children and family interactions: substantive findings and methodological issues', *Journal of Studies in Alcohol* 39: 1231–51.

Jahanshahi, M. and Marsden, C.D. (1989) 'Motor disorders', in G. Turpin (ed.) *Handbook of Clinical Psychophysiology*, Chichester: Wiley.

Jamrozic, K., Fowler, G., Vessey, G. and Wald, N. (1984) 'Placebo controlled trial of nicotine chewing gum in general practice', *British Medical Journal* 289: 794–7.

Janis, I.L. (1958) *Psychological Stress – Psychoanalytic and Behavioural Studies of Surgical Patients*, New York: John Wiley.

Janis, I.L. (1969) *Stress and Frustration*, New York: Harcourt Brace and Jovanovich.

Janz, N.K. and Becker, M.H. (1984) 'The health belief model: a decade later', *Health Education Quarterly* 11: 1–47.

Jarvis, M.J., Raw, M., Russell, M.A.H. and Feyerabend, C. (1982) 'Randomised controlled trial of nicotine chewing gum', *British Medical Journal* 285: 537–40.

Jarvis, M.J., Hajek, P., Russell, M.A.H., West, R.J. and Feyerabend, C. (1986) 'Nasal nicotine solution as an aid to cigarette withdrawal: a pilot clinical trial', *British Journal of Addiction* 82: 983–8.

Jemmott, J.B. and Magloire, K. (1988) 'Academic stress, social support and secretory immunoglobulin A', *Journal of Personality and Social Psychology* 55: 803–10.

Jenkins, C.D. (1971) 'Psychologic and social precursors of coronary heart disease', *New England Journal of Medicine* 284: 244–55, 307–17.

Jenkins, C.D. (1976) 'Recent evidence supporting psychologic and social risk factors for coronary heart disease', *New England Journal of Medicine* 294: 987–94, 1033–8.

Jennings, G., Nelson, L., Nestel, P., Esler, M., Korner, P., Burton, D. and Bazem, M. (1986) 'The effects of changes in physical activity on major cardiovascular risk factors, haemodynamics, sympathetic function and glucose utilisation in man: a controlled study of four levels of activity', *Circulation* 73: 30–40.

Jick, H., Miettenen, O.S., Neff, R.K., Shapiro, S., Heinonen, O.P. and Slone, D. (1973) 'Coffee and myocardial infarction', *New England Journal of Medicine* 289: 63–7.

Johnson, J.E. and Leventhal, H. (1974) 'Effects of accurate expectations and behavioural instructions on reactions during a noxious medical examination', *Journal of Personality and Social Psychology* 29: 710–18.

Johnson, J.E., Leventhal, H. and Dabbs, J.M. (1971) 'Contribution of emotional and instrumental response processes in adaptation to surgery', *Journal of Personality and Social Psychology* 20: 55–64.

Johnson, J.E., Rice, V.H., Fuller, S.S. and Endress, M.P. (1978) 'Sensory information, instruction in coping strategy and recovery from surgery', *Research in Nursing and Health* 1: 4–17.

Johnson, S.B. (1984) 'Knowledge, attitudes and behavior: correlates of health in childhood diabetes', *Clinical Psychology Review* 4: 503–24.

Johnsson, A. and Hansen, L. (1977) 'Prolonged exposure to a stressful stimulus (noise) as a cause of raised blood pressure in man', *Lancet* 1: 86–7.

Johnston, D.W. (1984) 'Biofeedback, relaxation and related procedures in the treatment of psychophysiological disorders', in A. Steptoe and A. Mathews (eds) *Health Care and Human Behaviour*, London: Academic Press.

Johnston, D.W. (1987) 'The behavioural control of high blood pressure', *Current Psychological Research and Reviews* 6: 99–114.

Johnston, D.W. (1989) 'Will stress management prevent coronary heart disease?', *The Psychologist: Bulletin of the British Psychological Society* 2: 275–8.

Johnston, L.M. (1942) 'Tobacco smoking and nicotine', *Lancet* ii: 742.

Johnston, M. (1980) 'Anxiety in surgical patients', *Psychological Medicine* 10: 145–52.

Johnston, M. (1982) 'Recognition of patients' worries by nurses and by other patients', *British Journal of Clinical Psychology* 21: 255–61.

Johnston, M. (1987) 'Emotional and cognitive aspects of anxiety in surgical patients', *Communication and Cognition* 20: 261–76.

Johnston, M. (1988) 'Health psychology: an integrated discipline?', *Health Psychology Update* 1 (Newsletter of the Health Section of the British Psychological Society).

Johnston, M. and Carpenter, L. (1980) 'Relationship between pre-operative anxiety and post-operative state', *Psychological Medicine* 10: 361–7.

Jones, D.R., Goldblatt, P.O. and Leon, D.A. (1984) 'Bereavement and cancer: some data on deaths of spouses from the longitudinal study of office of population censuses and surveys', *British Medical Journal* 3: 461–4.

Joyce, E.M. (1987) 'The neurochemistry of Korsakoff's syndrome', in S.M. Stahl and S.D. Iversen (eds) *Cognitive Neurochemistry*, Oxford: Oxford University Press.

Julien, R.M. (1985) *A Primer of Drug Action*, 4th edition, New York: Freeman.

Justice, A. (1985) 'Review of the effects of stress on cancer in laboratory animals', *Psychological Bulletin* 98: 108–38.

Kane, J.M. and Lieberman, J.A. (1987) 'Maintenance therapy in schizophrenia', in H.Y. Meltzer (ed.) *Psychopharmacology. The Third Generation of Progress*, New York: Raven.

Kannel, W.B. and Schatzkin, A. (1983) 'Risk factor analysis', *Progress in Cardiovascular Diseases* 26: 309–32.

Kantner, J. and Zelnick, M. (1972) 'Sexual experiences of young unmarried women in the US', *Family Planning Perspectives* 4: 9–18.

Kaplan, N.M. (1982) *Clinical Hypertension*, 3rd edition, Baltimore: Williams & Wilkins.

Karacan, I., Thornby, J.A., Anch, M., Booth, G.H., Williams, R.L. and Sallis, P.J. (1976) 'Dose-related sleep disturbances induced by coffee and caffeine', *Clinical Pharmacology and Therapeutics* 20: 682–9.

Karmel, M. (1972) 'Total institutions and models of adaptation', *Journal of Clinical Psychology* 28: 574–6.

Kasl, S.V. and Cobb, S. (1966) 'Health behaviour and illness behaviour: I. Health and illness behaviour', *Archives of Environmental Health* 12: 246–66.

Katzman, R. (1986) 'Alzheimer's disease', *New England Journal of Medicine* 314: 964–73.

Keefe, F.J. (1975) 'Conditioning changes in differential skin temperature', *Perceptual and Motor Skills* 40: 283–8.

Keefe, F.J. (1982) 'Behavioural assessment and treatment of chronic pain: current status and future directions', *Journal of Consulting and Clinical Psychology* 50: 896–911.

Kegeles, S.M., Allen, N.E. and Irwin, C.E. (1988) 'Sexually active adolescents and condoms: changes over one year in knowledge, attitudes and use', *American Journal of Public Health* 78: 460–1.

Kellerman, J., Zeltzer, L., Ellenberg, L., Dash, J. and Rigler, D. (1980) 'Psychological effects of illness in adolescence. 1. Anxiety, self-esteem, and perception of control', *Journal of Pediatrics* 97: 126–31.

Kelley, A.J. (1979) 'A media role for public health compliance?' in R.B. Haynes, D.W. Taylor and D.L. Sackett (eds) *Compliance in Health Care*, Baltimore: Johns Hopkins University Press.

Kellmer Pringle, M. (1980) *A Fairer Future for Children*, London: Macmillan Press.

Kemeny, M.E., Cohen, F., Zegans, L.S. and Conant, M.A. (1989) 'Psychological and immunological predictors of genital herpes recurrence', *Psychosomatic Medicine* 51: 195–208.

Kemmer, F.W., Baar, H., Hardtman, F., Bisping, R., Steingrum, H.J. and Berger, M. (1984) 'Acute psychological stress does not disturb metabolic control in type 1 diabetic patients', *Diabetologia* 27: A295.

Kempner, W. (1948) 'Treatment of hypertensive vascular disease with rice diet', *American Journal of Medicine* 4: 545–77.

Kendrick, R. and Bayne, J.R.D. (1982) 'Compliance with prescribed medication by elderly patients', *Canadian Medical Association Journal* 127: 961–2.

Kenny, M. and Darragh, A. (1986) 'Central effects of caffeine in man', in S.D. Iversen (ed.) *Psychopharmacology: Recent Advances and Future Prospects*, Oxford: Oxford University Press.

Kent, G. (1985) 'Memory of dental pain', *Pain* 21: 187–94.

Kerns, R.D., Turk, D.C. and Rudy, T.E. (1985) 'The West Haven-Yale Multi-dimensional Pain Inventory (WHYMPI)', *Pain* 23: 345–56.

Kerr, W. and Thompson, M. (1972) 'Acceptance of disability of sudden onset in paraplegia', *International Journal of Paraplegia* 10: 94–102.

Kiecolt-Glaser, J.K. and Glaser, R. (1986) 'Psychological influences on immunity', *Psychosomatics* 27: 621–4.

Kiecolt-Glaser, J.K., Garner, W., Speicher, C., Penn, G.M. Holliday, J. and Glaser, R. (1984) 'Psychosocial modifiers of immunocompetence in medical students', *Psychosomatic Medicine* 46: 7–14.

Kiecolt-Glaser, J.K., Glaser, R., Williger, D., Stout, J., Messick, G., Sheppard, S., Ricker, D., Romisher, S.C., Briner, W. and Bonnel, G. (1985) 'Psychosocial enhancement of immunocompetence in a geriatric population', *Health Psychology* 4: 25–41.

Killen, J.D., Maccoby, N. and Taylor, C.B. (1984) 'Nicotine gum and self regulation therapy in smoking relapse prevention', *Behaviour Therapy* 15: 234–48.

Kirley, B. (1982) 'Behavioral and social antecedents of non-compliance with nutritional management of diabetes', unpublished doctoral dissertation, Washington University.

Kirscht, J.P., Kirscht, J.L. and Rosenstock, I.M. (1981) 'A test of interventions to increase adherence to hypertension regimens', *Health Education Quarterly* 8: 261–72.

Klesges, R.C., Cigrang, J. and Glasgow, R.E. (1987) 'Worksite smoking modification programs: a state of the art review and directions for future research', *Current Psychological Research and Reviews* 6: 26–56.

Knight, R.G., Godfrey, H.P.D. and Shelton, E.J. (1988) 'The psychological deficits associated with Parkinson's disease', *Clinical Psychology Review* 8: 391–410.

Kobasa, S.C., Maddi, S.R. and Kahn, S. (1982) 'Hardiness and health: a prospective study', *Journal of Personality and Social Psychology* 42: 168–77.

Kochanska, G., Radke-Yarrow, M., Kuczynski, L. and Friedman, S.L. (1987) 'Normal and affectively ill mothers' beliefs about their children', *American Journal of Orthopsychiatry* 57: 345–50.

Koenig, W., Ruther, E. and Filipiak, B. (1987) 'Psychotropic drug utilisation in a metropolitan population', *European Journal of Clinical Pharmacology* 32: 43–51.

Kohl, R.L. and Homick, J.L. (1983) 'Motion sickness: a modulatory role for the central cholinergic nervous system', *Neurosciences and Biobehavioural Reviews* 7: 73–85.

Koolhaas, J. and Bohus, B. (1989) 'Social control in relation to neuroendocrine and immunological responses', in A. Steptoe and A. Appels (eds) *Stress, Personal Control and Health*, Chichester: John Wiley and Sons.

Kornfeld, D.S., Zimberg, S. and Malm, J.R. (1965) 'Psychiatric complications of open heart surgery', *New England Journal of Medicine* 278: 273–87.

Korsch, B.M., Gozzi, E.K. and Francis, V. (1968) 'Gaps in doctor–patient communication', *Pediatrics* 42: 855–71.

Krantz, D.S. and Manuck, S.B. (1984) 'Acute psychophysiological reactivity and risk of cardiovascular disease: a review and methodological critique', *Psychological Bulletin* 96: 435–64.

Kristt, D.A. and Engel, B.T. (1975) 'Learned control of blood pressure in patients with high blood pressure', *Circulation* 51: 370–8.

Kuhn, R. (1970) 'The imipramine story', in F.J. Ayd and B. Blackwell (eds) *Discoveries in Biological Psychiatry*, Philadelphia: Lippincott.

Lader, M. (1983) 'Benzodiazepine withdrawal states', in M.R. Trimble (ed.) *Benzodiazepines Divided: A Multidisciplinary Review*, Chichester: Wiley.

Lader, M. (1989) 'The psychopharmacology of addiction: benzodiazepine tolerance and dependence', in M. Lader (ed.) *The Psychopharmacology of Addiction*, Oxford: Oxford University Press.

Laing, S.P., Greenhalgh, R.M. and Taylor, G.W. (1981) 'The prevalence of smoking in patients with peripheral arterial disease', in R.M. Greenhalgh (ed.) *Smoking and Arterial Disease*, London: Pitman.

Landis, T., Graves, R., Benson, D.F. and Hebben, N. (1982) 'Visual recognition through kinaesthetic medication', *Psychological Medicine* 12: 515–31.

Lando, H.A. (1981) 'Effect of preparation, experimenter contact, and a maintained reduction alternative, on a broad spectrum program for eliminating smoking', *Addictive Behaviours* 6: 123–33.

Landrey, M.J. and Smith, D.E. (1988) 'AIDS and chemical dependency: an overview', *Journal of Psychoactive Drugs* 20: 141–7.

Lane Committee (1974) *Report of the Committee on the Working of the Abortion Act*, 1, Cmnd. 5579, London: Her Majesty's Stationery Office.

Laragh, J.H. and Pecker, M.S. (1983) 'Dietary sodium and essential hypertension: some myths, hopes and truths', *Annals of Internal Medicine* 98: 735–43.

Larbi, E.B., Cooper, R.S. and Stamler, J. (1983) 'Alcohol and hypertension', *Archives of Internal Medicine* 143: 28–9.

Lask, B. (1975) 'Short-term psychiatric sequelae to therapeutic termination of pregnancy', *British Journal of Psychiatry* 128: 173–7.

Lasky, P.A. and Eichelberger, K.M. (1985) 'Health-related views and self-care behaviors of young children', *Family Relations* 34: 13–18.

Last, J. (1963) 'The iceberg: Completing the clinical picture in general practice', *Lancet* ii: 28–31.

Lavallee, Y.J., Lamontagne, Y., Pinard, G., Annable, L. and Tetreault, L. (1977) 'Effects of EMG feedback, diazepam and their combination on chronic anxiety', *Journal of Psychosomatic Research* 21: 65–71.

Lawes, C. (1986) *Health Education and Spinal Cord Injury*. Report to Health Education Research Council.

Lawson, N.C. (1976) 'Depression after spinal cord injury: a multi-measure longitudinal study', doctoral dissertation, University of Houston, Texas.

Lawson, N.C. (1978) 'Significant events in rehabilitation process: spinal cord patients' point of view', *Archives of Physical Medicine and Rehabilitation* 59: 573–9.

Lazarus, R.S. (1974) 'Psychological stress and coping in adaptation and illness', *International Journal of Psychiatry in Medicine* 5: 321–33.

Lazarus, R.S. and Folkman, S. (1984) *Stress, Appraisal and Coping*, New York: Springer.

Lee, K., Moller, L. and Hardt, F. (1979) 'Alcohol induced brain damage and liver damage in young males', *Lancet* ii: 759–61.

Lee, P.N. (1980) 'Correspondence: Smoking and mortality of male doctors', *British Medical Journal* 280: 562.

Lefebvre, M.F. (1981) 'Cognitive distortion and cognitive errors in depressed psychiatric and low back pain patients', *Journal of Consulting and Clinical Psychology* 49: 517–25.

Lefebvre, R.C. and Flora, J.A. (1988) 'Social marketing and public health intervention', *Health Education Quarterly*, 15: 299–315.

Leff, J., Kuipers, L., Berkowitz, R., Eberlein Vries, R. and Sturgeon, D. (1982) 'A controlled trial of social intervention in the families of schizophrenic patients', *British Journal of Psychiatry* 141: 121–34.

Leonard, B.E. (1989) 'Animal models in psychopharmacology', in I. Hindmarch and P.D. Stonier (eds) *Human Psychopharmacology: Measures and Methods, Vol.2*, Chichester: Wiley.

Lethem, J., Slade, P.D., Troup, J.D.G. and Bentley, G. (1983) 'Outline of a fear-avoidance model of exaggerated pain perception – I', *Behaviour Research and Therapy* 21: 401–8.

Leventhal, H. and Cameron, L. (1987) 'Behavioral theories and the problem of compliance', *Patient Education and Counseling* 10: 117–38.

Levesque, L. and Charlesbois, M. (1977) 'Anxiety, locus of control and the effect of pre-operative teaching on patients' physical and emotional state', *Nursing Papers* 8: 11–26.

Ley, P. (1972)' Complaints made by hospital staff and patients: a review of the literature', *Bulletin of the British Psychological Society* 25: 115–20.

Ley, P. (1988) *Communicating with Patients: Improving Communication, Satisfaction and Compliance*, London: Croom Helm.

Ley, P. and Spelman, M.S. (1965) 'Communications in an outpatient setting', *British Journal of Social and Clinical Psychology* 4: 114–16.

Ley, P. and Spelman, M.S. (1967) *Communicating with the Patient*, London: Staples Press.

Libow, J.A. and Schreier, M.D. (1986) 'Three forms of fictitious illness in children. When is it Munchausen by proxy?', *American Journal of Orthopsychiatry* 56: 602–11.

Lieberman, H.R., Wurtman, R.J., Emde, G.G., Roberts, C. and Coviella, I.L.G. (1987) 'The effects of low doses of caffeine on human performance and mood', *Psychopharmacology* 92: 308–12.

Liebeskind, J.C. and Paul, L.A. (1977) 'Psychological and physiological mechanisms of pain', *Annual Review of Psychology* 28: 41–60.

Light, K.C. and Obrist, P.A. (1983) 'Task difficulty, heart rate reactivity and cardiovascular response to an appetitive reaction time task', *Psychophysiology* 20: 301–12.

Linn, B.S., Linn, M.W. and Klimas, N.G. (1988) 'Effects of psychophysical stress on surgical outcome', *Psychosomatic Medicine* 50: 230–44.

Linton, S.J. (1982) 'A critical review of behavioural treatments for chronic benign pain other than headache', *British Journal of Clinical Psychology* 21: 321–37.

Linton, S.J. (1985) 'The relationship between activity and chronic back pain', *Pain* 21: 289–94.

Locker, D. (1981) *Symptoms and Illness: The Cognitive Organization of Disorder*, London: Tavistock Publications.

Loke, W.H., Hinrichs, J.V. and Ghoneim, M.M. (1985) 'Caffeine and diazepam: separate and combined effects upon mood, memory, and psychomotor performance', *Psychopharmacology* 87: 344–50.

Lowe, G. (1984) 'Alcohol and alcoholism', in D.J. Sanger and D.E. Blackman (eds) *Aspects of Psychopharmacology*, London: Methuen.

Lowe, J. and Carroll, D. (1985) 'The effects of spinal cord injury on the intensity of emotional expression', *British Journal of Clinical Psychology* 24: 135–6.

Lowe, R. and McGrath, J.E. (1971) *Stress, Arousal, and Performance: Some Findings Calling for a New Theory*, Project Report AF 1161–7 AFOSR.

Lowery, D.J. and DuCette, J.P. (1976) 'Disease-related learning and disease control in diabetics as a function of locus of control', *Nursing Research* 25: 358–62.

Lucki, I., Rickels, K. and Geller, A.M. (1986) 'Chronic use of benzodiazepines and psychomotor and cognitive test performance', *Psychopharmacology* 88: 426–33.

Luker, K. (1975) *Taking Chances: Abortion and the Decision not to Contracept*, Berkeley: University of California Press.

Luker, K. (1977) 'Contraceptive risk-taking and abortion: results and implications of a San Francisco Bay study', *Studies in Family Planning* 8: 190–6.

Lukomskya, N.A. and Nikolskay, M.I. (1974) *Search for Drugs against Motion Sickness*, Leningrad: Sechenov Institute. English translation from the Civil Institute of Environmental Medicine, Ontario, Canada.

McAnarney, E.R., Lawrence, R.A., Ricciuti, H.N., Polley, J. and Szilagyi, M. (1986) 'Interactions of adolescent mothers and their 1-year-old children', *Pediatrics* 78: 585–90.

Maccoby, E.E. and Martin, J.A. (1983) 'Socialisation in the context of the family: parent–child interaction', in P.H. Mussen (ed.) *Handbook of Child Psychology, Volume IV*, New York: John Wiley and Sons.

McConachie, H. (1982) 'Fathers of mentally handicapped children', in N. Beail and J.McGuire (eds) *Fathers. Psychological Perspectives*, London: Junction Books.

McCusker, J. and Morrow, G.R. (1977) 'The relationship of health locus of control to preventive health behaviours and health beliefs', *Patient Counseling and Health Education* 1: 146–50.

McDonald, R.J. (1982) 'Drug treatment of senile dementia', in D. Wheatley (ed.) *Psychopharmacology of Old Age*, Oxford: Oxford University Press.

McDonnell, R. and Maynard, A. (1985) 'The costs of alcohol misuse', *British Journal of Addiction* 80: 27–36.

Machover, S. (1957) 'Rorschach study on the nature and origin of common factors in the personalities of parkinsonians', *Psychosomatic Medicine* 19: 332–8.

McGrath, J.E. (1976) 'Stress and behaviour in organisations', in M.D. Dunnette (ed.) *Handbook of Industrial and Organisational Psychology*, Chicago: Rand McNally College Publishing Co.

McIntyre-Kingsolver, K., Lichtenstein, E. and Mermelstein, R.J. (1986) 'Self efficacy and relapse in smoking cessation', *Journal of Consulting and Clinical Therapy* 51: 632–3.

Mackay, C.J., Cox, T., Burrows, C.G. and Lazzerini, A.J. (1978) 'An inventory for the measurement of self-reported stress and arousal', *British Journal of Social and Clinical Psychology* 17: 283–4.

McKenzie, R.E. and Elliott, L.L. (1965) 'Effects of secobarbital and d-amphetamine on performance during a simulated air mission', *Aerospace Medicine* 36: 774–9.

McNeil, B.J., Pauker, S.G., Sox, H.C. and Tversky, A. (1982) 'On the elicitation of preferences for alternative therapies', *New England Journal of Medicine* 306: 1259–62.

Maeland, J.G. and Havik, O.E. (1987) 'Psychological predictors for return to work after a myocardial infarction', *Journal of Psychosomatic Research* 31: 471–81.

Mair Report (1972) *Medical Rehabilitation: The Pattern for the Future.* Report for a sub committee of the Standing Medical Advisory Committee, Scottish Home and Health Department, London: Her Majesty's Stationery Office.

Malec, J. and Neimeyer, R. (1983) 'Psychologic prediction of duration of inpatient spinal cord injury rehabilitation and performance of self-care', *Archives of Physical Medicine and Rehabilitation* 64: 359–63.

Mander, A.J., Norton, B. and Hoare, P. (1987) 'The effect of maternal psychotic illness on a child', *British Journal of Psychiatry* 151: 848–50.

Mangan, G.L. and Golding, J.F. (1984) *The Psychopharmacology of Smoking*, Cambridge: Cambridge University Press.

Mann, A.H. (1977) 'Psychiatric morbidity and hostility in hypertension', *Psychological Medicine* 7: 653–9.

Mann, A.H. (1986) 'The psychological aspects of essential hypertension', *Journal of Psychosomatic Research* 30: 527–41.

Mann, A.H. and Brennan, P.J. (1987) 'Type A behavior score and the incidence of cardiovascular disease: a failure to replicate the claimed associations', *Journal of Psychosomatic Research* 31: 685–92.

Manuck, S.B. and Proietti, J.M. (1982) 'Parental hypertension and cardiovascular response to cognitive and isometric challenge', *Psychophysiology* 19: 481–9.

Markova, I. and Wilkie, P. (1987) 'Representations, concepts and social change: the phenomenon of AIDS', *Journal for the Theory of Social Behaviour* 17: 389–409.

Marks, J. (1978) *The Benzodiazepines: Use, Overuse, Misuse, Abuse,* Lancaster: MTP Press.

Marlatt, G.A. and Gordon, J.R. (1980) 'Determinants of relapse: implications for the maintenance of behavior change', in P.O. Davidson and S.M. Davidson (eds) *Behavioral Medicine: Changing Health Lifestyles,* New York: Brunner/Mazel.

Marmot, M.G. (1984) 'Geography of blood pressure and hypertension', *British Medical Bulletin* 40: 380–6.

Marmot, M.G., Rose, G., Shipley, M. and Hamilton, P.J.S. (1978) 'Employment grade and coronary heart disease in British civil servants', *Journal of Epidemiology and Community Health* 3: 244–9.

Marsh, G.G. and Markham, C.H. (1973) 'Does levodopa alter depression and psychopathology in parkinsonism patients?', *Journal of Neurology, Neurosurgery and Psychiatry* 36: 925–35.

Marteau, T.M. and Baum, J.D. (1984) 'Doctors' views of diabetes', *Archives of Diseases of Childhood* 59: 566–70.

Marteau, T.M. and Johnston, M. (1986) 'Determinants of beliefs about illness: a study of parents of children with diabetes, asthma and epilepsy and no chronic illness', *Journal of Psychosomatic Research* 30: 673–83.

Marteau, T.M. and Johnston, M. (1987) 'Health psychology: the danger of neglecting psychological models', *Bulletin of the British Psychological Society* 40: 82–5.

Marteau, T.M., Johnston, M., Baum, J.D. and Bloch, S. (1987) 'Goals of treatment in diabetes: a comparison of doctors and parents of children with diabetes', *Journal of Behavioral Medicine* 10: 33–48.

Martin, I. and Venables, P.H. (eds) (1980) *Techniques in Psychophysiology*, Chichester: John Wiley and Sons.

Masterson, J., Dunworth, R. and Williams, N. (1988) 'Extreme illness exaggeration in pediatric patients: a variant of Munchausen's by proxy?', *American Journal of Orthopsychiatry* 58: 188–95.

Matarazzo, J.D. (1980) 'Behavioral health and behavioral medicine. Frontiers for a new health psychology', *American Scientist* 35: 807–17.

Matarazzo, J.D. (1983) 'Behavioural immunogens and pathogens in health and illness', in B.L. Hammonds and C.J. Scheirer (eds) *Psychology and Health*, The Master Lecture Series, Volume 3. Washington, DC: American Psychological Association.

Mathews, A. and Ridgeway, V. (1981) 'Personality and surgical recovery: a review', *British Journal of Clinical Psychology* 20: 243–60.

Mathews, A. and Ridgeway, V. (1984) 'Psychological preparation for surgery', in A. Steptoe and A. Mathews (eds) *Health Care and Human Behaviour*, London: Academic Press.

Matthews, K.A. (1982) 'Psychological perspectives on the Type A behavior pattern', *Psychological Bulletin* 91: 293–323.

Matthews, K.A. (1988) 'Coronary heart disease and Type A behaviors: update on and alternative to the Booth-Kewley and Friedman (1987) quantitative review', *Psychological Bulletin* 104: 373–80.

Matthews, K.A., Glass, D.C., Rosenman, R.H. and Bortner, R.W. (1977) 'Competitive drive, pattern A, and coronary heart disease: a further analysis of some data from the Western Collaborative Group Study', *Journal of Chronic Diseases* 30: 489–98.

Mattson, A. (1972) 'Long-term physical illness in childhood: a challenge to psychosocial adaptation', *Pediatrics* 50: 801–11.

May, B. (1988) 'Do diabetic children and their parents learn from each other?', *Diabetic Medicine* 5: 283–94.

May, R.A. (1968) 'Anti-psychotic drugs and other forms of therapy', in D.H. Efron (ed.) *Psychopharmacology: A Review of Progress*, Washington, DC: US Government Printing Office.

Mayall, B. (1986) *Keeping Children Healthy*, London: Allen & Unwin.

Mayes, B.T., Sime, W.E. and Ganster, D.C. (1984) 'Convergent validity of Type A behavior pattern scales and their ability to predict physiological responsiveness in a sample of female public employees', *Journal of Behavioural Medicine* 7: 83–108.

Meadow, R. (1977) 'Munchausen syndrome by proxy: the hinterland of child abuse', *Lancet* ii: 343–5.

Mechanic, D. (1978) *Medical Sociology*, 2nd edition, New York: Free Press.

Melamed, B.G. (1974) *Ethan has an Operation* (Film), Cleveland, O.: Case Western Reserve University, Health Sciences Communication Center.

Melamed, B.G. (1984) 'Health intervention: collaboration for health and science', in B.L. Hammonds and C.J. Scheier (eds) *Psychology and Health* Master Lecture Series, Volume 3. Washington, DC: American Psychological Association.

Melamed, B.G. (1988) 'Section overview: Current approaches to hospital preparation', in B.G Melamed, K.A. Matthews, D.K. Routh, B. Stabler and N. Schneiderman (eds) *Child Health Psychology*, Hillsdale, NJ: Lawrence Erlbaum Associates.

Melamed, B.G., Dearborn, M. and Hermecz, D.A. (1983) 'Necessary considerations for surgery preparation: age and previous experience', *Psychosomatic Medicine* 45: 517–25.

Melamed, B.G., Yurcheson, R., Fleece, L., Hutcherson, S. and Hawes, R. (1978) 'Effects of film modelling on the reduction of anxiety-related behaviours in individuals varying in level of previous experience in the stress situation', *Journal of Consulting and Clinical Psychology* 46: 1357–67.

Melton, G. (1988) 'Adolescents and prevention of AIDS', *Professional Psychology: Research and Practice* 19: 403–8.

Melzack, R. (1973) *The Puzzle of Pain*, New York: Basic Books

Melzack, R. (1975) 'The McGill Pain Questionnaire: major properties and scoring methods', *Pain* 1: 277–99.

Melzack, R. and Dennis, S.G. (1978) 'Neurophysiological foundations of pain', in R.A. Sternbach (ed.) *The Psychology of Pain*, New York: Raven Press.

Melzack, R. and Wall, P.D. (1965) 'Pain mechanisms: a new theory', *Science* 150: 971–9.

Meyer, D., Leventhal, H. and Guttman, M. (1985) 'Common-sense models of illness: the example of hypertension', *Health Psychology* 4: 115–35.

Miller, E. (1984) *Recovery and Management of Neuropsychological Impairments*, London: John Wiley and Sons.

Miller, N.E. (1969) 'Learning of visceral and glandular response', *Science* 153: 434–45.

Miller, N.E. and Dworkin, B.R. (1977) 'Critical issues in therapeutic applications of biofeedback', in G.E.Schwartz and J. Beatty (eds) *Biofeedback: Theory and Research*, New York: Academic Press.

Miller, S.M. (1979a) 'Coping with impending stress: psychophysiological and cognitive correlates of choice', *Psychophysiology* 16: 572–81.

Miller, S.M. (1979b) 'Controllability and human stress: method, evidence and theory', *Behavior Research and Therapy* 17: 287–304.

Miller, S.M. and Mangan, C.E. (1983) 'Interacting effects of information and coping style in adapting to gynecologic stress: should the doctor tell all?', *Journal of Personality and Social Psychology* 45: 223–36.

Miller, W.R. (1983) 'Controlled drinking: a history and a critical review', *Journal of Studies on Alcohol* 44: 68–83.

Mills, D.E. and Ward, R.P. (1986) 'Attenuation of stress-induced hypertension by exercise independent of training effects: an animal model', *Journal of Behavioral Medicine* 9: 599–605.

Mills, M., Puckering, C., Pound, A. and Cox, A. (1985) 'What is it about depressed mothers that influences their child's functioning?', in J.E. Stevenson (ed.) *Recent Research in Developmental Psychopathology*, Oxford: Pergamon Press.

Mills, S., Campbell, M.J. and Waters, W.E. (1986) 'Public knowledge of AIDS and the DHSS advertisement campaign', *British Medical Journal* 293: 1089–90.

Minuchin, S., Rosman, B.L. and Baker, E.R.L. (1978) *Psychosomatic Families*, Cambridge, Mass.: Harvard University Press.

Mirowsky, J. and Ross, C.E. (1983) 'Patient satisfaction and visiting the doctor: a self-regulating system', *Social Science and Medicine* 17: 1353–61.

Mischel, W. (1974) 'Processes in delay of gratification', in L. Berkowitz (ed.) *Advances in Experimental Social Psychology No. 7*, New York: Academic Press.

Moatti, J.P., Manesse, L., Le Gales, C., Pages, J.P. and Fagnani, F. (1988) 'Social perception of AIDS in the general public: a French study', *Health Policy* 9: 1–8.

Moffic, H.S. and Paykel, E.S. (1975) 'Depression in medical inpatients', *British Journal of Psychiatry* 126: 346–53.

Mok, J. (1988) 'Children born to women with HIV infection', *Royal Society of Medicine. The AIDS Letter* 7 (June/July): 1–2.

Montgomery, S.A. and Pinder, R.M. (1987) 'Do some antidepressants promote suicide?', *Psychopharmacology* 92: 265–6.

Morisky, D.E., Green, L.W. and Levine, D.M. (1986) 'Concurrent and predictive validity of a self-reported measure of medication adherence', *Medical Care* 24: 67–74.

Morrell, D.C. and Wade, C.J. (1976) 'Symptoms perceived and recorded by patients', *Journal of the Royal College of General Practitioners* 26: 398–403

Morris, J.B. and Beck, A.T. (1974) 'The efficacy of antidepressant drugs', *Archives of General Psychiatry* 30: 667–74.

Morrison, D.M. (1985) 'Adolescent contraceptive behavior: a review', *Psychological Bulletin* 98: 538–68.

Moss, E. and Hooper, M.B. (1987) 'Morbidity following day case surgery', in I. Hindmarch, J.G. Jones and E. Moss (eds) *Aspects of Recovery from Anaesthesia*, Chichester: Wiley.

Mrazek, D.A. (1986) 'Childhood asthma: two central questions for child psychiatry', *Journal of Child Psychology and Psychiatry* 27: 1–5.

Mrazek, D.A., Anderson, I. and Strunk, R. (1985) 'Disturbed emotional development of severely asthmatic pre-school children', in J.E. Stevenson (ed.) *Recent Research in Developmental Psychopathology*, Oxford: Pergamon Press.

MRC (Medical Research Council Working Party) (1981) 'Adverse reactions to benedrofluazide and propranolol for the treatment of mild hypertension', *Lancet* ii: 539–43.

MRC (Medical Research Council Working Party) (1985). 'MRC trial of treatment of mild hypertension: principal results', *British Medical Journal* 291: 97–104.

Mulleady, G. (1987) 'A review of drug abuse and HIV infection', *Psychology and Health* 1: 149–63.

Mulleady, G. and Sher, L. (1989) 'Lifestyle factors for drug users in relation to risks for HIV', *AIDS Care* 1: 45–50.

Mulleady, G., Phillips, K.C. and White, D.G. (1989) 'Issues in sexual counselling for HIV positive injecting drug users', paper presented to International Conference on Health Psychology, Cardiff.

Mumford, E. Schlesinger, H.J., and Glass, G.V. (1982) 'The effects of psychological intervention on recovery from surgery and heart attacks. An analysis of the literature', *American Journal of Health* 72: 141–51.

Mutch, W.J. and Dingwell-Fordyce, I. (1985) 'Is it a hypo? Knowledge of the symptoms of hypoglycaemia in elderly diabetic patients', *Diabetic Medicine* 2: 54–6.

Myers, M.G. (1987) 'Caffeine as a possible cause of ventricular arhythmias during the healing phase of acute myocardial infarction', *American Journal of Cardiology* 59: 1024–8.

Nabarro, J.D.N. (1988) 'Diabetes in the United Kingdom: some facts and figures', *Diabetic Medicine* 5: 816–22.

Najman, J.M., Klein, D. and Munro, C. (1982) 'Patient characteristics negatively stereotyped by doctors', *Social Science and Medicine* 16: 1781–9.

Newton, R.W. (1985) 'Social integration of the adolescent diabetic', *Practical Diabetes* 2: 25–8.

Nichols, S. (1983) 'The Southampton breast study – implications for nurses', *Nursing Times* 14 December 24–7.

Nicholson, A.N. (1985) 'Central effects of H1 and H2 antihistamines', *Aviation Space and Environmental Medicine* 56: 293–8.

NIMH (1964) 'Phenothiazone treatment in acute schizophrenia: National Institute of Mental Health psychopharmacology collaborative study', *Archives of General Psychiatry* 10: 246–61.

Norbeck, J.S., Lindsey, A.M. and Carrieri, V.L. (1981) 'The development of an instrument to measure social support', *Nursing Research* 30: 264–9.

NRC (1989) *National Research Council Report of the Committee on AIDS Research and the Behavioral, Social and Statistical Sciences*, Washington, DC.; National Academy Press.

Nyquist, R. and Bors, E. (1967) 'Mortality and survival in traumatic myelopathy during 19 years from 1946–1965', *International Journal of Paraplegia* 5: 22–48.

Obrist, P.A. (1981) *Cardiovascular Psychophysiology: A Perspective*, New York: Plenum Press.

Ogg, T.W. (1972) 'An assessment of post-operative outpatient cases', *British Medical Journal* 4: 573–6.

Ogg, T.W. (1987) 'An anaesthetist's view of day case surgery', in I. Hindmarch, J.G. Jones and E. Moss (eds) *Aspects of Recovery from Anaesthesia*, Chichester: Wiley.

O'Hanlon, J.F. (1988) 'Explaining the common effects of sedative drugs on driving using performance models', in I. Hindmarch, B. Aufdembrinke and Ott, H. (eds) *Psychopharmacology and Reaction Time*, Chichester: Wiley.

Ojehagen, A. and Berglund, M. (1989) 'Changes of drinking goals in a two year outpatient alcoholic treatment programme', *Addictive Behaviours* 14: 1–9.

OPCS (1986) *Office of Population Censuses and Surveys Abortion Statistics Series AB, 13*, London: Her Majesty's Stationery Office.

OPCS (1987) *Office of Population Censuses and Surveys Abortion Statistics Series AB, 14*, London: Her Majesty's Stationery Office.

OPCS (1989) *Office of Population Censuses and Surveys Monitor, PP2 89/1*, London: Her Majesty's Stationery Office.

Orenstein, D.M. and Wasserman, A.L. (1986) 'Munchausen syndrome by proxy simulating cystic fibrosis', *Pediatrics* 78: 621–4.

Orogozo, J.M. and Spiegel, R. (1987) 'Critical review of clinical trials in senile dementia', *Postgraduate Medical Journal* 63: 237–40, 337–43.

Owens, R.G. and Ashcroft, J.B. (1982) 'Functional analysis in applied psychology', *British Journal of Clinical Psychology* 21: 181–9.

Owens, R.G., Daly, J., Heron, K. and Leinster, S.J. (1987) 'Psychological and social characteristics of attenders for breast screening', *Psychology and Health* 1: 303–13.

Pacey, L. and Parrott, A.C. (unpublished) 'Coffee for 24 hours: effects upon alertness and headache in high and low caffeine users', submitted for publication.

Page, P., Verstraete, D.G., Robb, J.R. and Etzwiler, D.D. (1981) 'Patient recall of self-care recommendations in diabetes', *Diabetes Care* 4: 96–8.

Pagel, M.D. and Davidson, A.R. (1984) 'A comparison of three social-psychological models of attitude and behavioral plan: prediction of contraceptive behavior', *Journal of Personality and Social Psychology* 47: 517–33.

Parrish, J.M. (1986) 'Parent compliance with medical and behavioral recommendations', in N.A. Krasnegor, J.D. Arateh and M.F. Cataldo (eds) *Child Health Behavior. A Behavioral Pediatrics Perspective*, New York: John Wiley and Sons.

Parrott, A.C. (1985) 'Clobazam, personality, stress and performance', *Royal Society of Medicine International Symposium Series* 74: 47–58.

Parrott, A.C. (1986) 'The effects of transdermal scopolamime and four doses of oral scopolamine (0.15, 0.3, 0.6, 1.2mg) upon psychological performance', *Psychopharmacology* 89: 347–54.

Parrott, A.C. (1987) 'Assessment of psychological performance in applied situations', in I. Hindmarch and P.D. Stonier (eds) *Human Psychopharmacology Measures and Methods, Volume 1*, Chichester: Wiley.

Parrott, A.C. (1989) 'Transdermal scopolamine: a review of its effects upon motion sickness, psychological performance, and physiological functioning', *Aviation Space and Environmental Medicine* 60: 1–9.

Parrott, A.C. and Kentridge, R. (1982) 'Personal constructs of anxiety under the 1.5

benzodiazepine derivative clobazam related to trait anxiety levels of the personality', *Psychopharmacology* 78: 353–7.

Parrott, A.C. and Wesnes, K. (1987) 'Promethazine, scopolamine and cinnarizine: comparative time course of psychological performance effects', *Psychopharmacology* 92: 513–19.

Parrott, A.C. and Winder, G. (1989) 'Nicotine chewing gum (2mg, 4mg) and cigarette smoking: comparative effects upon vigilance and heart rate', *Psychopharmacology* 97: 257–61.

Parry, H.J., Balter, M.B., Mellinger, G.D., Cisin, I.H. and Manheimer, D.I. (1973) 'National patterns of psychotropic drug use', *Archives of General Psychiatry* 28: 769–83.

Patel, C. and North, W. (1975) 'Randomised controlled trial of yoga and biofeedback in the management of hypertension', *Lancet* ii: 93–5.

Patel, C., Marmot, M.G. and Terry, D.J. (1981) 'Controlled trial of biofeedback-aided behavioural methods in reducing mild hypertension', *British Medical Journal* 282: 2005–8.

Patel, C., Marmot, M.G., Terry, D.J., Carruthers, M., Hunt, B. and Patel, M. (1985) 'Trial of relaxation in reducing coronary risk: four year follow up', *British Medical Journal* 290: 1103–6.

Paul, G.L. (1969) 'Physiological effects of relaxation training and hypnotic suggestion', *Journal of Abnormal Psychology* 74: 425–37.

Paul, O., MacMillan, A., McKean, H. and Park, H. (1968) 'Sucrose intake and coronary heart disease', *Lancet* ii: 1049–51.

Paykel, E.S. (1974) 'Life stress and psychiatric disorder: applications of the clinical approach', in B.S. Dohrenwend and B.P. Dohrenwend (eds) *Stressful Life Events: Their Nature and Effects*, New York: Wiley.

Pearl, R. (1939) *Natural History of Population*, Oxford: Oxford University Press.

Peele, S. (1985) *The Meaning of Addiction*, Lexington, Mass.: D.C. Heath and Co.

Pennebaker, J.W. (1982) *The Psychology of Physical Symptoms*, New York: Springer.

Pennebaker, J.W. and Watson, D. (1988) 'Blood pressure estimation and beliefs among normotensives and hypertensives', *Health Psychology* 7: 309–28.

Perkins, K.A., Dubbert, P.M., Martin, J.E., Faulstich, M.E. and Harris, J.K. (1986) 'Cardiovascular reactivity to psychological stress in aerobically trained versus untrained mild hypertensives and normotensives', *Health Psychology* 5: 407–21.

Perlick, D., Stastny, P., Katz, I., Mayer, M. and Mattis, S. (1986) 'Memory deficits and anticholinergic levels in chronic schizophrenia', *American Journal of Psychiatry* 143: 230–2.

Peterson, J.L. and Bakeman, R. (1989) 'AIDS and iv drug use among ethnic minorities', *Journal of Drug Issues* 19: 27–37.

Pettingale, K.W., Philatithis, A., Tee, D.E.H. and Greer, H.S. (1981) 'The biological correlates of psychological response to breast cancer', *Journal of Psychosomatic Research* 25: 453–8.

Philips, H.C. (1987) 'The effects of behavioural treatment on chronic pain', *Behaviour Research and Therapy* 25: 365–77.

Philips, H.C. and Jahanshahi, M. (1986) 'The components of pain behaviour report', *Behaviour Research and Therapy* 24: 117–25.

Phillips, G.T., Gossop, M. and Bradley, B. (1986) 'The influence of psychosocial factors on the opiate withdrawal syndrome', *British Journal of Psychiatry* 149: 235–8.

Phillips, K.C. (1979) 'Biofeedback as an aid to autogenic training', in B.A. Stoll (ed.) *Mind and Cancer Prognosis*, Chichester: Wiley.

Phillips, K.C. (1987) 'Psychophysiology: a discipline in search of its paradigm?', *Journal of Psychophysiology* 1: 101–4.

Phillips, K.C. (1988) 'Strategies against AIDS', *The Psychologist: Bulletin of the British*

Psychological Society 1: 46–7.

Phillips, K.C. (1989a) 'Psychophysiological consequences of behavioural choice in aversive situations', in A. Steptoe and A. Appels (eds) *Stress, Personal Control and Health*, Chichester: John Wiley and Sons.

Phillips, K.C. (1989b) 'The psychology of AIDS', in A. Colman and J.G. Beaumont (eds) *Psychology Survey No. 7*, Leicester: British Psychological Society.

Pickering, T.G. and Gorham, G. (1975) 'Learned heart rate control by a patient with a ventricular parasystolic rhythm', *Lancet* ii: 252–3.

Pickering, T. G. and Miller, N.E. (1977) 'Learned voluntary control of heart rate and rhythm in two subjects with premature ventricular contractions', *British Heart Journal* 39: 152–9.

Pickett, C. and Clum, G.A. (1982) 'Comparative treatment strategies and their interaction with locus of control in the reduction of post-surgical pain and anxiety', *Journal of Consulting and Clinical Psychology* 50: 439–41.

Pinder, R.M. (1988) 'The benefits and risks of antidepressant drugs', *Human Psychopharmacology* 3: 73–86.

Piot, P., Plummer, F., Mhalu, F., Lamboray, J-L., Chin, J. and Mann, J.M. (1988) 'AIDS: an international perspective', *Science* 239: 573–9.

Pittner, M.S. and Houston, B.K. (1980) 'Response to stress, cognitive coping strategies and the Type A behavior pattern', *Journal of Personality and Social Psychology* 39: 147–57.

Pitts, M.K. and Jackson, H. (1989) 'AIDS and the press: an analysis of the coverage of AIDS by Zimbabwe newspapers', *AIDS Care* 1: 77–83.

Podboy, J.W. and Mallory, W.A. (1977) 'Caffeine reduction and behaviour change in the severely retarded', *Mental Retardation* 15: 40.

Pomerleau, O.F., Fertig, J.B., Streyler, L.E. and Jaffe, J. (1983) 'Neuroendocrine reactivity to nicotine in smokers', *Psychopharmacology* 81: 61–7.

Potkin, S.G., Shen, Y.C., Pardes, H., Zhou, D.F., Phelps, B., Shu, L., and Poland, R. (1984) 'Failure of insulin coma and presence of a therapeutic window for haloperidol in Chinese schizophrenics', *Collegium Internationale Neuro-Psychopharmacologicum, 14th Congress, Florence, Italy. Proceedings*, New York: Raven Press.

Potter, J.F. and Beevers, D.G. (1984) 'Pressor effects of alcohol in hypertension', Lancet i: 119–22.

Potter, R. (1963) 'Additional measures of use effectiveness', *Millbank Memorial Fund Quarterly* 41: 400.

Potts, M., Diggory P. and Peel, J. (1977) *Abortion*, Cambridge: Cambridge University Press.

Pound, A., Cox, A., Puckering, C. and Mills, M. (1985) 'The impact of maternal depression on young children', in J.E. Stevenson (ed.) *Recent Research in Developmental Psychopathology*, Oxford: Pergamon Press.

Pramming, S., Thorsteinsson, B., Theilgaard, A., Pinner, E.M. and Binder, C. (1986) 'Cognitive function during hypoglycaemia in type 1 diabetes mellitus', *British Medical Journal* 292: 647–50.

Pratt, L. (1973) 'Child-rearing methods and children's health behavior', *Journal of Health and Social Behavior* 14: 61–9.

Price, V. (1982) *Type A Behavior Pattern: A Model for Research and Practice*, New York: Academic Press.

Puente, A.E. and Beiman, I. (1980) 'The effects of behavior therapy, self-relaxation, and transcendental meditation on cardiovascular stress response', *Journal of Clinical Psychology* 36: 291–5.

Rachman, S. and Hodgson, R. (1974) 'Synchrony and desynchrony in fear and avoidance', *Behaviour Research and Therapy* 12: 311–18.

Radcliffe Richards, J. (1982) *The Sceptical Feminist*, Harmondsworth: Penguin.

Ragland, D.R. and Brand, R.J. (1988) 'Type A behavior and mortality from coronary heart disease', *New England Journal of Medicine* 318: 65–9.

Rahe, R.H. and Lind, E. (1971) 'Psychosocial factors and sudden cardiac death: a pilot study', *Journal of Psychosomatic Research* 15: 19–24.

Raskin, M., Johnson, G. and Rondestvedt, T. (1973) 'Chronic anxiety treated by feedback-induced muscle relaxation', *Archives of General Psychiatry* 28: 263–6.

Rasmussen, H. (1974) 'Organisation and control of endocrine systems', in R. H. Williams (ed.) *Textbook of Endocrinology* 5th edition. Philadelphia: Saunders.

Reading, A. (1983) *Psychological Aspects of Pregnancy*, London: Longman.

Reading, A.E., Cox, D.N. and Sledmere, C.M. (1982) 'Issues arising from the development of new male contraceptives', *Bulletin of the British Psychological Society* 35: 369–71.

Reading, A.E., Everritt, B.S. and Sledmore, C.M. (1982) 'The McGill Pain Questionnaire: a replication of its construction', *British Journal of Clinical Psychology* 21: 339–49.

Reason, J.T. and Brand, J.J. (1975) *Motion Sickness*, London: Academic Press.

Redmond, G.P.and Gordon, K. (1982) 'Pediatricians' attitudes regarding controversial aspects of diabetes management', *Diabetes* 31: 16.

Regina, E.G., Smith, G.M., Keiper, C.G. and McKelvey, R.K. (1974) 'Effects of caffeine on alertness in simulated automobile driving', *Journal of Applied Psychology* 59: 483–9.

Richman, N. (1978) 'Depression in mothers of young children', *Journal of the Royal Society of Medicine* 71: 489–93.

Richman, N., Stevenson, J.E. and Graham, P. (1982) *Preschool to School: A Behavioural Study*, London: Academic Press.

Rickels, K., Case, G.W., Downing, R.W. and Winokur, A. (1983) 'Long term diazepam therapy and clinical outcome', *Journal of the American Medical Association* 250: 767–71.

Ridgeway, V. and Mathews, A. (1982) 'Psychological peparation for surgery: a comparison of methods', *British Journal of Clinical Psychology* 21: 243–60.

Riggio, R.E., Singer, R.D., Hartman, K. and Sneider, R. (1982) 'Psychological issues in the care of critically ill respirator patients: differential perceptions of patients, relatives and staff', *Psychological Reports* 51: 363–9.

Rigotti, N.A. (1989) 'Cigarette smoking and body weight', *New England Journal of Medicine* 320: 931–3.

Rime, B., Ucros, C.G., Bestgen, Y. and Jeanjean, M. (1989) 'Type A behaviour pattern: specific coronary risk factor or general disease-prone condition?', *British Journal of Medical Psychology* 62: 229–40.

Robertson, D. and Curatolo, P.W. (1984) 'The cardiovascular effects of caffeine', in P.B. Dews (ed.) *Caffeine. Perspectives from Recent Research*, Berlin: Springer-Verlag.

Robertson, J.R., Bucknall, A., Welsby, P., Inglis, J., Peutherer, J. and Brettle, R. (1986) 'Epidemic of AIDS related virus (HTLV III/LAV) infection among intravenous drug users', *British Medical Journal* 292: 527–9.

Robinson, J.O. (1964) 'A possible effect of selection on the test scores of a group of hypertensives', *Journal of Psychosomatic Research* 8: 239–43.

Robinson, J.O. and Granfield, A.J. (1986) 'The frequent consulter in primary medical care', *Journal of Psychosomatic Research* 30: 589–600.

Rogers, E.M. (1987) 'The diffusions of innovation perspective', in N.D. Weinstein (ed.) *Taking Care: Understanding and Encouraging Self-Protective Behavior*, Cambridge: Cambridge University Press.

Rogers, M.F. (1985) 'AIDS in children: a review of the clinical, epidemiologic and public health aspects', *Pediatric Infectious Diseases* 4: 230–6.

Romano, J.M., Syrjala, K.L., Levy, R.L., Turner, J.A. and Evans, P. (1988) 'Overt pain behaviours: relationship to patient functioning and treatment outcome', *Behaviour Therapy* 19: 191–201.

Rose, M.I., Firestone, P., Heick, H.M.C. and Faught, A.K. (1983) 'The effects of anxiety management training on the control of juvenile diabetes mellitus', *Journal of Behavioral Medicine* 6: 381–95.

Rosenberg, S.J., Peterson, R.A., Hayes, J.R., Hatcher, J. and Headen, S. (1988) 'Depression in medical in-patients', *British Journal of Medical Psychology* 61: 245–54.

Rosenfeld, J. and Shohat, J. (1983) 'Obesity and hypertension', in F. Gross and T. Strasser (eds) *Mild Hypertension: Recent Advances*, New York: Raven Press.

Rosenman, R.H., Brand, R.J., Jenkins, C.D., Friedman, M., Straus, R. and Wurm, M. (1975) 'Coronary heart disease in the Western Collaborative Group Study: final follow-up experience of eight and a half years', *Journal of American Medical Association* 233: 872–7.

Rosensteil, A.K. and Keefe, F.J. (1983) 'The use of cognitive coping strategies in chronic low back pain patients. Relationship to patient characteristics and current adjustment', *Pain* 17: 33–44.

Rosenstock, I.M. (1966) 'Why people use health services', *Millbank Memorial Fund Quarterly* 44: 94.

Rosenstock, I.M. (1974) 'Historical origins of the health belief model', *Health Education Monographs* 2: 409–19.

Ross, D.M. and Ross, S.A. (1982) *Hyperactivity: Research, Theory, Action*, New York: Wiley.

Roth, H.P. (1987) 'The measurement of compliance', *Patient Education and Counseling* 10: 107–16.

Rotter, J.B. (1966) 'Generalised expectancies for internal versus external control of reinforcement', *Psychological Monographs* 80: 1–28.

Rovinsky, J.J. (1972) 'Abortion recidivism', *Journal of Obstetrics and Gynaecology* 39: 649–59.

Royal College of Physicians (1983) *Health or Smoking: Follow-up Report*, London: Pitman.

Royal College of Psychiatrists (1986) *Alcohol: Our Favourite Drug*, London: Tavistock Publications.

Royal College of Surgeons of England (1985) *Guidelines for Day Case Surgery*, London: Royal College of Surgeons.

Ruesch, S. (1948) 'The infantile personality – the core problem of psychosomatic medicine', *Psychosomatic Medicine* 10: 134–49.

Russell, M.A.H. (1989) 'The addiction research unit at the Institute of Psychiatry – II. The work of the unit's smoking section', *British Journal of Addiction* 84: 853–64.

Rutledge, D.N. (1987) 'Factors related to women's practice of breast self-examination', *Nursing Research* 36: 117–21.

Rutter, M. and Quinton, D. (1984) 'Parental psychiatric disorder: effects on children', *Psychological Medicine* 14: 853–80.

Ryan, G.M. and Sweeney, P.J. (1980) 'Attitudes of adolescents toward pregnancy and contraception', *American Journal of Obstetrics and Gynecology* 137: 358–66.

Sackett, D.L. and Haynes, R.B. (1976) *Compliance with Therapeutic Regimens*, Baltimore, Md.: Johns Hopkins University Press.

Sackett, D.L. and Snow, J.C. (1979) 'The magnitude of compliance and noncompliance', in R.B. Haynes, D.W. Taylor, and D.L. Sackett (eds) *Compliance in Health Care*, Baltimore, Md.: Johns Hopkins University Press.

Samora, J., Saunders, L. and Larson, M. (1961) 'Medical vocabulary knowledge among hospital patients', *Journal of Health and Human Behaviour* 2: 83–9.

Scambler, G. and Scambler, A. (1984) 'The illness iceberg and aspects of consulting behaviour', in R. Fitzpatrick, J. Hinton, S. Newman, G. Scambler and J. Thompson (eds) *The Experience of Illness*, London: Tavistock Publications.

Schachter, S. (1971) *Emotion, Obesity, and Crime*, New York: Academic Press.

Schafer, L.C., Glasgow, R.E. and McCaul, K.D. (1982) 'Increasing the adherence of diabetic adolescents', *Journal of Behavioral Medicine* 5: 353–62.

Schiffrin, A., Desrosiers, M.T. and Belmonte, M. (1983) 'Evaluation of two methods of self blood glucose monitoring by trained insulin-dependent diabetic adolescents outside the hospital', *Diabetes Care* 6: 166–9.

Schilling, R.F., Schinke, S.P., Nichols, S.E., Zayas, L.H., Miller, S.O., Orlandi, M.A. and Botvin, G.J. (1989) 'Developing strategies for AIDS prevention research with black and hispanic drug users', *Public Health Reports* 104: 2–11.

Schinke, S.P. (1984) 'Preventing teenage pregnancy', in M. Hersen, R.M. Eisler and R.M. Miller (eds) *Progress in Behavior Modification 16*, New York: Academic Press.

Schleifer, S.J., Keller, S.E., Camerino, M., Thornton, J.C. and Stein, M. (1983) 'Suppression of lymphocyte stimulation following bereavement', *Journal of American Medical Association* 250: 374–7.

Schneider, N.G., Jarvik, M.E., Forsythe, A.B., Read, L.L. and Elliott, M.L. (1983) 'Nicotine gum in smoking cessation: a placebo controlled trial', *Addictive Behaviours* 8: 256–61.

Schooler, N.R. and Hogarty, G.E. (1987) 'Medication and psychological strategies in the treatment of schizophrenia', in H.Y. Meltzer (ed.) *Psychopharmacology: The Third Generation of Progress*, New York: Raven Press.

Schradle, S.B. and Dougher, M.J. (1985) 'Social support as a mediator of stress: theoretical and empirical issues', *Clinical Psychology Review* 5: 641–61.

Schwab, J.J., Bialow, M.R., Brown, J. and Holzer, C.F. (1967) 'Diagnosing depression in medical inpatients', *Annals of Internal Medicine* 67: 695–707.

Schwartz, G.E. (1977) 'Psychosomatic disorders and biofeedback: a psychobiological model of disregulation', in J.D. Maser and M.E.P. Seligman (eds) *Psychopathology: Experimental Models*, San Francisco: W.H. Freeman.

Schwartz, S.K. and Rutherford, G.W. (1989) 'Acquired immunodeficiency syndrome in infants, children and adolescents', *Journal of Drug Issues* 19: 75–92.

Scott, R.W., Blanchard, E.B., Edmundson, E.B. and Young, L.D. (1973) 'A shaping procedure for heart rate control in chronic tachycardia', *Perceptual and Motor Skills* 37: 327–38.

Seashore, R.H. and Ivy, A.C. (1953) 'The effects of analeptic drugs in relieving fatigue', *Psychological Monographs* 67(15): 1–16.

Seeburg, K.N. and DeBoer, K.P. (1980) 'Effects of EMG biofeedback on diabetes', *Biofeedback and Self-Regulation* 5: 289–93.

Segall, A. and Roberts, L.W. (1980) 'A comparative analysis of physician estimates and levels of medical knowledge among patients', *Sociology of Health and Illness* 2: 317–34.

Seligman, M.E.P. (1975) *Helplessness. On Depression, Development and Death*, San Francisco: W.H. Freeman.

Selye, H. (1956) *The Stress of Life*, New York: McGraw-Hill.

Shapiro, A.K. (1978) 'The placebo effect', in W.G. Clark and J. Del Giudice (eds) *Principles of Psychopharmacology*, New York: Academic Press.

Shapiro, D. and Goldstein, I.B. (1982) 'Biobehavioral perspectives on hypertension', *Journal of Consulting and Clinical Psychology* 50: 841–58.

Shapiro, D., Schwartz, G.E. and Tursky, B. (1972) 'Control of diastolic blood pressure in man by feedback and reinforcement', *Psychophysiology* 9: 296–304.

Shearn, D.W. (1962) 'Operant conditioning of heart rate', *Science* 137: 530–1.

Shedivy, D.I. and Kleinman, K.M. (1977) 'Lack of correlation between frontalis EMG and either neck EMG or verbal ratings of tension', *Psychophysiology* 14: 182–6.

Shekelle, R.B., Gale, M., Ostfeld, A.M. and Paul, O. (1983) 'Hostility, risk of coronary heart disease and mortality', *Psychosomatic Medicine* 45: 109–14.

Shekelle, R.B., Raynor, W.J., Ostfeld, A.M., Garron, D.C., Bieliauskas, L.A., Liu, S.C., Maliza, C. and Paul, O. (1981) 'Psychological depression and 17 year risk and death from cancer', *Psychosomatic Medicine* 43: 117–25.

Shentag, J.J., Culleri, G., Rose, J.Q., Cerra, F.B., DeGlopper, E. and Bernhard, H. (1979) 'Pharmacokinetic and clinical studies in patients with cimetidine-associated mental confusion', *Lancet* ii: 177.

Sher, L. (1987) 'An evaluation of the UK Government health education campaign on AIDS', *Psychology and Health* 1: 61–72.

Sherlock, S. (ed.) (1982). 'Alcohol and disease', *British Medical Bulletin* 38 (whole issue).

Siegel, L. (1988) 'AIDS: Perceptions versus realities', *Journal of Psychoactive Drugs* 20: 149–52.

Silver, B.V. and Blanchard, E.B. (1978) 'Biofeedback and relaxation training in the treatment of psychophysiological disorders: or are the machines really necessary?', *Journal of Behavioral Medicine* 1: 217–39.

Silver, R.L. and Wortman, C.B. (1980) 'Coping with undesirable events', in J. Garber and M.E.P. Seligman (eds) *Human Helplessness: Theory and Application*, New York: Academic Press.

Sims, E. (1982) 'Mechanisms of hypertension in the overweight', *Hypertension* 4 (Suppl. 3): 43–9.

Singer, E. (1974) 'Premature social ageing: the social-psychological consequences of a chronic illness', *Social Science and Medicine* 8: 143–51.

Singer, E., Rogers, T.F. and Corcoran, M. (1987) 'The polls. A report – AIDS', *Public Opinion Quarterly* 51: 580–95.

Sirota, A.D., Schwartz, G.E. and Shapiro, D. (1974) 'Voluntary control of human heart rate: effect on reaction to aversive stimulation', *Journal of Abnormal Psychology* 83: 261–7.

Sirota, A.D., Schwartz, G.E. and Shapiro, D. (1976) 'Voluntary control of human heart rate: effect on reaction to aversive stimulation: a replication and extension', *Journal of Abnormal Psychology* 85: 473–6.

Skegg, D.C.G., Doll, R. and Perry, J. (1977) 'Use of medicines in general practice', *British Medical Journal* i: 1561–3.

Smetana, J.G. and Adler, N.E. (1979) 'Decision-making regarding abortion: a value x expectancy analysis', *Journal of Population* 2: 338–57.

Smith, G.M, and Beecher, H.K. (1959) 'Amphetamine sulfate and athletic performance. 1: objective effects', *Journal of the American Medical Association* 170: 542–7.

Smith, P., Weinman, M. and Nenny, S.W. (1984) 'Desired pregnancy during adolescence', *Psychological Reports* 54: 227–31.

Smith, T.W., Houston, B.K. and Zurawski, R.M. (1985) 'The Framingham Type A scale: cardiovascular and cognitive-behavioral responses to interpersonal challenge', *Motivation and Emotion* 9: 123–34.

Somani, S.M. and Gupta, P. (1988) 'Caffeine: a new look at an age old drug', *International Journal of Clinical Pharmacology Therapy and Toxicology* 26: 521–33.

Sorensen, R.C. (1973) *Adolescent Sexuality in Contemporary America*, New York: World Press.

Southam, M.A., Agras, W.S., Taylor, C.B., and Kraemer, H.C. (1982) 'Relaxation training: blood pressure lowering during the working day', *Archives of General Psychiatry* 39: 715–17.

Spiegel, R. (1989) *Psychopharmacology: An Introduction*, 2nd edition, Chichester: Wiley.

Stabler, B., Surwit, R.S., Lane, J.D., Morris, M.A., Litton, J. and Feinglos, M.N. (1987) 'Type A behavior pattern and blood glucose control in diabetic children',

Psychosomatic Medicine 49: 313–16.

Stall, R., McKusick, L., Wiley, J., Coates, T.J. and Ostrow, D.G. (1986) 'Alcohol and drug use during sexual activity and compliance with safe sex guidelines for AIDS: the AIDS Behavioral Research Project', *Health Education Quarterly* 13: 359–71.

Steel, J.M. (1985) 'Evolution of diabetic care in Edinburgh', *Practical Diabetes* 2: 29–30.

Steptoe, A. (1981) *Psychological Factors in Cardiovascular Disease*, London: Academic Press.

Steptoe, A. (1983) 'Stress, helplessness and control: the implications of laboratory studies', *Journal of Psychosomatic Research* 27: 361–7.

Steptoe, A. (1989) 'Psychophysiological interventions in behavioural medicine', in G. Turpin (ed.) *Handbook of Clinical Psychophysiology*, Chichester: Wiley.

Steptoe, A. and Appels, A. (eds) (1989) *Stress, Personal Control and Health*, Chichester: John Wiley and Sons.

Steptoe, A. and Sawada, Y. (1989) 'Assessment of baroreceptor reflex function during mental stress and relaxation', *Psychophysiology* 26: 140–7

Steptoe, A., Melville, D. and Ross, A. (1984) 'Behavioural response demands, cardiovascular reactivity, and essential hypertension', *Psychosomatic Medicine* 46: 33–48.

Steptoe, A., Patel, C., Marmot, M. and Hunt, B. (1987) 'Frequency of relaxation practice, blood pressure reduction, and the general effects of relaxation following a controlled trial of behaviour modification for reducing coronary risks', *Stress Medicine* 3: 101–7.

Sterling, P. and Eyer, J. (1988) 'Allostasis: a new paradigm to explain arousal pathology', in S. Fisher and J. Reason (eds) *Handbook of Life Stress, Cognition and Health*, Chichester: John Wiley and Sons.

Sternbach, R.A. (1968) *Pain: A Psychophysiological Analysis*, New York: Academic Press.

Sternbach, R.A. (ed.) (1978) *The Psychology of Pain*, New York: Raven Press.

Stewart, D.C. and Sullivan, T.J. (1982) 'Illness behaviour and the sick role in chronic disease: the case of multiple sclerosis', *Social Science and Medicine* 16: 1397–1404.

Stillman, M.J. (1977) 'Women's health beliefs about breast cancer and breast self examination', *Nursing Research* 26: 121–7.

Stimson, G.V. and Webb, B. (1975) *Going to See the Doctor: The Consultation Process in General Practice*, London: Routledge & Kegan Paul.

Stimson, G.V., Alldritt, L., Dolan, K. and Donoghoe, M. (1988) *Injecting Equipment Exchange Schemes: A Preliminary Report on Research*, London; University of London, Monitoring Research Group.

Stoll, B.A. (1988) 'Neuroendocrine and psychoendocrine influences on breast cancer growth', in C.L. Cooper (ed.) *Stress and Breast Cancer*, Chichester: John Wiley and Sons.

Stollerman, I.P., Fink, R. and Jarvik, M.E. (1973) 'Influencing cigarette smoking with nicotine antagonists', *Psychopharmacologia* 28: 247–59.

Stone, A.A., Bruce, R. and Neale, J.M. (1988) 'Changes in daily event frequency precede episodes of physical symptoms', *Journal of Human Stress* 13: 70–4.

Stoyva, J. and Budzynski, T. (1974) 'Cultivated low arousal – an anti-stress response?', in L.V. DiCara (ed.) *Recent Advances in Limbic and Autonomic Nervous System Research*, New York: Plenum.

Stroebel, C.F. and Glueck, B.C. (1973) 'Biofeedback treatment in medicine and psychiatry: an ultimate placebo?', *Seminars in Psychiatry* 5: 379–93.

Strunin, L. and Hingson, R. (1987) 'Acquired immunodeficiency syndrome and adolescents: knowledge, beliefs, attitudes and behaviors', *Pediatrics* 79: 825–8.

Surgeon General (1980) *The Health Consequences of Smoking for Women*, Washington,

DC: US Government Printing Office.

Surgeon General (1986) *The Health Consequences of Involuntary Smoking*, Washington, DC: US Government Printing Office.

Surgeon General (1988) *Nicotine Addiction: The Health Consequences of Smoking*, Washington, DC: US Government Printing Office.

Swift, C.G. (1988) 'Prescribing in old age', *British Medical Journal* 296: 913–15.

Tapper-Jones, L., Smail, S.A., Pill, R. and Harvard Davis, R. (1988) 'General practitioners' use of written materials during consultations', *British Medical Journal* 296: 908–9.

Taub, E. (1977) 'Self-regulation of human tissue temperature', in G.E. Schwartz and J. Beatty (eds) *Biofeedback: Theory and Research*, San Francisco: Academic Press.

Taylor, B., Wadsworth, J. and Butler, N.R. (1983) 'Teenage mothering: admission to hospital and accidents during the first five years', *Archives of Diseases in Childhood* 58: 6–11.

Taylor, C.B., Sheikh, J., Agras, W.S., Roth, W.T., Margraf, J., Ehlers, A., Maddock, R.J. and Gossard, D. (1986) 'Ambulatory heart rate changes in patients with panic attacks', *American Journal of Psychiatry* 143: 478–82.

Taylor, D. (1987) 'Current usage of benzodiazepines in Britain', in H. Freeman and Y. Rue (eds) *The Benzodiazepines in Current Clinical Practice*, London: Royal Society of Medicine Publication.

Taylor, G. (1967) 'Predicted versus actual response to spinal cord injury: a psychological study', doctoral dissertation, University of Minnesota.

Taylor, S.E. (1979) 'Hospital patient behaviour: reactance, helplessness or control?', *Journal of Social Issues* 35: 156–84.

Taylor, S.E. (1983) 'Adjustment to threatening events: a theory of cognitive adaptation', *American Psychologist* 38: 1161–73.

Tessler, R.C., Mechanic, D. and Diamond, M. (1976) 'The effect of psychological distress on physician utilization: a prospective study', *Journal of Health and Social Behaviour* 17: 353.

Theorell, T. (1974) 'Life events before and after the onset of premature myocardial infarction', in B.S. Dohrenwend and B.P. Dohrenwend (eds) *Stressful Life Events: Their Nature and Effects*, New York: Wiley.

Theorell, T. (1976) 'Selected illnesses and somatic factors in relation to two psychosocial stress indices – a prospective study on middle-aged construction building workers', *Journal of Psychosomatic Research* 20: 7–20.

Theorell, T. (1982) 'Review of research on life events and cardiovascular illness', *Advances in Cardiology* 29: 140–7.

Theorell, T. (1989) 'Personal control at work and health: a review of epidemiological studies in Sweden', in A. Steptoe and A. Appels (eds) *Stress, Personal Control and Health*, Chichester: John Wiley and Sons.

Thompson, J. (1984) 'Compliance', in R. Fitzpatrick, J. Hinton, S. Newman, G. Scambler and J. Thompson (eds) *The Experience of Illness*, London: Tavistock Publications.

Thompson, S.C. (1981) 'Will it hurt less if I can control it? A complex answer to a simple question', *Psychological Bulletin* 90: 89–101.

Tibblin, G and Wilhelmsen, L. (1975) 'Risk factors for myocardial infarction and death due to ischemic heart disease', *American Journal of Cardiology* 35: 514–22.

Totman, R.G. and Kiff, J. (1980) 'Life stress and susceptibility to colds', in D.J. Oborne (ed.) *Research in Psychology and Medicine Volume 1*, London: Academic Press.

Toubas, P.L., Duke, J.C., McCaffree, M.A., Mattice, C.D., Bendell, D. and Orr, W.C. (1986) 'Effects of maternal smoking and caffeine habits on infantile apnea: a retrospective study', *Pediatrics* 78: 159–63.

Trelawny-Ross, C. and Russell, O. (1987) 'Social and psychological responses to myocardial infarction: multiple determinants of outcome at six months', *Journal of Psychosomatic Research* 31: 125–30.

Tucker, S.J. (1980) 'The psychology of spinal cord injury: patient–staff interaction', *Rehabilitation Literature* 41: 114–21.

Turk, D.C. and Rudy, T.E. (1986) 'Assessment of cognitive factors in chronic pain: a worthwhile enterprise?', *Journal of Consulting and Clinical Psychology* 54: 760–8.

Turk, D.C., Rudy, T.E. and Salovey, P. (1985) 'The McGill Pain Questionnaire in the clinical assessment of pain', *Pain* 21: 385–97.

Turner, C., Anderson, P., Fitzpatrick, R., Fowler, G. and Mayon-White, R. (1988) 'Sexual behaviour, contraceptive practice and knowledge of AIDS of Oxford University students', *Journal of Biosocial Science* 20: 445–51.

Turnquist, D.C., Harvey, J.H. and Anderson, B.L. (1988) 'Attributions and adjustment to life-threatening illness', *British Journal of Clinical Psychology* 27: 55–65.

Turpin, G. (1985) 'Ambulatory psychophysiological monitoring: techniques and applications', in D. Papakostopoulos, S. Butler and I. Martin (eds) *Clinical and Experimental Neuropsychophysiology*, London: Croom Helm.

Turpin, G. (1989) 'An overview of clinical psychophysiological techniques: tools or theories?', in G. Turpin (ed.) *Handbook of Clinical Psychophysiology*, Chichester: John Wiley and Sons.

Turpin, G., Tarrier, N. and Sturgeon, D. (1988) 'Social psychophysiology and the study of biopsychosocial models of schizophrenia', in H.L. Wagner (ed.) *Social Psychophysiology and Emotion: Theory and Clinical Applications*, Chichester: John Wiley and Sons.

Tversky, A. and Kahnemann, D. (1974) 'Judgement under uncertainty: heuristics and biases', *Science* 185: 1124–31.

Tyrer, P. (1988) 'Prescribing psychotropic drugs in general practice', *British Medical Journal* 296: 588–9.

Uzan, A., Le Fur, G. and Malgouris, C. (1979) 'Are antihistamines sedative via a blockade of brain H1 receptors', *Journal of Pharmacy and Pharmacology* 31: 701–2.

Van der Ploeg, H.M. (1988) 'Stressful medical events: a survey of patients' perceptions', in S. Maes, C.D. Spielberger, P.B. Defares and I.G. Sarason (eds) *Topics in Health Psychology*, New York: John Wiley and Sons.

Van Toller, C. (1979) *Nervous Body: An Introduction to the Autonomic Nervous System and Behaviour*, Chichester: John Wiley and Sons.

Veleber, D.M. and Templer, D.I. (1984) 'Effects of caffeine on anxiety and depression', *Journal of Abnormal Psychology* 93: 120–2.

Victor, R., Mainardi, J.A. and Shapiro, D. (1978) 'Effects of biofeedback and voluntary control procedures on heart rate and perception of pain during the cold pressor test', *Psychosomatic Medicine* 40: 216–25.

Visitainer, M.A. and Wolfer, J.A. (1975) 'Psychological preparation for surgical pediatric patients', *Pediatrics* 56: 187–202.

Volicier, B.J. and Bohannon, M.W. (1975) 'A hospital rating scale', *Nursing Research* 24: 352–9.

Waal-Manning, H.J., Knight, R.G., Spears, G.F. and Paulin, J.M. (1986) 'The relationship between blood pressure and personality in a large unselected adult sample', *Journal of Psychosomatic Research* 30: 361–8.

Wadden, T.A. (1984) 'Relaxation therapy for essential hypertension: specific or nonspecific effects?', *Journal of Psychosomatic Research* 28: 53–61.

Wadsworth, J., Taylor, B., Osborn, A. and Butler, N.R. (1984) 'Teenage mothering: child development at five years', *Journal of Child Psychology and Psychiatry* 25: 305–13.

Wallace, L.M. (1984) 'Psychological preparation as a method of reducing the stress of surgery', *Journal of Human Stress* 10: 62–77.

Wallston, K.A. and Wallston, B.S. (1981) 'Health locus of control scales', in H. Lefcourt (ed.) *Research with the Locus of Control Construct. Volume 1*, New York: Academic Press.

Wallston, T.S. (1978) *Three Biases in the Cognitive Processing of Diagnostic Information*, Chapel Hill: Psychometric Laboratory, University of North Carolina.

Warburton, D.M. (1975) *Brain, Behaviour and Drugs*, Chichester: Wiley.

Warwick, I., Aggelton, P. and Homans, H. (1988) 'Constructing commonsense – young people's beliefs about AIDS', *Sociology of Health and Illness* 10: 213–33.

Washington, A.C., Rosser, P.L. and Cox, E.P. (1983) 'Contraceptive practices of teenage mothers', *Journal of the National Medical Association* 75: 1059–63.

Wason, P.C. and Johnson-Laird, P.N. (eds) (1972) *Thinking and Reasoning*, Harmondsworth: Penguin.

Watkins, J.D., Roberts, D.E., Williams, T.F., Martin, D.A. and Coyle, V. (1967) 'Observation of medication errors made by diabetic patients in the home', *Diabetes* 16: 882–5.

Watkins, J.D., Williams, F.T., Martin, D.A., Hogan, M.D. and Anderson, E. (1967) 'A study of diabetic patients at home', *American Journal of Public Health* 37: 452–9.

Watters, J.K. (1988) 'Meaning and context: the social facts of intravenous drug use and HIV transmission in the inner city', *Journal of Psychoactive Drugs* 20: 173–7

Watters, J.K. (1989) 'Observations on the importance of social context in HIV transmission among intravenous drug users', *Journal of Drug Issues* 19: 9–26.

Watters, W.W. (1980) 'Mental health consequences of abortion and refused abortion', *Canadian Journal of Psychiatry* 25: 68–73.

Watts, F.N. (1980) 'Behavioral aspects of the management of diabetes mellitus: education, self-care and metabolic control', *Behavior Research and Therapy* 18: 171–80.

Weiner, H. (1977) *Psychobiology and Human Disease*, New York: Elsevier.

Weinman, J. (1981) *An Outline of Psychology as Applied to Medicine*, Bristol: John Wright and Sons Ltd.

Weinman, J. and Johnston, M. (1988) 'Stressful medical procedures: an analysis of the effects of psychological interventions and of the stressfulness of the procedures', in S. Maes, C.D. Spielberger, P.B. Defares and I.G. Sarason (eds) *Topics in Health Psychology*, New York: John Wiley and Sons.

Weinstein, N.D. (1987) 'Unrealistic optimism about susceptibility to health problems: conclusions from a community wide sample', *Journal of Behavioural Medicine* 10: 481–500.

Weinstein, N.D. (1988) 'The precaution adoption process', *Health Psychology* 7: 355–86.

Weiss, J.M. (1977) 'Psychological and behavioral influences on gastrointestinal lesions in animal models', in J.D. Maser and M.E.P. Seligman (eds) *Psychopathology: Experimental Models*, San Francisco: Freeman.

Weiss, T. and Engel, B.T. (1971) 'Operant conditioning of heart rate in patients with premature ventricular contractions', *Psychosomatic Medicine* 33: 301–21.

Wellings, K. (1988) 'Perceptions of risk – media treatments of AIDS', in P. Aggleton and H. Homans (eds) *Social Aspects of AIDS*, London: Falmer Press.

Wesnes, K. and Warburton, D.M. (1983) 'Smoking, nicotine, and human performance', *Pharmacology and Therapeutics* 21: 189–208.

West, M.O. and Prinz, R.J. (1987) 'Parental alcoholism and childhood psychopathology', *Psychological Bulletin* 102: 204–18.

West, R.J. and Russell, M.A.H. (1985) 'Effects of withdrawal from long term nicotine gum use', *Psychological Medicine* 15: 891–3.

Westbrook, M.T. and Nordholm, L.A. (1986) 'Effects of diagnosis on reactions to patient optimism and depression', *Rehabilitation Psychology* 31: 79–94.

White, D.G., Phillips, K.C., Clifford, B.R., Davies, M., Elliott, J.R. and Pitts M.K. (1989) 'AIDS and intimate relationships: adolescents' knowledge and attitudes', *Current Psychology: Research and Reviews* 8: 130–43.

White, D.G., Phillips, K.C., Pitts, M.K., Clifford, B.R., Elliott, J. and Davies, M.M. (1988) 'Adolescents' perceptions of AIDS', *Health Education Journal* 47: 117–19.

WHO (1978) *Induced Abortion*, Technical Report Series No. 623, Geneva: World Health Organisation.

WHO (1983) *Primary Prevention of Essential Hypertension*, Report of WHO Scientific Group, Technical Report series 686. Geneva: World Health Organisation.

Wilcox, N. and Stauffer, E. (1972) 'Follow-up of 423 consecutive patients admitted to the spinal cord center, Rancho Los Amigos Hospital, January 1 to 31 December, 1967', *International Journal of Paraplegia* 10: 115–22.

Williams, R.B. (1978) 'Psychophysiological processes. The coronary prone behaviour pattern, and coronary heart disease', in T.M. Dembroski, S.M. Weiss, J.L. Shields, S.G. Haynes and M.Feinleib (eds) *Coronary Prone Behavoiur*, New York: Springer-Verlag.

Williams, G.D. (1980) 'Effect of cigarette smoking on immediate memory and performance in different kinds of smoker', *British Journal of Psychology* 71: 83–90.

Williams, G., Pickup, J. and Keen, H. (1988) 'Psychological factors and metabolic control: time for re-appraisal?', *Diabetic Medicine* 5: 211–15.

Williams, R.B. (1989) *The Trusting Heart: Great News about Type A Behavior*, New York: Random House.

Williams, T.F., Anderson, E., Watkins, J.D. and Coyle, V. (1967) 'Dietary errors made at home by patients with diabetes', *Journal of the American Diabetic Association* 51: 19–25.

Williams, W.O. (1970) *A Study of General Practitioners' Workload in South Wales. 1965–1966*, Reports from General Practice No. 12, Royal College of General Practitioners.

Wilson, D.P. and Endres, R. (1986) 'Compliance with blood glucose monitoring in children with type 1 diabetes mellitus', *Journal of Pediatrics* 108: 1022–4.

Wilson-Barnett, J. (1976) 'Patients' emotional reactions to hospitalisation', *Journal of Advanced Nursing* 1: 351–8.

Wing, R.R., Epstein, L.H., Nowalk, M.P. and Lamparski, D.M. (1986) 'Behavioral self-regulation in the treatment of patients with diabetes mellitus', *Psychological Bulletin* 99: 78–89.

Winkelstein, W., Samuel, M., Padian, N.S. and Wiley, J.A. (1987) 'The San Francisco men's health study III: reduction in human immunodeficiency virus transmission among homosexual/bisexual men, 1982–1986', *American Journal of Public Health* 76: 685–9.

Wise, T. and Rosenthal, J. (1982), 'Depression, illness beliefs, and severity of illness', *Journal of Psychosomatic Research* 26: 247–53.

Wittenborn, J.R. (1981) 'Pharmacotherapy for age-related behavioural difficulties', *Journal of Nervous and Mental Diseases* 19: 139–56.

Wold, D.A. (1968) 'The adjustment of siblings to childhood leukaemia', unpublished medical thesis, University of Washington, Seattle.

Wolf, M.W., Putnam, S.M., James, S.A. and Stiles, W.B. (1978) 'The medical interview satisfaction scale: development of a scale to measure patient perceptions of physician behaviour', *Journal of Behavioural Medicine* 1: 391–401.

Wolf, S.L. (1983) 'Electromyographic biofeedback applications to stroke patients: a critical review', *Physical Therapy* 63: 1448–59.

Wood, C.D. and Graybiel, A. (1968) 'Evaluation of 16 anti-motion sickness drugs under controlled motion conditions', *Aerospace Medicine* 39: 1341–4.

Woods, P.J. and Burns, J. (1984) 'Type A behaviour and illness in general', *Journal of Behavioural Medicine* 7: 411–15.

Wooldridge, C.P. and Russell, G. (1976) 'Head position training with the cerebral palsied child: an application of biofeedback techniques', *Archives of Physical Medicine and Rehabilitation* 57: 407–14.

Wright, L. (1979) 'Health care psychology. Prospects for the well-being of children', *American Psychologist* 34: 1001–6.

Yates, A.J. (1980) *Biofeedback and the Modification of Behavior*, New York: Plenum Press.

Young, J.S., Burns, P.E., Bowen, A.M., and McCutchen, R. (1982) *Spinal Cord Injury Statistics*, Phoenix, Ariz.: Good Samaritan Medical Center.

Zapka, J.G. and Mamon, J.A. (1982) 'Integration of theory, practitioner standards, literature findings, and baseline data: a case study in planning breast self-examination education', *Health Education Quarterly* 9: 330–57.

Zeanah, C.H., Keener, M.A., Anders, T.F. and Vieira-Baker, C.C. (1987) 'Adolescent mothers' perceptions of their infants before and after birth', *American Journal of Orthopsychiatry* 57: 351–60.

Zelnick, M. and Kantner, J.F. (1977) 'Sexual and contraceptive experience of young unmarried women in the United States, 1976 and 1971', *Family Planning Perspectives* 9: 55–71.

Zelnick, M. and Shah, F.K. (1983) 'First intercourse among young Americans', *Family Planning Perspectives* 15: 64–70.

Ziegler, J.B., Cooper, D.A., Johnson, R.O. and Gold, J. (1985) 'Postnatal transmission of AIDS-associated retrovirus from mother to infant', *Lancet* i: 896–8.

Zuckerman, A.J. (1989) 'The enigma of AIDS vaccines', *Royal Society of Medicine: The AIDS Letter* 10 (Dec. 88/Jan. 89): 1–3.

Name index

Subject index

abortion 156, 170; Abortion Act 1967 165; accidents 237; contraception following 169; decision making by professionals 167; decision making by women 166; effects of 166; moral attitudes to 167; and social policy 165
adrenalin 19, 24, 32–3
adrenocortical-immune system 44
adrenocortico-trophic hormone (ACTH) 19, 33
AIDS 21, 139, 140, 144, 149–51, 232 *see also* HIV; campaigns, costs, benefits 161; ecology of 152; intravenous drug users (ivdus) 141–2, 144, 153; paediatric 142; policies for protecting against 147; sexual behaviours and 143
alcohol 174, 177, 183–4, 205, 207–8
alcoholism 245; parental 244
allostasis 27
ambulatory recording 23
anaesthesia 82, 87–8
anatomical reorganization 122
anger 125, 127, 175, 197
angina pectoris 187
anticholinergic effects 78, 80, 85–6
antidepressants 75–7, 79–80, 89, 212
antihistamines 75, 85, 89, 242
antipsychotic (neuroleptic) drugs 75–6
anxiety 65, 67–9, 72–4, 77, 81–3, 88–90, 123, 125–6, 130, 196, 207, 209, 232, 238, 240, 245; management training 219; maternal 234; measures of 68; parental 238; pre-operative 68; trait 71
anxiolytic 77, 81–2
arteriosclerosis *see* atherosclerosis
arthritis 133

artifact theories of recovery 122
asthma 239, 241–2, 245
atherosclerosis 187, 192–3, 196–7, 201
attributions 227
attribution theory 134
autogenic training 111, 119
autonomic nervous system (ANS) 16–19, 27, 32
avoidance behaviour 94–7, 104, 134
avoidance spiral 95

back pain 101, 112
barbiturates 81, 88
baroreceptor reflex sensitivity 178
Beck Depression Inventory (BDI) 66, 126
behavioural medicine 106, 111
behavioural pathogens 4
benzodiazepines 76, 81–3, 84, 88–90, 212
bereavement 40, 43, 82, 123
bioelectrical responses, recording 22–4
biofeedback 106, 108, 111–12, 118; clinical applications of 109, 118; clinical effectiveness of 110, 116; in combined therapies 119; for direct symptom control 113; efficacy of 109; and reactions to stressors 115; thermal and electrodermal 112; training 107–10, 112–20, 179–80
biopsychosocial models 26, 27, 29
blunters 39
breast cancer 11–13, 20–1, 44, 159; adjustment to 134
breast-feeding 140
breast self-examination (BSE) 11–13
buffering 42
burns 124